Textbook of
Veterinary Pathology

Quick Review and Self Assessment

Prof RS Chauhan
MVSc, PhD (Path), FNAVS, FSIIP, FIAVP, Diplomat ICVP

Director
Indian Veterinary Research Institute
Izatnagar-243122, Bareilly (UP)
India

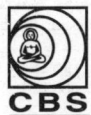

CBS Publishers & Distributors Pvt Ltd

New Delhi • Bengaluru • Chennai • Kochi • Kolkata • Mumbai
Hyderabad • Jharkhand • Nagpur • Patna • Pune • Uttarakhand

Textbook of Veterinary Pathology

ISBN: 978-93-88327-51-0

© Publisher

All Rights Reserved

First Edition: 2010
CBS Reprint: 2019, 2021, 2024

All rights reserved. No part of this publication may be reproduced, stored in a retrieval system, or transmitted, in any form or by any means, electronic, mechanical, photocopying, or otherwise, without the prior permission of the publisher.

This book is sold subject to the condition that it shall not, by way of trade or otherwise be lent, re-sold, hired out, or otherwise circulated without the publisher's prior conset in any form of binding or cover other than that in which it is published and without a similar condition including this condition being imposed on the subsequent purchaser.

Published by Satish Kumar Jain and produced by Varun Jain for
CBS Publishers & Distributors Pvt Ltd
4819/XI Prahlad Street, 24 Ansari Road, Daryaganj, New Delhi 110 002, India.
Ph: 011-23289259, 23266861, 23266867 Fax: 011-23243014
Website: www.cbspd.com
e-mail: delhi@cbspd.com; cbspubs@airtelmail.in.
Corporate Office: 204 FIE, Industrial Area, Patparganj, Delhi 110 092
Ph: 011-4934 4934 Fax: 011-4934 4935 e-mail: publishing@cbspd.com; publicity@cbspd.com

Branches

- **Bengaluru:** Seema House 2975, 17th Cross, K.R. Road, Banasankari 2nd Stage, Bengaluru 560 070, Karnataka
  Ph: +91-80-26771678/79 Fax: +91-80-26771680 e-mail: bangalore@cbspd.com
- **Chennai:** 7, Subbaraya Street, Shenoy Nagar, Chennai 600 030, Tamil Nadu
  Ph: +91-44-26260666, 26208620 Fax: +91-44-42032115 e-mail: chennai@cbspd.com
- **Kochi:** 42/1325, 1326, Power House Road, Opp KSEB Power House, Ernakulam 682 018, Kochi, Kerala
  Ph: +91-484-4059061-65 Fax: +91-484-4059065 e-mail: kochi@cbspd.com
- **Kolkata:** 6/B, Ground Floor, Rameswar Shaw Road, Kolkata-700014 (West Bengal), India
  Ph: +91-33-2289-1126, 2289-1127, 2289-1128 e-mail: kolkata@cbspd.com
- **Mumbai:** PWD Shed, Gala no 25/26, Ramchandra Bhatt Marg, Next to JJ Hospital Gate no. 2, Opp. Union Bank of India, Noorbaug Mumbai-400009, Maharashtra
  Ph: +91-22-66661880/89 e-mail: mumbai@cbspd.com

Representatives

• Hyderabad	0-9885175004	• Jharkhand	0-9811541605	• Nagpur	0-9421945513
• Patna	0-9334159340	• Pune	0-9623451994	• Uttarakhand	0-9716462459

Printed at Rashtriya Printers, Dilshad Garden, Delhi, India

PREFACE

Veterinary Pathology is an important discipline of Veterinary sciences which makes a bridge in between the basic and clinical sciences. The knowledge of Veterinary Pathology makes the veterinarian a perfect diagnostician particularly when his patient (animal) can't speak his/her illness to the doctor. Keeping the need of study of Veterinary Pathology to become a good Veterinary doctor, two books "Illustrated Veterinary Pathology" and "Illustrated Special Veterinary Pathology" were published which were very much appreciated by Teachers, students and field Veterinarians. The complexity of the subject was presented in a simplified way particularly keeping the view of Indian geo-climatic conditions and animal population. However, students of Veterinary Science desire a compact text of Veterinary Pathology covering all four courses of Pathology which can be utilized during the examinations particularly competitive examinations. Hence, this textbook is prepared as a quick review material to all those who want to appear in any kind of examination or interview. It covers all four subjects of Veterinary Pathology viz. General Veterinary Pathology, Systemic Pathology, Special Pathology-I and Special Pathology-II. The text is described in a very simple format including definition, etiology, clinical manifestations, macroscopic and microscopic features and only salient features are mentioned avoiding detailed text. In order to make a self assessment key questions of each and every chapter are also given to understand the conditions in a better way.

Hope this textbook "Veterinary Pathology-Quick Review and Self Assessment" will find a place in the young fraternity of Veterinary Science. The help rendered by Mr. Himanshu Agarwal, Mr. Tasabber Khan and Mr. Manish Manohar in preparation and designing of this textbook is duly acknowledged. Readers' comments are welcome to further improve the textbook.

PROF. R.S. CHAUHAN
MVSc, PhD (Path), Diplomat, ICVP
FIAVP, FSIIP, FNAVS

ABOUT THE AUTHOR

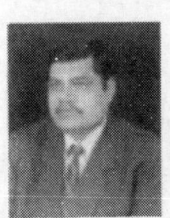

Prof. R.S. Chauhan is currently Director of Indian Veterinary Research Institute, Izatnagar, Bareilly (UP). He has worked as Joint Director (CADRAD), National Fellow, Associate Professor, Assistant Professor in IVRI, CCS HAU, Hisar and GB Pant University, Pantnagar. He has more than 600 publications to his credit that have appeared in various national and international journals of repute. He has authored 24 books including textbooks on Veterinary Pathology, Laboratory Diagnosis, Glossary, Manuals and Monographs. He was awarded with various national awards including Young Scientist Award, IAAVR Award, Shri Ram Lal Agrawal National Award, Dr. K.S. Nair Memorial Award, Dr. Rajendra Prasad Award of ICAR, Best Teacher Award of GB Pant University, etc. He has been widely travelled and attended several international conferences and visited Kenya, UAE, Egypt, France, UK, The Netherlands, Canada, and Germany. He is Fellow of National Academy of Veterinary Sciences and Society for Immunology and Immunopathology. He is also heading "Society for Immunology and Immunopathology" as Secretary-General. He is President of The Cow Therapy Society and Vice-President of the Indian Association of Veterinary Educators. Earlier he has been in executive committee member of IAAVR, Joint Secretary, Indian Virology Society and Zonal Secretary, Indian Association of Veterinary Pathologists. He is Managing-Editor of the *Journal of Immunology and Immunopathology*, Editor in Chief of the *International Journal on Cow Science* and Editor of *The Indian Cow*. He has been Task Force member of WHO on EHC and Temporary Advisor, WHO/ IPCS. He was Chief Editor, Indian Journal of Veterinary Pathology and honoured as Fellow, Indian Association of Veterinary Pathologists. He has been elected as Vice President, IAVP and awarded Diplomat, Indian College of Veterinary Pathologists.

Contents

SECTION-A: GENERAL VETERINARY PATHOLOGY

Chapter 1	Introduction	1
Chapter 2	Etiology	13
Chapter 3	Genetic Disorders, Developmental Anomalies and Monsters	39
Chapter 4	Disturbances in Growth	49
Chapter 5	Disturbances in Circulation	53
Chapter 6	Disturbances in Cell Metabolism	61
Chapter 7	Necrosis, Gangrene and Post-mortem Changes	67
Chapter 8	Disturbances in Calcification and Pigment Metabolism	77
Chapter 9	Inflammation and Healing	85
Chapter 10	Concretions	121
Chapter 11	Immunity and Immunopathology	125

SECTION-B: SYSTEMIC PATHOLOGY

Chapter 12	Pathology of Cutaneous System	141
Chapter 13	Pathology of Musculoskeletal System	149
Chapter 14	Pathology of Cardiovascular System	159
Chapter 15	Pathology Respiratory System	171
Chapter 16	Pathology of Digestive System	189
Chapter 17	Pathology of Hemopoitic and Immune System	209
Chapter 18	Pathology of Urinary System	221
Chapter 19	Pathology of Genital System	233
Chapter 20	Pathology of Nervous System	247
Chapter 21	Pathology of Endocrine System, Eyes and Ear	253

SECTION-C: SPECIAL PATHOLOGY-I

Chapter 22	Neoplasm	263
Chapter 23	Viral Diseases	307
Chapter 24	Bacterial Diseases	349
Chapter 25	Chlamydial Diseases	381
Chapter 26	Rickettsial Diseases	383
Chapter 27	Mycoplasmal Diseases	385
Chapter 28	Spirochaetal Diseases	389
Chapter 29	Prion Diseases	391
Chapter 30	Fungal Diseases	393
Chapter 31	Parasitic Diseases	403

SECTION-D: SPECIAL PATHOLOGY II, DISEASES OF POULTRY, WILD, ZOO AND LABORATORY ANIMALS

Chapter 32	Avian Inflammation	433
Chapter 33	Pathology of Nutritional Disorders	435
Chapter 34	Viral Diseases	439
Chapter 35	Bacterial Diseases	463
Chapter 36	Chlamydial Disease	477
Chapter 37	Mycoplasmal Diseases	479
Chapter 38	Spirochaetal Disease	483
Chapter 39	Fungal Diseases	485
Chapter 40	Parasitic Diseases	493
Chapter 41	Vices and Miscellaneous Disease Conditions	501
Chapter 42	Pathology of Diseases of Wild and Zoo Animals	505
Chapter 43	Pathology of Diseases of Laboratory Animals	509
Chapter 44	Cytopathology	515
Chapter 45	Appendices	519
Chapter 46	Self Assessment – MCQ	575
Index		641

Chapter 1
Introduction

DEFINITIONS

Pathology

Pathology is the study of the anatomical, chemical and physiological alterations from normal as a result of disease in animals. It is a key subject because it forms a vital bridge between preclinical sciences (Anatomy, Physiology, Biochemistry) and clinical branches of medicine and surgery. Pathology is derived from a Greek word *pathos* = disease, *logos*= study. It has many branches, which are defined as under:

General Pathology

General Pathology concerns with basic alterations of tissues as a result of disease. *e.g.* Fatty changes, Thrombosis, Amyloidosis, Embolism, Necrosis.

Systemic Pathology

Systemic Pathology deals with alterations in tissues/ organs of a particular system. *e.g.* Respiratory system, Genital system etc.

Specific Pathology

Specific Pathology is the application of the basic alterations learned in general pathology to various specific diseases. It involves whole body or a part of body. *e.g.* Tuberculosis, Rinderpest.

Experimental Pathology

Experimental Pathology concerns with the production of lesion through experimental methods. *e.g. Rotavirus* → calves → enteritis/ diarrhoea in calves.

Clinical Pathology

Clinical Pathology includes certain laboratory methods which helps in making the diagnosis using animal excretions/ secretions/ blood/ skin scrapings/ biopsy etc. *e.g.* Urine examination, Blood examination.

Post-mortem Pathology

Post-mortem Pathology is examination of an animal after death. Also known as *Necropsy* or *Autopsy*. It forms the base for study of pathology.

Microscopic Pathology

Microscopic Pathology deals with examination of cells/ tissues/ organs using microscope. It is also known as histopathology/ cellular pathology. *e.g.* Microscopy, Electronmicroscopy.

Humoral Pathology

Humoral Pathology is the study of alterations in fluids like antibodies in serum.

Chemical Pathology

Chemical Pathology is the study of chemical alterations of body fluids/ tissues. *e.g.* Enzymes in tissue.

Physiological Pathology

Physiological Pathology deals with alteration in the functions of organ/ system. It is also known as Pathophysiology. *e.g.* Indigestion, Diarrhoea, Abortion.

Nutritional Pathology

Nutritional Pathology is the study of diseases occurred due to deficiency or excess of nutrients. *e.g.* Vit.-A deficiency induced nutritional roup, rickets due to calcium deficiency.

Comparative Pathology

Comparative Pathology is the study of diseases of animals with a comparative study in human beings and other animals. *e.g.* Zoonotic diseases such as Tuberculosis.

Introduction

Oncology

Oncology is the study of cancer/ tumor/ neoplasms.

Immunopathology

Immunopathology deals with the study of diseases mediated by immune reactions. It includes Immunodeficiency diseases, autoimmunity and hypersensitivity reactions.

Cytopathology

Cytopathology is the study of cells shed off from the lesions for diagnosis.

Health

Health is a state of an individual living in complete harmony, with his environment/ surroundings.

Disease

Disease is a condition in which an individual shows an anatomical, chemical or physiological deviation from the normal. (Discomfort with environment & body).

Illness

Illness is the reaction of an individual to disease in the form of illness.

Forensic Pathology

Forensic Pathology includes careful examination and recording of pathological lesions in case of veterolegal cases.

Homeostasis

Homeostasis is the mechanism by which body keeps equilibrium between health and disease. *e.g.* Adaptation to an altered environment.

Toxopathology

Toxopathology or Toxic Pathology deals with the study of tissue/ organ alterations due to toxins/ poisons.

Etiology

Etiology is the study of causation of disease.

Diagnosis

Diagnosis is an art of precisely knowing the cause of a particular disease (*Dia*= thorough, *gnosis*= knowledge)

Symptoms

Any subjective evidence of disease of animal characterized by an indication of altered bodily or mental state as told by owner (Complaints of the patients).

Signs

Indication of the existence of something, any objective evidence of disease, perceptible to veterinarian (Observations of the clinicians).

Syndrome

A combination of symptoms caused by altered physiological process.

Lesion

Lesion is a pathological alteration in structure/ function that can be detectable.

Pathogenesis

Pathogenesis is the progressive development of a disease process. It starts with the entry of cause in body and ends either with recovery or death. It is the mechanism by which the lesions are produced in body.

Incubation period

Incubation period is the time elapses between the action of a cause and manifestation of disease.

Course of disease

Course of disease is the duration for which the disease process remains till fate either in the form of recovery or death.

Prognosis

Prognosis is an estimate by a clinician of probable severity/ out come of disease.

Morbidity rate

Morbidity rate is the percentage/ proportions of affected animals out of total population in a particular disease outbreak. *e.g.* Out of 100 animals, 20 are suffering from diarrhoea. The morbidity rate of diarrhoea will be 20%.

Mortality rate

Mortality rate is the percentage/ proportions of animals out of total population died due to disease in a particular disease outbreak. *e.g.* In a population of 100 animals, 20 falls sick and 5 died. The mortality rate will be 5%.

Case fatality rate

Case fatality rate is the percentage/ proportions of animals died among the affected animals. In a population of 100 animals, 20 falls sick and 5 died. The case fatality rate will be 25%.

Biopsy

Biopsy is the examination of tissues received from living animals.

Infection

Infection is the invasion of the tissues of the body by pathogenic organisms resulting in the development of a disease process.

Infestation

Infestation is the superficial attack of any parasite/ organisms on the surface of body.

Pathogenicity

Pathogenicity is the capability of an organism for producing a disease.

Virulence

Virulence is the degree of invasiveness of pathogenic organism.

HISTORICAL MILESTONES

2500-1500 BC	Shalihotra (India)	• First known veterinarian of the world • Written "Haya Ayurved"/ "Ashwa- Ayurved" in Sanskrit, 8 volumes on equine medicine with diagnosis, treatment, effect of planetary forces and evils on health
	Muni Palkapya (India)	• Written a treatise on elephants "Gaj Ayurved"
2100 BC	Hammurabi	• Conduct of Veterinary Practitioners "Laws of Hammurabi"
1000 BC	Krishna (India)	• Mathura is known for best cattle production/ milk production
	Nakul (4th Pandav) (India)	• Written "Ashwa- Chikitsa" a book on equine medicine. • He is considered as an expert of equine management
	Sahdev (5th Pandav) (India)	• Expert in cattle rearing and disease management.
800 BC	Charak (India)	• Written "Charak Sanhita" with details of cause of diseases and impact of environment.
500 BC	Jeevak (India)	• Described the Pathology of brain.
460-375 BC	Hippocrates (Greek)	• Physician, Studied Malaria, pneumonia "Father of Medicine"

Introduction

384-323 BC	Aristotle (Greek)	• Humoral theory of disease • Father of Zoology • Originator of Modern Anatomy & Physiology
300 BC	Chandra Gupta Maurya period	• In Kautilya Arthshashtra description on "Animal Husbandry and Veterinary Sciences", rules on animal ethics and jurisprudence
	Samrat Ashok	• First Veterinary Hospital established for treatment of animal diseases • Prevention of cruelty on animals advertised through wall posters
53 BC-37 AD	Cornelius Celsus (Roman)	• Written 8 volumes of pathology (1st special pathology) Cardinal signs of inflammation (Redness, swelling, heat and pain)
131-206 AD	Claudius Galen (Roman)	• Meat inspection • 5th cardinal sign of inflammation "Loss of function"
450-500 AD	Renatus Vegetius (Roman)	• Father of Veterinary Medicine • Disregard divine pleasure • Disease of animals influence man
600 AD	Madhav	• Described pathology of diarrhoea, dysentery, icterus, tuberculosis and various toxic conditions.
980-1037 AD	Avicenna	• Cause of disease are minute organism • Spreads through air, food, water.
1578-1657 AD	William Harvey	• Blood vascular system and its impact on Pathology

1564 AD-1642 AD	Galileo Galilei	• Developed single microscope
1617 AD-1619 AD	Drebbel	• Developed double lens microscope
1632 AD-1723 AD	Antony van Leeuwenhoek	• Saw microbes first • Book "little animals"
1497 AD-1558 AD	Jean Fernel	• Compiled the information of his time"First to attempt to codify the knowledge of Pathology".
1682-1771 AD	G.B. Morgagni (Italian)	• Conducted 700 autopsies • Began modern pathology • Book "The seats and causes of disease"
1771-1802 AD	Bichat (French)	• Father of pathological anatomy • Foundation for the study of histology • Father of histology
1617-1680 AD	Solleysel (French)	• Book on 'Le Parfact Marechal'
1712-1779 AD	Bourgelat, C (French)	• New Knowledge of equine medicine
1762 AD	Bourgelat, C (French)	• 1st Veterinary School established "Ecole Veterinaire Nationale'd Alfort"
1753-1793 AD	Saint-Bel (French)	• Teacher at Alfort Established Vet School in England 1791 and in 1793 died due to glanders.
1728-1793 AD	John Hunter (English)	• First experimental Pathologist
1804-1878 AD	Carl Rokitanskey (German)	• Supreme descriptive Pathologist

1801-1858 AD	Mueller. J. (German)	• Cellular Pathology, his work "The fine structure and form of morbid tumors"
1821-1902 AD	R. Virchow (German)	• Journal "Virchow's Archives" • Great work on cellular Pathology "Father of modern Pathology"
1818-1865 AD	Semmelwiss (Hungarian)	• Surgery/ autopsy • Started hospital sanitation.
1822-1895 AD	Louis Pasteur (France)	• Bacteria cause of disease
1843-1890 AD	R. Koch (German)	• Koch's postulates, • Identified Tuberculosis, Staphylococcus and Vibrio as cause of disease
1839-1884 AD	J. Cohnheim (German)	• Originator of modern experimental Pathology • Detected leucocytes at the site of inflammation • This forms the basis for the pathology of inflammation. • Introduced frozen sections
1889 AD		• Establishment of Imperial Bacteriological laboratory at Pune (Now IVRI)
1893 AD		• Imperial Bacteriology Laboratory relocated to Mukteshwar in Kumaon Hills
1850-1934 AD	W.H. Welch (U.S.A)	• Professor Pathology • Started Pathology in USA.
1869 AD	Bruck Muller (USA)	• Textbook of Pathological anatomy of domestic and zoo animals.

1884 AD	E. Metchnikoff	•	Phagocytosis (microphages/ macrophages)
1913 AD		•	Imperial Bacteriological Laboratory (now IVRI) established at new campus at Izatnagar- Bareilly
1924 AD		•	The Publication of Indian Veterinary Journal started.
1926 AD	E. Joest	•	Wrote 5 volume of Veterinary Pathology
1931 AD		•	The publication of Indian Journal of Veterinary Sciences and Animal Husbandry (Presently Indian Journal of animal Sciences) started
1933 AD	Ruska and Lorries	•	First developed electronmicroscope.
1936 AD	Bittner	•	Milk transmission of cancer
1938 AD	R.A. Runnels	•	Written book on "Animal Pathology"
1884-1955 AD	Robert Feulgen (Germany)	•	Founder of Histochemistry
1883-1962 AD	G.N. Papanicolaou	•	Father of exfoliative cytology
1953 AD	Watson and Crick	•	Structure of DNA
1885-1979 AD	William Boyd (Canada)	•	Author of Textbook of Pathology

Introduction

1968 AD	G.A. Sastry (India)	•	Author of "Veterinary Pathology" textbook.
1973 AD		•	The Publication of Indian Veterinary Medical Journal started from Lucknow
1974 AD		•	The publication of Indian Journal of Veterinary Pathology started from Izatnagar
1976 AD		•	"Indian Association of Veterinary Pathologist" established under the persidentship of Dr. S. Damodaran.
1989 AD		•	"Veterinary Council of India" established
		•	Dr. C.M. Singh became 1st President of VCI
		•	1st Veterinary and Animal Sciences University established in Madras (now Chennai).
1905-1993 AD	L. Ackerman (USA)	•	Authority on interpretation of frozen sections.
1998 AD		•	Establishment of "Society for Immunology and Immunopathology" at Pantnagar.
		•	Publication of "Journal of Immunology and Immunopathology" started from Pantnagar
2008		•	Indian Association of Veterinary Pathologists celebrated Silver Jubilee
		•	Indian College of Veterinary Pathologists established and First batch of 22 Nos. of Charter Member and Diplomats, ICVP passed out.

Chapter 2
Etiology

Etiology is the study of cause of disease. It gives precise causal diagnosis of any disease. Broadly, the cause of diseases can be divided into two:

a. Intrinsic causes, b. Extrinsic causes

INTRINSIC CAUSES

Those causes, which determine the type of disease present within an individual over which he has no control. These causes are further divided into following subgroups:

Genus

Specific diseases occur in a particular genus or species of animals. *e.g.* Hog cholera in pigs, Canine distemper in dogs

Breed/Race

Diseases do occur in particular breed of animals such as: Dairy cattle are more prone for mastitis. Brain tumors common in Bull dog/ Boxer.

Family

Genetic relationship plays a role in occurrence of diseases in animals. *e.g.* some chickens have resistance of leucosis; hernia in pigs due to weak abdominal wall.

Age

Age of animal may also influence the occurrence of diseases such as:

- In young age diarrhoea/ pneumonia.
- Old age- Tumor
- Canine distemper- Young dogs
- Strangles- Young horse
- Prostatic hyperplasia- Old dogs
- Coccidiosis- Young chickens

Sex

Reproductive disorders are more common in females
- Milk fever, mastitis and metritis in females.
- Nephritis is more in male dogs than female, but Bovine nephritis is more common in females.

Colour

Colour may also play role in occurrence of diseases. *e.g.* Squamous cell carcinoma in white coat colour cattle, melanosarcoma in gray and white horses

Idiosyncrasy

An unusual reaction of body to some substances such as:
- Drug reaction, small dose of drug may produce reaction.
- Individual variations.

EXTRINSIC CAUSES

The etiological factors which are present in the out side environment and may cause/ influence the occurrence of disease. These are also known as exciting cause/ acquired cause. Majority of cause of diseases falls under this group which are further classified as physical, chemical, biological and nutritional causes.

PHYSICAL CAUSES

TRAUMA

Traumatic injury occurs due to any force or energy applied on body of animal *e.g.* During control/ restraining, shipping or transport of animal.

Etiology

Contusions/ Bruises

Contusions or bruises arise from rupture of blood vessel with disintegration of extravassated blood.

Abrasions

Abrasions are circumscribed areas where epithelium has been removed by injury and it may indicate the direction of force.

Erosions

Partial loss of surface epithelium on skin or mucosal surface is termed as erosion.

Incised wounds/ cuts

Incised wounds are produced by sharp edged instrument. They are longer than deep

Stab wound

Stab wounds are deeper than longer produced by sharp edged instrument.

Laceration

Severance of tissue by excessive stretching and is common over bony surfaces or are produced by cut through a dull instrument.

Compression

Compression injury is produced as a result of force applied slowly *e.g.* During parturition.

Blast injury

Force of compression waves against surfaces followed by a wave of reduced pressure. It can rupture muscles/ viscera.

Bullet wound

Hitting at 90° by firearms to produce uniform margins of abrasion. Exit wounds are irregular and lacerated.

ELECTRICAL INJURY

High voltage currents induce tetanic spasms of respiratory muscles and hits the respiratory centre of brain. It also produce flash burns. Lightning causes cyanotic carcass, postmortem bloat, congestion of viscera, tiny haemorrhage and skin damage.

TEMPERATURE

Burns

I degree burns

There is only congestion and injury to the superficial layers of epidermis *e.g.* sun burn on hairless parts or white skinned animal.

II degree burns

Epidermis is destroyed; hair follicles remain intact and provide a nidus for healing of epithelium.

III degree burns

Epidermis and dermis both are destroyed leading to fluid loss, local tissue destruction, laryngeal and pulmonary oedema, renal failure, shock and sepsis. Till 20 hrs of burn, the burn surface remains sterile then bacterial contamination occurs. After 72 hrs millions of bacteria enters in the affected tissue. Bacteria such as staphylococci, streptococci and *Pseudomonas aeruginosa* invade the deeper layers of skin and cause sepsis. There is a state of immunosuppression in severe burns leading to impaired phagocytosis by neutrophils.

Hyperthermia

Hyperthermia means increased body temperature due to high environmental temperature *e.g.* Pets in hot environment without water. Hyperthermia leads to increased respiration (hyperpnoea), rapid heart beat (tachycardia), and degeneration in myocardium, renal tubules and brain.

Etiology

Hypothermia

Hypothermia means decreased body temperature and includes freeze induced necrosis of tissues at extremities

RADIATION INJURY

Radiation as a result of exposure to X-rays, Gamma rays or UV rays leads to cell swelling, vacuolation of endoplasmic reticulum, swelling of mitochondria, nuclear swelling and chromosomal damage resulting in mutation. The impact of radiation is more on dividing cells of ovary, sperm, lymphocytes, bone marrow tissue, and intestinal epithelium. It is characterized by vomiting, leucopenia, bone marrow atrophy, anemia, oedema, lymphoid tissue and epithelial necrosis.

BIOLOGICAL CAUSES

Virus

Viruses are smallest organisms, which have only one type of nucleic acid DNA or RNA in their core covered by protein capsid.

Viruses of Veterinary Importance with their classification

(International Committee on taxonomy of viruses, 2005)

DNA Viruses

S.No.	Family	Genus	Virus species	Disease
Group I - ds DNA viruses (Double stranded DNA virus)				
1.	Adenoviridae	Aviadenovirus Atadenovirus Mastadenovirus	Fowl adenovirus Ovine adenovirus A Canine adenovirus 1	IBH, EDS, HPS in birds Pneumonia in Sheep ICH in Dog
2.	Herpesviridae	Alphaherpes virus	Herpes suis	Pseudorabies in pigs
			Bovine herpes virus - 1 (BHV-1)	IBR, IPV in cattle
			Equine herpes virus - 1 (EHV-1)	Equine viral abortion
			Equine herpes virus - 4 (EHV-4)	Rhinopneumonitis in equines
			Equine herpes virus - 3 (EHV-3)	Coital exanthema
			Avian herpes virus type-1 (AHV-1)	ILT in birds

		Betaherpes virus	Porcine cytomegalo virus	Inclusion body rhinitis in pigs
		Gammaherpes virus	Malignant catarrhal fever virus	MCF in cattle
			Marek's disease virus	Marek's disease in birds
3.	Papillomaviridae	Papillomavirus	Bovine papillomavirus	Cutaneous papilloma in cattle
			Canine oral papillomavirus	Oral papilloma in dogs
			Rabbit papillomavirus	Cutaneous papilloma in rabbits
4.	Poxviridae	Orthopox virus	Vaccinia virus, Cowpox virus, Buffalopox virus, Monkeypox virus, Rabbitpox virus Camelpox virus	Pox in animals
		Avipox virus	Fowlpox virus, Pigeonpox virus, Turkeypox virus, Canarypox virus	Fowl pox, Pigeon pox, Turkeypox, Canarypox
		Capripox virus	Sheeppox virus, Goatpox virus	Sheep pox, Goat pox
		Leporipox virus	Myxoma virus	Myxomatosis in Rabbits
		Suipox virus	Swinepox virus	Swine pox
		Parapox virus	Orfpox virus	Orf in sheep
Group II - ss DNA viruses (Single stranded DNA virus)				
1.	Circoviridae	Circovirus	Porcine circovirus	-
		Gyrovirus	Chicken anemia virus	Chicken infectious anemia
2.	Parvoviridae	Parvovirus	Murine minute virus	
		Bocavirus	Bovine parvovirus	Diarrhoea in cattle
			Canine parvovirus	Enteritis, myocarditis in dogs
			Porcine parvovirus	Infertility, fetal death in pigs

Etiology

RNA Viruses

S.No	Family	Genus	Virus species	Disease
	Group III - ds RNA virus (Double stranded RNA virus)			
1.	Birnaviridae	Avibirnavirus	IBD virus	IBD in birds
		Aquabirnavirus	Infectious pancreatic necrotic virus	Infectious pancreatic necrosis
2.	Reoviridae	Orthoreovirus	Mammalian orthoreo virus	Pneumoenteritis in calves
		Orbivirus	Blue tongue virus	Blue tongue in sheep
		Rotavirus	Rotavirus	Diarrhoea in neonates
	Group IV - (+ve) ss RNA virus (Positive single stranded RNA or M RNA like)			
1.	Arteriviridae	Arterivirus	Equine arteritis virus	Equine viral arteritis
2.	Coronaviridae	Coronavirus	Infectious bronchitis virus	Infectious bronchitis in birds
			Bovine coronavirus	Diarrhoea in calves
3.	Astroviridae	Avastrovirus	Turkey astrovirus	-
4.	Calciviridae	Vesivirus	Swine vesicular exanthema virus	Vesicular exanthema in pigs
		Lagovirus	Rabbit haemorrhagic disease virus	Haemmorhagic disease in rabbit
		Norovirus	Norwalk virus	-
5.	Flaviviridae	Flavirus	Yellow fever virus	Yellow fever in man
		Hepacivirus	Hepatitis C virus	Hepatitis in man
		Pestivirus	BVD virus, CSF virus	BVD, CSF
6.	Picornaviridae	Enterovirus	Poliovirus	Polio in man
		Rhinovirus	Rhinovirus	Rhinitis
		Hepatovirus	Hepatitis A virus	Hepatitis
		Cardiovirus	Encephalomyocarditis virus	Encephalomyocarditis
		Aphthovirus	FMD virus	FMD
		Erbovirus	Equine rhinitis B virus	Respiratory disease in equines
7.	Togaviridae	Alphavirus	Equine Encephalomyelitis virus	Equine encephalomyelitis
		Rubivirus	Rubellavirus	
	Group V – (-ve) ss RNA virus (Negative single stranded RNA)			
1.	Paramyxoviridae	Paramyxovirus	Parainfluenza virus 1 (PI-1)- Pigs,	Respiratory diseases in pigs
			Parainfluenza virus 2 (PI-2)- Dogs,	Kennel cough in dogs
			Parainfluenza virus 3 (PI-3)- Cattle	Respiratory disease in cattle

		Avulavirus	Ranikhet disease virus	Ranikhet disease in birds
		Morbillivirus	Canine Distemper virus, Rinderpest virus, PPR virus	CD in dogs, RP- in animals, PPR – sheep, goat
2.	Bornaviridae	Borna disease virus	Borna disease virus	Borna disease in sheep
3.	Filoviridae	Ebolavirus	-	-
		Filovirus	-	-
4.	Rhabdoviridae	Vesiculovirus	Vesicular stomatitis virus	Vesicular stomatitis in bovines
		Lyssavirus	Rabies virus	Rabies
		Ephemerovirus	Ephemeral fever virus	Ephemeral fever in animals
5.	Bunyaviridae	Hantavirus	Hantaanvirus	Hantavirus pulmonary syndrome, Korean haemorragic fever
		Phlebovirus	Nairobi sheep disease virus, Rift valley fever virus, Akabana disease virus	Nairobi Sheep disease, RVF Akabana disease
6.	Orthomyxoviridae	Influenza virus A, Influenza virus B, Influenza virus C	Influenza virus A, Influenza virus B, Influenza virus C	Influenza in animals

Group VI ss RNA-RT virus (Single stranded RNA virus with reverse transcriptase)

1.	Retroviridae	Alpharetrovirus	Avian leucosis virus	ALC in birds
		Betaretrovirus	Mouse mammary tumour virus	Cancer in mice
		Gammaretrovirus	Murine leukemia virus	Leukemia in mice
			Feline leukemia virus	Leukemia in cats
		Deltaretrovirus	Bovine leukemia virus	Bovine leukemia
		Lentivirus	Bovine immunodeficiency virus	Bovine immunodeficiency syndrome
			Feline immunodeficiency virus	Feline immunodeficiency syndrome

Group VII ds DNA-RT virus (Double stranded DNA virus with reverse transcriptase)

1.	Hepadnaviridae	Orthohepadnavirus	Hepatitis B virus	Hepatitis
		Avihepadna virus	Duck hepatitis B virus	Duck hepatitis

Sub viral agents

- Prion proteins are infectious proteins without any nucleic acid. *e.g.* Bovine spongiform encephalopathy.
- Viroids are having only nucleic acid without proteins. They do not cause any disease in animals. However, they are associated with plant diseases.

Rickettsia

Coxiella burnetti causes Q-fever

Mycoplasma

Mycoplasma mycoides is responsible for pneumonia, joint ailments and genital disorders

Chlamydia

Chlamydia trachomatis, C. psittaci cause abortions, pneumonia, and eye ailments.

Spirochaete

Leptospira sp. causes abortion, icterus.

Borrelia ansarina causes fowl spirochetosis in chickens.

Bacteria

Bacteria are classified as Gram positive and Gram negative on the basis of Gram's staining. Gram positive bacteria include Staphylococci, Streptococci, Corynebacterium, Listeria, Bacillus Clostridia. Gram negative bacteria are *E. coli*, Salmonella, Proteus, Klebsiella, Pasteurella, Pseudomonas, Brucella, Yersinia, Campylobactor etc. Besides, there are certain organisms stained with Zeihl Neelson stain and are known as acid fast bacilli *e.g.Mycobacterium tuberculosis* and *M. paratuberculosis*.

Fungi

Fungi pathogenic for animals are mostly belongs to fungi imperfecti. *e.g.* Histoplasmosis

Fungi cause three type of disease- Mycosis *e.g.* Actinomycosis; Allergic disease *e.g.* Ringworm; Mycotoxicosis *e.g.* Aflatoxicosis.

Parasites

Parasites are classified mainly in 3 groups:

Protozoan Parasites

Trypanosoma evansi, Theileria annulata, Babesia bigemina, Toxoplasma gondii, Eimeria Spp.

Helminths

Nematodes- Roundworms *e.g.* Ascaris,

Trematod- Flat worms *e.g.* Liverfluke

Cestodes- Tapeworms *e.g Taenia* spp.

Arthropods

Ticks, Mites, Flies, Lice

TRANSMISSION

Biological agents are transmitted from one animal to another through horizontal or vertical transmission.

Horizontal Transmission

Horizontal transmission of biological causes occurs through direct contact or indirectly via animal or inanimate (fomites) objects. It is also known as lateral transmission as it occurs in a population from one to another. Various methods of horizontal transmission are as under:

Ingestion: Food, water, faecal-oral route *e.g.* Salmonellosis, Johne's disease, Rotavirus infection.

Inhalation: Air borne infections, droplet infection *e.g.* R.P., FMD, Tuberculosis.

Contact: Fungal infection, Bacterial dermatitis, Flu, Brucellosis, Rabies through bite.

Inoculation: Introduction of infection in body through puncture either mechanically through needles or by arthropods such as by ticks. Ticks transmit diseases through transovarian (one generation to next generation) or transstadial (through developmental stages) transmission.

Iatrogenic: Transmission of infection during surgical practice or it is created by doctor, through dirty instrument and contaminated preparations.

Coitus: Through sexual contact of animals, biological agents spread from one to another animals. *e.g.* Campylobacteriosis, Trichomoniasis.

Vertical Transmission

Vertical transmission occurs from one generation to another generation *in ovo*/ *in utero* or through milk. These include:

Hereditary

Infection/ disease carried in the genome of either parent *e.g.* Retrovirus

Congenital

Diseases acquired either *in utero*/ *in ovo*
- Infection in ovary/ ovum (Germinative transmission) *e.g.* ALC in chickens, lymphoid leukemia in mice, Salmonellosis in poultry.
- Infection through placenta. *e.g.* Feline panleukopenia virus (Transmission to embryo)
- Ascending infection from lower genital canal to amnion/ placenta *e.g.* Staphylococci.
- Infection at Parturition: Infection from lower genital tract during birth. *e.g.* Herpex simplex virus.

MAINTENANCE OF INFECTION

Biological agents face difficulty of survival at both places in environment or in host. Two types of hazards which create problem to agent.

Internal hazards e.g. Host immune system

External hazards e.g. Desiccation, UV light

Agents try to maintain themselves by adopting following maintenance strategies:
- Avoidance of a stage in the external environment.
- Resistant forms *e.g.* Anthrax spores.
- Rapidly in-rapidly out strategy *e.g.* Viruses of respiratory tract.
- Persistence within the host *e.g. Mycobacterium tuberculosis*, Slow viral diseases.
- Extension of host range.
- Infection in more than one host *e.g.* Foot and mouth disease.

CHEMICAL CAUSES

Biological Toxins

Snake venom

Snake venom have phospholipase A_2 which causes lytic action on membranes of RBC and platelets.

The presence of hyaluronidase, phosphodiesterase and peptidase in snake venom are responsible for oedema, erythema, haemolytic anemia, swelling of facial/ laryngeal tissues, haemoglobinurea, cardiac irregularities, fall in blood pressure, shock and neurotoxicity.

Microbial toxins

Microbial toxins are those toxins/ poisons that are produced by microbial agents particularly by bacteria and fungi.

Bacterial toxins

Bacterial toxins include structural proteins (endotoxins) and soluble peptides/ secretary toxins (exotoxins). Endotoxins are present in cell wall of Gram-negative bacteria and are found to be responsible for septicemia and shock. Exotoxins are secreted by bacteria outside their cell wall and are found responsible for protein lysis and damage of cell membrane. *e.g.* Clostridium toxins suppress metabolism of cell. Most potent clostridial toxins

Etiology

are botulinum and tetanus, which are the cause of hemolysis and are powerful neurotoxin. Besides, *Clostridium chauvei* toxins are responsible for black leg disease in cattle.

Fungal Toxins (Mycotoxins)

There are several fungi known for production of toxins. Such toxins are known as mycotoxins and they are mostly found in food/ feed items, which causes disease in animals through ingestion.

Aflatoxins

Aflatoxins are produced by several species of fungi including mainly *Aspergillus flavus, A. parasiticus* and *Penicillium puberlum*. These aflatoxins are classified as B_1, B_2, G_1, G_2, M_1, M_2, B_2a, G_2a and aspertoxin. Aflatoxins are produced in moist environment in grounded animal/ poultry feed on optimum temperature and are more common in tropical countries where storage conditions are poor and provide suitable environment for the growth of fungi. These toxins are known to cause immunosuppression, formation of malignant neoplasms and hepatopathy.

Ergot

Ergot is produced by *Claviceps purpura* in grains which causes blackish discoloration. It produces gangrene by chronic vasoconstriction, ischemia and capillary endothelium degeneration. It is also associated with summer syndrome in cattle characterized by gangrene of extremities.

Fusarium toxins

Fusarium toxins are produced by *Fusarium tricinctum* in paddy straw, which are found to cause gangrene in extremities. Zearalenone toxin is the cause of ovarian abnormality in sow.

Ochratoxins

Ochratoxins are produced by *Aspergillus ochracheous* and *A. viridicatum* fungi in grounded feed on optimum temperature and moisture and are found to cause renal tubular necrosis in chickens and pigs.

Plant toxins

Over 700 plants are known to produce toxin. *e.g.* Braken fern which causes haematuria and enccphalomalacia. Strychnine from *Strychnos nuxvomica* is highly toxic and causes death in animals with nervous signs. It is used for dog killing in public health operations to control rabies. HCN is found in sorghum which is known to cause clonic convulsions and death in animals characterized by haemorrhage in mucous membranes.

Drug toxicity

- *Antibiotics:* Cause direct toxicity by destroying gut microflora. Oxytetracyline, sulfonamides are nephrotoxic. Neomycin and Lincomycin cause Mal-absorption diarrhoea and Immunosuppression.
- *Anti-inflammatory drugs:* like acetaminophen causes hepatic necrosis, icterus and hemolytic anemia.
- *Anticoccidiostate drug:* Monensin is responsible for necrosis of cardiac and skeletal muscles.
- *Trace elements:* There are various trace elements; excess of which may cause poisoning in animals. *e.g.* Selenium poisoning "Blind staggers" or "Alkali Disease" in cattle characterized by chronic debilitating disease. It also causes encephalomalacia in pigs.

Environmental Pollutants

Environment is polluted due to presence of unwanted materials in food, water, air and surroundings of animals, particularly by agrochemicals including pesticides and fertilizers. The environmental pollutants exert their direct or indirect effect on the animal health and production. The main pollutants are:
- Heavy metals such as mercury, lead, cadmium are found in industrial waste, automobile and generator smoke, soil, water and also found as contaminants of pesticides and fertilizers, are responsible for damage in kidneys, immune system and neuropathy. They are also associated with immune complex mediated glomerulonephritis.

- Sulpher dioxide is produced by automobiles, industries and generators. It is responsible for loss of cilia in bronchiolar epithelium.
- Hydrogen sulfide is produced by animal's decay and in various industries. It inhibits mitochondrial cytochrome oxidase leading to death.
- Pesticides are agrochemicals used in various agricultural, animal husbandry and public health operations. They are classified as insecticides, herbicides, weedicides and rodenticides. Chemically, insecticides are grouped mainly as organochlorine organophosphates, carbamates and synthetic pyrethroids. Acute poisoning of pesticides causes death in animals after nervous clinical signs of short duration. Chronic toxicity is characterized by immunosuppression, nephropathy, neuropathy, hypersensitivity and autoimmunity in animals.

NUTRITIONAL CAUSES

Nutrition causes disease in animals either due to deficiency or excess of nutrients. It is very difficult to diagnose the nutritional causes and sometimes it is not possible to find a precise cause as in case of infectious disease because functions of one nutrient can be compensated by another in cell metabolism. Experimental production of nutritional deficiency is not identical to natural disease. When tissue concentration of nutrient falls down to the critical level, it leads to abnormal metabolism and the abnormal metabolites present in tissues can be detected in urine and faeces. First changes of nutritional deficiency are recorded in rapidly metabolizing tissues *e.g.* skeletal muscle, myocardium and brain. Immature animals are more susceptible to nutritional disease. *e.g.* calves, chicks, piglets etc.

Types of deficiency
- Acute/ chronic *e.g.* Thiamine deficiency in pigs
- Multiple deficiencies: *e.g.* Poor quality food.
- Nutritional imbalance: *e.g.* Imbalance in calcium: phosphorus (2:1) ratio.

- Protein malnutrition: *e.g.* Malabsorption
- Calorie deficiency: *e.g.* Loss of fat/ Muscle wasting.

Factors responsible for nutritional deficiency
- Interference with intake *e.g.* Anorexia, G.I. tract disorders.
- Interference with absorption *e.g.* Intestinal hypermotility, Insoluble complexes in food (Fat/ Calcium)
- Interference with storage *e.g.* Hepatic disease leads to deficiency of vit. A.
- Increased excretion *e.g.* Polyuria, Sweating and Lactation
- Increased requirement *e.g.* Fever, Hyperthyroidism and Pregnancy
- Natural inhibitors *e.g.* Presence of thiaminases in feed, leads to thiamine deficiency.

Calorie deficiency

Calorie deficiency in animals occurs due to food deprivation or starvation.

Food deprivation

Dietary deficiency of food in terms of quantity/ quality leads to emaciation, loss of musculature, atrophy of fat, subcutaneous oedema, cardiac muscle degeneration and atrophy of viscera including liver and pancreas. The volume of hepatocytes reduced by 50% and mitochondrial total volume is also reduced 50%.

Starvation

Starvation is the long continued deprivation of food. It is characterized by fatty degeneration of liver, anemia and skin diseases. Young and very old animals are more susceptible to starvation while in pregnant animals it causes retarded growth of foetus. In animals, following changes can be seen due to starvation.

Intestinal involution

Absorptive surface is reduced with shrunken cells and pyknotic nuclei. Villi becomes shorter and shows atrophy.

Etiology

Atrophy of muscles

There is decrease in muscle mass.

Lipolysis

Increased cortisol leads to increased lipolysis resulting in formation of fatty acids in liver which in turn converts into ketones used by brain.

Gluconeogenesis

In early fasting blood glucose level drops down. The insulin level becomes low while glucagon goes high in starvation. The glucose comes from skeletal muscle, adipose tissue and lymphoid tissue during starvation. Twenty four hours of food deprivation causes reduction in liver glycogen and blood glucose. Fatty acids from adipose tissue forms glucose and in mitochondria after oxidation it forms acetoacetate, hydroxybutyrate and acetone. Which are also known as ketone bodies and are present in blood stream during starvation. It is also known as ketosis *e.g.* Ketosis/ Acetonemia in bovines. Lack of glucose in blood leads to oxidation of fatty acids which forms ketone bodies as an alternate source of energy. They are normal/ physiological at certain level but may become pathological when their level is high.

Clinically it is characterized by anorexia, depression, coma, sweet smell in urine, concentration of acetone increases in milk, blood and urine along with hyperlipimia and acidosis. A similar condition also occurs in sheep known as pregnancy toxaemia which is characterized by depression, coma and paralysis. This situation occurs when many children/ foetuses are there in uterus. There are fatty changes in liver, kidneys, and heart, with subepicardial petechiae or echymosis.

Protein deficiency

Generally, protein deficiency does not occur. However, the deficiency of essential amino acids has been reported in animals when certain ingredients are deficient in certain amino acids. *e.g.* maize is deficient in lysine, and tryptophan that leads to slow growth; peanuts and soybean are deficient in methioine. Protein deficiency is characterized by hypoproteinemia, anemia, poor growth, delayed healing, decreased or cesation of cell proliferation, failure of collagen formation, atrophy of testicles and ovary, atrophy of thymus and lymphoid tissue.

Deficiency of Lipids

Generally, there is no deficiency of fat in animals. However, essential fatty acids including linolenic acid, linoleic acid and arachidonic acid deficiency may occur which causes dermatoses in animals. Fat has high calorie value and it is required in body because there are certain vitamins soluble in fat only.

Deficiency of Water

Deficiency of water may lead to dehydration and slight wrinkling in skin. Deficiency may occur due to fever, vomiting, diarrhoea, haemorrhage and polyuria, which can be corrected through adequate water supply for drinking or through intravenous fluid therapy.

Deficiency of Vitamins

Vitamin deficiency may occur due to starvation. There are two types of vitamins viz., fat soluble and water soluble. Fat soluble vitamins are vit. A, D, E and K and water soluble are vit B complex and C.

Vitamin A

It is also known as retinol. It is derived from its precursor carotene. It is found in abundant in plants having yellow pigment, animal fat, liver, cod liver oil, shark liver oil. b-carotene is cleaved in gut mucosa into two molecules of retinol (Vit. A aldehyde) which after absorption is stored in liver. Bile salts and pancreatic juice are responsible for absorption of vit. A from gut. Deficiency of Vit. A occurs due to damage in liver.

Vit. A deficiency may lead to following disease conditions:

Squamous metaplasia of epithelial surfaces in esophagus, pancreas, bladder and parotid duct, which is considered

Etiology

pathognomonic in calves. Destruction of epithelium/ goblet cell in respiratory mucosa is generally replaced by keratin synthesizing squamous cells in vit. A deficient animals. There are *abnormal teeth* in animals due to hypoplasia of enamel and its poor mineralization. Vitamin A deficiency is also associated with *still birth* and *abortions* in pigs. It causes night blindness (*Nyctalopia*) in animals. Due to deficiency of Vit. A there is recurrent episodes of conjunctivitis/ keratitis. In poultry, there is distention of mucous glands, which opens in pharynx and esophagus because of metaplasia of duct epithelium leading to enlargement of esophageal glands due to accumulation of its secretions. The glands become spherical, 1-2 mm dia. over mucosa. It is considered pathognomonic for hypovitaminosis A. and is known as *Nutritional roup*. Inflammation of upper respiratory tract lead to coryza. Urinary tract of cattle, sheep and goat suffers due to formation of calculi, which may cause obstruction in sigmoid flexure of urethra in males. Such calculi are made up of desquamated epithelial cells and salts and the condition is known as *urolithiasis*. Deficiency of vit. A may also lead to in abnormal bone growth of cranial bones and there is failure of foramen ovale to grow leading to constriction of optic nerves which results in blindness in calves, increased CSF pressure, blindness at birth and fetal malformations. In sows, piglets are born without eyes (*Anophthalmos*) or with smaller eyes- (*Microphthalmos*).

Vitamin D

Vitamin D occurs in 3 forms viz. vitamin D_2 or calciferol, Vit. D_3 or cholecaliciferol and Vit D_1 impure mixture of sterols. About 80% Vit. D is synthesized in body skin through UV rays on 7-hydrocholesterol. In diet containing egg butter, it is found in abundant quantity in milk, plants, grains etc. Active forms of vit. D are 25-hydroxy vit. D and 1, 25 dihydroxy vit D. (Calcitriol) which is 5 to 10 times more potent than former. Vit D is stored in adipose tissue in body. The main functions of vit D are absorption of Ca and P from intestines and kidneys, mineralization of bones, maintains blood levels of Ca and P and in immune regulation as it activates lymphocytes and macrophages.

- The deficiency of vitamin D is associated with rickets in young animals, osteomalacia in adult animals and hypocalcemic tetany.
- Excess of vitamin D leads to the formation of renal calculi, metastatic calcification and osteoporosis in animals.

Vitamin E (α- tocopherol)

Source of vitamin E is grains, oils, nuts, vegetables, and in body it is stored in adipose tissue, liver and muscles. It has antioxidant activity and prevents oxidative degradation of cell membrane.
- Deficiency of vit E causes degeneration of neurons in peripheral nerves. There is denervation of muscles leading to muscle dystrophy e.g. *White muscle disease* in cattle and *Stiff lamb disease* in sheep and *Myoglobinuria* in horses. Deficiency of vit. E causes degeneration of pigments in retina reduces life span of RBC, leading to anemia and sterility in animals. Crazy chick disease (*Encephalomalacia*) is also caused by vit E deficiency; the chicks become sleepy with twisting of head and neck. There is muscular dystrophy in chickens due to vit. E deficiency.

Vitamin K

Vit. K occurs in two forms namely Vit. K_1 or Phylloquinone found in green leaf and vegetables and Vit- K_2 or Menadione which is produced by gut microflora. Its main function is coagulation of blood. Deficiency of vit K may leads to hypoprothrombinemia and haemorrhages.

Vitamin B

Vitamin B is a water soluble vitamin which has at least 9 sub types including B_1 or thiamine, B_2 or riboflavin, B_6 or pyridoxine, B_{12} or cyanocobalamin, niacin or nicotinic acid, folate or folic acid, choline, biotine and pantothenic acid.

Thiamine

In ruminants synthesis of thiamine occurs in rumen. Source of vit. B are pea, beans, pulses, green vegetables, roots, fruits,

Etiology

rice, wheat bran etc. Strong tea, coffee have antithiamine action. It is stored in muscles, liver, heart, kidneys and bones of animals. Thiamine plays active role in carbohydrate metabolism.

- Deficiency of thiamine may lead to *Beri beri disease* characterized by Ataxia and neural/ lesions. *Chastek paralysis* in cats, fox and mink and *stargazing* attitude of chicks due to thiaminase (thiamine deficiency) in meal may be observed. Bracken fern poisoning in cattle and horses may cause deficiency of thiamine due to presence of thiaminase enzyme in bracken fern. Toxicity of thiamine splitting drugs like amprolium, a coccidiostate, may cause polioencephalomalcia in cattle and sheep. Cardiac dialation in pigs has also been observed due to vit. B_1 deficiency.

Riboflavin

Riboflavin is a component of several enzymes and is found in plants, meat, eggs and vegetables.

- Deficiency of riboflavin may cause *Curled Toe Paralysis* in chicks and swelling of sciatic and brachial nerves.

Niacin

Role of niacin (NAD/ NADP, nicotinamide adenine dinueotide) is in electron transport in mitochondria of cells. It is found in grains, cereals, meat, liver, kidneys, vegetables and plants.

- Deficiency of niacin is associated with skin disorders in man *Pellegra*; anorexia, diarrhoea, anemia in pigs and mucous hyperplasia, haemorrhage in gastrointestinal tract and black tongue in dogs which is also known as *Canine pellegra*.

Pyridoxine

It is found in egg, green vegetables, meat, liver etc.

- Deficiency of pyridoxine causes uremia, convulsions, dermatitis and glossitis.

Pantothenic acid

- Pantothenic acid deficiency is associated with stunted growth of chicks.

Folate
- Folic acid is required in formation of erythrocytes and hence its deficiency leads to anemia.

Cyanocobalamin
Deficiency of cyanocobalamin may also lead to anemia, as it is also needed in RBC formation.

Biotin
Biotin deficiency causes paralysis of hind legs in calves.

Choline
Choline deficiency is associated with fatty changes in liver and perosis.

Vitamin C (Ascorbic acid)
It is found in green plants and citrus fruits.

Deficiency of vit. C may cause retardation of fibroplasia, scurvy in G. pigs, haemorrhage, swelling, ulcers and delayed wound healing in animals.

MINERALS
Various minerals are also necessary for survival of animals. Deficiency of any one of them or in combination may cause serious disease in animals. Some of the important minerals are:

- Sodium chloride
- Calcium
- Phosphorus
- Magnesium
- Iodine
- Iron
- Copper
- Cobalt
- Manganese
- Potassium
- Fluorine
- Sulfur
- Selenium
- Zinc

Etiology

Sodium chloride

Sodium chloride is an essential salt which maintains osmotic pressure in blood, interstitial tissue and the cells because 65% of osmotic pressure is due to sodium chloride. Chloride ions of hydrochloric acid present in stomach also comes from sodium chloride.

- The excess of sodium chloride causes gastroenteritis in cattle, gastroenteritis and eosinophilic meningoencephalitis in pigs and ascites in poultry.
- Deficiency of sodium chloride is characterized by anorexia, constipation, loss of weight in sows and pica, weight loss, decreased milk production and polyurea in cattle. Deficiency of salt occurs due to diarrhoea, dehydration and vomiting.

Calcium

Normal range of calcium is 10-11 mg/ 100 ml blood in body of animals. If it increases above 12 mg/ 100 ml blood, metastatic calcification occurs, while its level less than 8 mg/ 100 ml blood may show signs of deficiency characterized by tetany.

Absorption of calcium from gut is facilitated by vit. D. Paratharmone stimulates to raise blood Ca level from bones while calcitonin from thyroid stimulates it's deposition in bones and thus reduces blood Ca levels.

- In pregnant cows, calcium deficiency occurs just after parturition. During gestation calcium goes to foetus from skeleton of cows, resulting in weak skeleton of dam. If calcium is not provided in diet, it may cause disease in dam characterized by locomotor disturbances, abnormal curvature of back, distortion of pelvis, tetany, incoordination, muscle spasms, unconsciousness and death. Such symptoms occur in animals when their blood calcium level falls below 6 mg/ 100 ml of blood and if it is less than 3 mg/ 100ml blood, death occurs instantly.
- Milk fever is a disease of cattle occurs due to deficiency of calcium just after parturition. Cow suddenly becomes recumbent and sits on sternum with head bending towards

flank and is unable of get up. No gross/ microscopic lesion reported in this disorder. The calcium therapy recovers the animal immediately.

- The excess of calcium may cause metastatic calcification leading to its deposition in soft tissue of kidney, lungs and stomach.

Magnesium

It acts as activator of many enzymes *e.g.* alkaline phosphatase. It requires for activation of membrane transport synthesis of protein, fat and nucleic acid and for generation/ transmission of nerve impulses. The normal blood levels are 2 mg/ 100 ml of blood.

- Dietary deficiency leads to hypomagnesaemia and a level below 0.7 mg/ 100 ml cause symptoms in calves characterized by nervous hyperirritability, tonic and clonic convulsions, depression, coma and death.
- The post-mortem lesions of magnesium deficiency includes haemorrhage in heart, intestines, mesentery and congestion of viscera.
- Microscopic lesions include calcification of intimal layer of heart blood vessels (metastatic) muscles and kidneys. *Grass tetany and Grass staggers* occurs due to hypomagne semia and characterized by hyperirritability, abnormal gait, coma and death.

Phosphorus

Normal level of phosphorus is 4-8 mg/ 100 ml of blood. In bones, it is in the form of calcium phosphate. Deficiency of phosphorus may lead to hypophosphatemia and characterized by pica, rheumatism and hemoglobinurea.

- Pica is licking/ eating of objects other than food. It mainly occurs in cattle, buffaloes and camels, who eats bones, mud and other earthern materials. Such animals have heavy parasitic load in their gut.
- Rheumatism like syndrome is characterized by lameness in hind legs particularly in camels and buffaloes.

Etiology

- Hemoglobinurea is characterized by the presence of coffee colour urine of animal due to extensive intravascular hemolysis Hemo globinurea thus known as postparturient hemoglobinurea.

Selenium

Deficiency of selenium causes hemolysis as it protects cell membrane of RBC and thus its deficiency leads to anemia. Blind Staggers occurs due to excess of selenium.

Iron

Deficiency of iron leads to anemia, which is hypochromic and microcytic but rarely occurs in animals.

Copper

Deficiency of copper results in anemia and steel wool disease in sheep, which is characterized by loss of crimp in wool. Enzootic ataxia with incoordination of posterior limb has been observed in goats.

Cobalt

Vit. B_{12} is synthesized by ruminal bacteria from cobalt in ruminants. Cobalt also stimulates erythropoiesis. Its deficiency may cause wasting disease, cachexia and emaciation in animals. The pathological lesions are comprised of anemia, hemosiderosis in liver, spleen and kidneys.

Manganese

Deficiency of manganese causes slipped tendon in chicken or perosis characterized by shortening of long bones in chickens. It occurs as the epiphyseal cartilage fails to ossify at 12 week of age and epiphysis becomes loose and thus gastrocnemious tendon slips medially and condition is known as *Slipped Tendon* or *Perosis*.

Zinc

Deficiency of zinc may cause parakeratosis in pigs at 10-20 weeks age. Calcium in diet with phytate or phosphate forms a complex with zinc making it unavailable for absorption leading to its deficiency, which is characterized by rough skin of abdomen, medial surface of thigh, which becomes horny. It also causes fascial eczema in cattle, thymic hypoplasia in calves and immunodeficiency in animals.

Iodine

Deficiency of iodine causes goiter in newborn pigs characterized by absence of hair on their skin. Other signs of iodine deficiency include abnormal spermatozoa, decreased spermatogenesis, loss of libido, reduced fertility, suboestrus, anoestrus, abortions, dystocia and hydrocephalus. Excess of iodine may lead to lacrimation and exfoliation of dandruff like epidermal scales from skin.

Fluorine

Excess of fluorine causes mottling in teeth and bones. The teeth become shorter, broader with opaque areas.

Chapter 3

Genetic Disorders, Developmental Anomalies and Monsters

GENETICS

Genetics is the branch of science deals with study of genes, chromosomes and transmittance of characters from one generation to another.

CHROMOSOMES

Chromosomes are thread like structures present in the form of short pieces in nucleus of a cell. They are in pairs; of which one pair is sex chromosome and others are autosomes.

Table 3.1: Number of chromosomes in different species of animals

Sl. No.	Animal	Chromosomes		Male	Female
		Pairs	Total		
1.	Cattle	30	60	XY	XX
2.	Buffalo (River)	25	50	XY	XX
3.	Sheep	27	54	XY	XX
4.	Goat	30	60	XY	XX
5.	Pig	19	38	XY	XX
6.	Dog	39	78	XY	XX
7.	Cat	19	38	XY	XX
8.	Horse	32	64	XY	XX
9.	Donkey	31	62	XY	XX
10.	Poultry	39	78	ZZ	ZW

- Each chromosome is composed of two chromatids connected at centromere.
- Chromosomes are grouped together on the basis of their

length, location of centromere and this procedure is known as *Karyotyping*.
- The study of Karyotyping is known as *cytogenetics*.
- Chromosomes are composed of 3 components:
- DNA - 20%
- RNA - 10%
- Nuclear Proteins - 70%

Deoxyribo nucleic acid (DNA)
- Double helix structure of polynucleotide chain.
- A nucleotide consists of phosphate, sugar and base of either purine (Adenine, Guanine) or pyrimidine (Thymine, Cytosine).
- A sequence of 3 nucleotide determines the synthesis of an amino acid and is known as *genetic code/ codon*.
- During cell division, one half of DNA molecule acts as template for the synthesis of other half by an enzyme DNA polymerase to transmit the genetic information which may also have some disorders to next progeny.

Gene
- Sequence of nucleotides which controls the synthesis of one specific protein is known as *gene*. It is a unit of function. Study of genes is termed as *Genetics*. In higher animals about 1.0 million genes are present.
- Genes located on X or Y chromosomes are termed as sex linked and all other genes are autosomal genes.
- When the genes at one locus are same from both parents they are termed as *homozygous* but when they are different at one locus they are known as *heterozygous*.
- In heterozygous, characters of one gene are manifested in phenotype and such gene is known as *dominant* while unexpressed gene is called as *recessive*.

Karyotyping

- Karyotyping is the study of chromosomes in cell.
- Collection of blood, separation of lymphocytes using Histopaque-1077 gradient.
- The lymphocytes are cultured with mitogen concanavalin A (ConA) or phytohemagglutinin - M (PHA-M) for 72 hrs.
- Colchicine is used after 72 hrs to arrest the cell division at metaphase stage.
- Hypotonic solution is added to allow cells for swelling which causes separation of chromosomes.
- Prepare glass slides and stain with Giemsa or other special stain.
- Identify the chromosomes and photograph them.
- Cut photographs having homologous chromo-somes and make pairs.

GENETIC DISORDERS

ABERRATION IN CHROMOSOMES

- A large number of chromosomal aberrations are removed due to death of gamete or zygote which is termed as *"species cleansing effect"*. Even though some aberrations do persist and expressed in phenotype leading to illness.

1. Aberration in number

- Chromosomes are in pairs (2n). When number of chromosomes are other than (n) or (2n). It is known as *heteroploidy*.

(a) Heteroploidy

- The number of chromosomes are other than (n) or (2n).
- When abnormal number is exact multiplies of the haploid set due to errors in mitosis. The polar body may fail to be extruded from ovum leaving diplod set to be fertilized by sperm (n) i.e. 2n + n = 3n (Triploid zygote).
- When abnormal number is not the exact multiplies of haploid set. It may have specific chromosome in triple number *(trisomy)* or in single number *(monosomy)*.

(b) Duplication and deficiencies

- Duplication or deficiency may occur in a section of chromosome and total number of chromosomes remains same.
- *Translocation* is the rearrangement of a part of chromosome in two non-homologous chromosomes. It may be reciprocal or non-reciprocal. Absence of a piece of chromosome is known as *deletion*.

(c) Mosaicism

- In mosaicism, there is more than one population of cells in body; each population differs in their chromosomes/ genes due to error during development.
- May be due to chromosomal non-disjunction e.g. XXY in some cells, XY in other cells.

(d) *Chimerism*

- In this, one type of cells are acquired *in utero* from a twin e.g. Bovine twin 1 male and 1 female with joint placenta. The blood cells of male may go in female counterpart. Then the female will have two type of cell population, one of its own and another acquired from twin. Similarly, male may also have XX leucocytes in its blood. Such chimeric bulls are sterile.

2. Abnormalities in sex chromosomes

(a) *Klinefelters syndrome*

- Male have sex chromatin i.e. XXY = 47(2n) in man.
- In some cells, different number of chromosomes i.e. XX, XXY, XXXY, XXYY
- It is recognized in adolscence by small testes, tall body, and low sexual characters, mostly infertile.
- May occur in sheep, cattle and horse.

(b) *Tortoiseshell male cat*

- Male cat has small testes, lack of libido and absence of spermatozoa in testes with 3n chromosomes (XXY).

Genetic Disorders, Developmental Anomalies and Monsters

(c) Turner's syndrome
- Mare are with XO karyotype having gonadal dysgenesis and such animals are sterile and do not have sex chromatin.

In mice XO karyotype is normal.

(d) Intersexes
- In this condition ambiguity occurs in genitalia or the secondary sex characters are present for both the sexes including male and female.
- Hermaphrodites have male and female genitalia while pseudohermaphrodites are having external genitalia of one sex and gonads of opposite sex.

(e) Freemartinism
- In bovine twins, one male with (XY) and one female (XX) karyotype but they share placental circulation so cells of embryo establish in other co-twin.

(f) Testicular feminization
- Animal is having female genitalia as external and internal organs but in place of ovaries, there are testes. It occurs due to single gene defect and makes tissues unresponsive to androgenic hormones.

3. Abnormalities in autosomal chromosomes

(a) Down's syndrome/ Mongolism
- It occurs as a result of trisomy, number of a particular chromosome increases leaving 2n, as 61 in bovines, 77 in dogs and 47 in man *e.g.* bovine lymphosarcoma occurs in animals with 2n=61. Male dog with 2n= 77 are prone to lymphoma.

(b) Sterility in hybrids
- Donkey has 2n=62 and horse has 2n= 64. Their cross mule has 2n=63.

- Sterility in mules, cause is not known, may be due to uneven number of chromosomes.

4. Abnormalities in genes
- Lethal genes are those genes, which are responsible for death of zygote.
- Sublethal genes
- X-linked or sex linked: Diseases transmitted by heterozygous carrier females only to male offsprings who are homozygous for X-chromosome.

ANOMALIES

Anomaly is a developmental abnormality occurs in any organ/tissue. It may be due to genetic disorder and may affect the zygote itself within few days after fertilization or may occur during any stage of pregnancy. It may be classified as under:

1. Imperfect development

(a) Agenesis

Agenesis is incomplete development of an organ or mostly it is associated with absence of any organ.
- **Acrania** is absence of cranium.
- **Anencephalia** is absence of brain.
- **Hemicrania** is absence of half of head.
- **Agnathia** is absence of lower jaw.
- **Anophathalmia** is absence of one or both eyes.
- **Abrachia** is absence of fore limbs.
- **Abrachiocephalia** is absence of forelimbs and head.
- **Adactylia** is absence of digits.
- **Atresia** is absence of normal opening e.g. *Atresia ani* is absence of anus opening.

(b) Fissures

Fissures are a cleft or narrow opening in an organ on the median line of head, thorax and abdomen.

Genetic Disorders, Developmental Anomalies and Monsters

- **Cranioschisis** is a cleft in skull.
- **Chelioschisis** is a cleft in lips also known as *harelip*.
- **Palatoschisis** is a cleft in palates; also known as *cleft palate*.
- **Rachischisis** is a cleft in spinal column.
- **Schistothorax** is a fissure in thorax.
- **Schistosomus** is a fissure in abdomen.

(c) Fusion

Fusion is joining of paired organs.
- **Cyclopia** is fusion of eyes.
- **Renarcuatus** is fusion of kidneys; also known as *horse shoe kidneys*.

2. Excess of development

- Congenital hypertrophy of any organ.
- Increase in the number of any organ or part/ tissue.
- **Polyotia** is increased number of ears.
- **Polyodontia** is increased number of teeth.
- **Polymelia** is increased number of limbs.
- **Polydactylia** is increased number of digits.
- **Polymastia** is increased number of mammary gland.
- **Polythelia** is increased number of teats.

3. Displacement during development

(a) Displacement of organ
- **Dextrocardia** is the transposition of heart into right side instead of left side of thoracic cavity.
- **Ectopia cordis** is the displacement of heart into neck.

(b) Displacement of tissues
- **Teratoma** is a tumor arising due to some embryonic defect and composed of two or more types of tissues. In this at least two tissues should be of origin.

- Dermoid cyst is a mass containing skin, hair, feathers or teeth depending on the species and often arranged as cyst. It mostly occurs in the subcutaneous tissues.

MONSTERS

Monster is a disturbance of development in several organs and causes distortion of the foetus *e.g.* Duplication of all or most of the organs.
- Monsters develop from a single ovum; these are the product of incomplete twinning.
- Monsters are classified as under:

1. Separate twins

One twin is well developed while another is malformed and lack the heart, lungs or trunk, head, limbs.

2. United twins

These twins are united with symmetrical development and are further classified as:

(a) Anterior twinning

Anterior portion of foetus is having double structures while posterior remains as single.
- **Pyopagus** is a monster twin united in the pelvic region with the bodies side by side.
- **Ischiopagus** is a monster twin united in the pelvic region with the bodies at more than a right angle.
- **Dicephalus** is a monster having two separate heads, neck, thorax, and trunk.
- **Diprosopus** is a monster having double organs in cephalic region without complete separation of heads and with double face.

(b) Posterior twinning

When in monsters, the anterior portion remains single and posterior parts become double.

- **Craniopagus** is a monster having separate brain with separate bodies arranged at an acute angle.
- **Cephalothoracopagus** is the monster having united head and thorax.
- **Dipygus** is the monster having double posterior extremities and posterior parts of body.

(c) **Almost complete twining**

In some monster, twins are having complete development with joining in thorax and abdomen.

- **Thoracopagus** is a monsters united in thorax region.
- **Prosopothoracopagus** is the monster twin united at thorax, head, neck and abdomen.
- **Rachipagus** is the monster in which thoracic and lumber portion of vertebral column are united in twin.

Chapter 4
Disturbances in Growth

APLASIA/ AGENESIS
Aplasia or agenesis is absence of any organ.

HYPOPLASIA
Hypoplasia is failure of an organ/ tissue to attain its full size.

Etiology
- Congenital anomalies *e.g.* Hypoplasia of kidneys in calves.
- Inadequate innervation.
- Inadequate blood supply.
- Malnutrition
- Infections *e.g.* Cerebral hypoplasia in Bovine viral diarrhoea.

Macroscopic and microscopic features
- Organ size, weight, volume reduced
- Reduced size of cells
- Reduced number of cells
- Connective tissue and fat is more

ATROPHY
- Atrophy is decrease in size of an organ that have reached their full size.

Etiology
- Physiological *e.g.* Senile atrophy.
- Pressure atrophy

- Disuse atrophy *e.g.* Atrophy of immobilized legs.
- Endocrine atrophy *e.g.* Atrophy of testicles.
- Environmental pollution *e.g.* Atrophy of lymphoid organs.
- Inflammation/ fibrosis

Macroscopic and microscopic features
- Size, weight, volume of organ decreased.
- Wrinkles in capsule of organ.
- Size of cell is smaller.
- Cell number is less.
- Fat and connective tissue cells are more.

HYPERTROPHY

Hypertrophy is increase in size of cells leading to increase in size of organ/ tissue without increase in the number of cells.

Etiology
- Increase metabolic activity *e.g.* Myometrium during pregnancy.
- Compensatory *e.g.* If one kidney is removed, another becomes hypertrophied due to compensatory effect.

Macroscopic and microscopic features
- Organ becomes large in size.
- Organ weight increases.
- Size of cells increases.

HYPERPLASIA

Hyperplasia is increase in number of cells leading to increase in size of organ/ tissue.

Etiology
- Prolonged irritation *e.g.* Fibrosis/ nodules in hands, pads.
- Nutritional disorders *e.g.* Iodine deficiency
- Infections *e.g.* Pox.
- Endocrine disorders *e.g.* Prostate hyperplasia.

Macroscopic and microscopic features
- Increase in size, weight of organ., Nodular enlargement of organ.
- Increased number of cells, Displacement of adjacent tissue, Lumen of ducts/ tubules obstructed.

METAPLASIA

Metaplasia is defined as transformation of one type of cells to another type of cells.

Etiology
- Prolonged irritation *e.g.* Gall stones cause metaplasia of columnar cells to stratified squamous epithelial cells in wall of gall bladder.
- Endocrine disturbances *e.g.* In dog columnar epithelium of prostate changes into squamous epithelium.
- Nutritional deficiency *e.g.* Nutritional roup. In poultry, cuboidal/ columnar epithelium of esophageal glands changed into stratified squamous epithelium.
- Infections *e.g.* Pulmonary adenomatosis

Macroscopic and microscopic features
- Mucous membrane becomes dry in squamous metaplasia.
- Presence of nodular glands on oesophageal mucous membrane due to vitamin A deficiency in chickens also known as "Nutritional roup".
- Change of one type of cells to another type,In place of columnar cells, there are squamous epithelial cells.
- In place of endothelial cells, cuboidal or columnar cells in alveoli *e.g.* pulmonary adenomatosis.

ANAPLASIA

Anaplasia is defined as reversion of cells to a more embryonic and less differentiated type. It is a feature in neoplasia. Neoplasia is uncontrolled new growth, serves no useful purpose, have no orderly structural arrangement and is of undifferentiated or less differentiated in nature with more embryonic characters of the cells.

Etiology
- Chemicals
- Radiation
- Viruses *e.g.* Oncogenic Viruses.

Macroscopic and microscopic features
- Enlargement of organ/ tissue.
- Nodular growth of tissue, hard to touch.
- Presence of pleomorphic cells and less or undifferentiated cells
- Hyperchromasia
- Size of cells increases
- Size of nucleus and nucleolus increases
- Presence of many mitotic figures
- Seen in neoplastic conditions.

DYSPLASIA

Abnormal development of cells/ tissues which are improperly arranged. It is the malformation of tissue during maturation.
1. Spermatozoa head and tailpiece are structurally abnormal or aligned in improper way.
2. Fibrous dysplasia in bones.
3. In gastrointestinal tract, disruption of cellular orientation, variation in size, and shape of cells, increase nuclear and cytoplasmic ratio and increased mitotic activity.

Chapter 5
Disturbances in Circulation

CONGESTION/ HYPEREMIA

Hyperemia is increased amount of blood in circulatory system. It is of two types, active and passive. In active hyperemia blood accumulates in arteries while in passive hyperemia the amount of blood increases in veins.

Etiology
- As a result of inflammation.
- Obstruction of blood vessels.

Macroscopic and microscopic features
- Organ becomes dark red/ cyanotic.
- Size of organ increases.
- Weight of organ increases.
- Blood vessels become distended due to accumulation of blood.
- Increased amount of blood in blood vessels.
- Veins/ capillaries/ arteries are distended due to accumulation of blood.
- Blood vessels become enlarged with blood and their number increases.

HAEMORRHAGE

Escape of all the constituents of blood from blood vessels. It may occur through two processes *i.e. rhexis*- break in wall of blood vessel or through *diapedesis* in which blood leaves through intact wall of blood vessel. It occurs only in living animals.

Etiology
- Mechanical trauma
- Necrosis of the wall of blood vessels
- Infections
- Toxins
- Neoplasm

Macroscopic and microscopic features
- Organ becomes pale due to escape of blood
- As per size, the haemorrhage is classified as under:
- Pinpoint haemorrhage of about one mm diameter or pinhead size is known as *petechiae*.
- More than one to 10 mm diameter haemorrhage are known as *ecchymoses*.
- Irregular, diffuse and flat areas of haemorrhage on mucosal or serosal surfaces are known as *suffusions*.
- Haemorrhage appear in line in crests or folds on mucous membrane are known as *linear haemorrhage*.
- *Hematoma* is the accumulation of blood in spherical shaped mass.
- According to location, the haemorrhage is classified as:
- **Hemothorax:** Blood in thoracic cavity.
- **Hemopericardium:** Blood in pericardial sac. When there is increased amount of blood in pericardial sac, it causes heart failure and is known as *cardiac temponade*.
- **Hemoperitonium:** Blood in peritoneal cavity.
- **Hemoptysis:** Blood in sputum.
- **Hematuria:** Blood in urine.
- **Epistaxis:** Blood from nose.
- **Metrorrhagia:** Blood from uterus.
- **Melena:** Bleeding in faeces.
- **Hematemesis:** Blood in vomitus.
- Blood constituents are seen outside the blood vessels.

- Break in blood vessels.
- Presence of red blood cells in tissues outside the blood vessels.

THROMBOSIS

Formation of clot of blood in vascular system in the wall of blood vessel. It occurs due to endothelial injury leading to accumulation of thrombocytes, fibrinogen, erythrocytes and leucocytes.

Etiology
- Injury in endothelium of blood vessels.
- Alteration in blood flow.
- Alteration in composition of blood.

Macroscopic and microscopic features
- Blood clot in wall of blood vessels.
- On removal of clot, rough surface exposed.
- Clot may be pale, red or laminated.
- *Occlusive thrombus* totally occlude blood vessels.
- *Mural thrombus* is on the wall of heart.
- *Valvular thrombus* is on valves of heart.
- *Cardiac thrombus* is in heart.
- *Saddle thrombus* is at the bifurcation of blood vessel just like saddle on back of horse.
- *Septic thrombus* contains bacteria.
- Blood clot in blood vessel.
- Attached with wall of blood vessel.
- Alternate, irregular, red and gray areas in thrombi.

EMBOLISM

Presence of foreign body in circulatory system which may cause obstruction in blood vessel.

Etiology
- Thrombus, Fibrin
- Bacteria
- Neoplasm
- Clumps of normal cells
- Fat, Gas
- Parasites

Macroscopic and microscopic features
- Emboli causing obstruction of blood vessels lead to formation of infarct in the area.
- Organ/ tissue becomes pale.
- Parasitic emboli *e.g. Dirofilaria immitis*
- Presence of foreign material in blood.
- Dependent area necrotic due to absence of blood supply.

ISCHEMIA

Ischemia is deficiency of arterial blood in any part of an organ. It is also known as *local anemia*.

Etiology
- External pressure on artery
- Narrowing/ obliteration of lumen of artery
- Thrombi/ emboli

Macroscopic and microscopic features
- Necrosis of dependent part.
- Occurrence of infarction.
- Dead tissue replaced by fibrous tissue.
- Lesions of infarction

INFARCTION

Local area of necrosis resulting from ischemia. Ischemia is the deficiency of blood due to obstruction in artery.

Disturbances in Circulation

Etiology
- Thrombi
- Emboli
- Poisons like Fusarium toxins

Macroscopic and microscopic features
- Necrosis in triangular area
- *Red infarct* is observed as red triangle bulky surface.
- *Pale infarct* is gray in colour and seen as triangle depressed surface.
- Necrosis in cone shaped area.
- Obstruction of blood vessels.

EDEMA

Accumulation of excessive fluid in intercellular spaces and/or in body cavity.

Etiology
- Deficiency of protein.
- Passive hyperemia.
- Increased permeability of capillaries.
- Obstruction of lymphatics.

Macroscopic and microscopic features
- Swelling of tissue/ organ/ body.
- Weight and size of organ increased.
- Colour becomes light.
- Pitting impressions on pressure.
- *Ascites* is accumulation of fluid in peritoneum. It is also known as *hydroperitonium*.
- *Hydropericardium* is fluid accumulation in pericardial sac.
- *Hydrocele* is fluid accumulation in tunica vaginalis of the testicles.
- *Anasarca* is generalized edema of body.

- *Hydrocephalus* is accumulation of fluid in brain.
- *Hydrothorax* is accumulation of fluid in thoracic cavity.
- Inter cellular spaces becomes enlarged.
- Serum/ fluid deposits (pink in colour on H&E. staining) in intercellular spaces.
- Cells separated farther.

SHOCK

Shock is a circulatory disturbance characterized by reduction in total blood volume, blood flow and by hemconcentration.

Etiology
Primary shock
- Occurs immediately after injury.
- Injury/ extensive tissue destruction.
- Emotional crisis.
- Surgical manipulation.

Secondary shock
- Crushing injury involving chest and abdomen.
- Occurs after several hours of incubation.
- Release of histamine and other substances by injured tissue.
- Extensive haemorrhage.
- Burns
- Predisposing factors like cold, exhaustion, depression.

Macroscopic and microscopic features
- Acute general passive hyperemia
- Dilatation of capillaries
- Cyanosis
- Numerous petechial haemorrhages
- Edema and loose connective tissue
- Capillaries and small blood vessels are distended due to accumulation of blood.

- Number of engorged blood vessels increased.
- Focal haemorrhage.
- Edema, cells separated farther due to accumulation of transudate in intercellular spaces.

SLUDGED BLOOD

Sludged blood is agglutination of erythrocytes in the vascular system of an animal.

Etiology
- Fluctuation in blood flow
- Slow rate of blood flow

Macroscopic and microscopic features
- Edema
- Emboli
- Infarction
- Necrosis
- Clumping of erythrocytes in pulmonary capillaries.
- Infarction, necrosis.
- Edema.
- Erythrophagocytosis by reticuloendothelial cells.

Chapter 6
Disturbances in Cell Metabolism

CLOUDY SWELLING

Swelling of cells occur with hazy appearance due to a mild injury. The cells take more water due to defect in sodium pump leading to swollen mitochondria which gives granular cytoplasmic appearance. It is the first reaction of cell to a mildest injury. Cloudy swelling is a reversible reaction.

Etiology
- Can be caused by any mildest injury.
- Any factor causing interference with metabolism of the cell like bacterial toxins, fever, diabetes, circulatory disturbances etc.

Macroscopic and microscopic features
- Organ becomes enlarged and rounded.
- Weight of organ increases.
- Bulging on cut surfaces.
- Amount of fluid increases in organ.
- Swelling of cells, edges become rounded.
- Increased size of cells.
- Cytoplasm of the cells becomes hazy/cloudy due to increased granularity.
- Can be seen in liver, kidney and muscles.

HYDROPIC DEGENERATION

Cells swell due to intake of clear fluid. Such cells may burst due to increased amount of fluid and form vesicle. Hydropic degeneration can be seen in epithelium of skin and/or mucous membranes of body.

Etiology
- Mechanical injury
- Burns
- Chemical injury
- Infections like foot and mouth disease virus, pox virus etc.

Macroscopic and microscopic features
- Vesicle formation
- Accumulation of fluid under superficial layer of skin/ mucus membrane.
- Heals rapidly within 2-4 days
- No scar formation
- **Pyogenic organisms may convert it into** *pustule*.
- Cell size increases due to accumulation of clear fluid in cytoplasm.
- Droplets in cytoplasm as vacuoles.
- Cell bursts and epithelium protrudes leading to blister.
- Mostly affects prickle cell layer (Stratum spinosum) of skin.

MUCINOUS DEGENERATION

Excessive accumulation of mucin in degenerating epithelial cells. Mucin is a glassy, viscid, stringy and slimy glycoprotein produced by columnar epithelial cells on mucus membranes. Such cells burst to release the mucin in lumen of organ and are called as *goblet cells*. When mucin is mixed with water, it is known as *mucus*.

Etiology
- Any irritant to mucus membrane like chemicals and infection.
- Bacteria *e.g. E. coli*

- Virus *e.g.* Rotavirus
- Parasite *e.g.* Ascaris

Macroscopic and microscopic features
- Over production of mucus in intestines which covers intestinal contents/ stool.
- Over production of mucus in genital tract during oestrus and is characterized by mucus discharge from vulva.
- Nasal discharge during respiratory mucosa involvement.
- Mucus is mucin mixed with water and slimy and stringy in nature.
- Increased number of goblet cells.
- Goblet cells are elliptical columnar cells containing mucus.
- Mucin in lumen stains basophilic through H & E staining.
- Seen on mucous surfaces only.

MUCOID DEGENERATION

Mucoid degeneration is mucin like glycoprotein deposits in connective tissue.

Etiology
- In embryonic tissue *e.g.* umblical cord.
- In connective tissue tumors *e.g.* Myxosarcoma.
- Myxedema due to thyroid deficiency.
- In cachexia due to starvation, parasitism or chronic wasting diseases.

Macroscopic and microscopic features
- Shrunken tissue giving translucent jelly like appearance.
- A watery, slimy and stringy material on cut surface.
- Mucoid degeneration tissue stains blue
- Nuclei are hyperchromatic.
- Fibrous tissue as pale blue.
- Usually accompanied by fat necrosis.

PSEUDOMUCIN

Pseudomucin is secretion of ovaries and is observed in cystadenomas. However, it is not a disturbance of cell metabolism.

Etiology
- Cystadenoma, cystadenocarcinoma
- Paraovarian cysts.

Macroscopic and microscopic features
- Transparent, slimy similar to mucin.
- It is not precipitated by acetic acid while mucin is precipitated.
- Homogenous like plasma stains pink with H&E stain
- Extracellular

AMYLOID INFILTRATION

Deposition of amyloid between capillary endothelium and adjacent cells. Amyloid is a starch like substance which stains brown/ blue/ black with iodine and chemically is protein polysaccharide.

Etiology
- Not exactly known.
- It is thought to be due to antigen-antibody reaction/ deposition of immune complexes in between capillary endothelium and adjacent cells.

Macroscopic and microscopic features
- Organ size increases with rounded edges, pits on pressure, cyanotic/ yellow in colour and fragile.
- *Sago spleen* due to deposition of gray, waxy sago like material.
- Amyloid stains pink on H& E stain.
- It is a permanent effect in body and remains in whole life without causing much adverse effects.

HYALINE DEGENERATION

Glossy substance (glass like) solid, dense, smoothly homogenous deposits in tissues. Tissue becomes inelastic. It is a permanent change. Hyaline is very difficult to distinguish macroscopically.

Etiology
- Disturbance in protein metabolism
- No specific cause

Macroscopic and Microscopic features

Connective tissue hyaline
- In old scars, due to lack of nutrients; homogenous, strong acidophilic and pink in colour. There are no nuclei and no fibrils.

Epithelial Hyaline
- Starch like bodies in prostate, lungs, kidneys.
- Microscopically characterized by round, homogeneous, pink, within an alveolus of lung.
- Homogenous, pink in kidney tubules/ glomeruli.

Keratohyaline
- Occurs due to slow death of stratified squamous epithelial cells and because of lack of nutrients. Keratinized epithelium is firm, hard and colourless. Microscopically, it is seen in epithelial pearls *e.g.* horn cancer, warts.

FATTY CHANGES

Intracellular accumulation of fat in liver, kidneys and heart. It is a reversible change.

Etiology
- Increased release of fatty acids.
- Decreased oxidation of fatty acids.
- Lipotrope deficiency.
- In ketosis, diabetes, pregnancy toxaemia.

Macroscopic and microscopic features
- Enlargement of organ.
- Cut surfaces are bulging and greasy.
- Organ colour becomes light.
- Intracellular deposition of fat droplets.
- In cytoplasm clear round/ oval spaces with eccentrically placed nucleus.
- Stains yellow orange with sudan III.

GLYCOGEN INFILTRATION (GLYCOGEN STORAGE DISEASE)

Glycogen accumulates when increased amount of glycogen enters in the cells of kidneys, muscles and liver.

Etiology
- Diabetes mellitus.
- Impaired carbohydrate metabolism due to drugs *e.g.* corticosteroid therapy.

Macroscopic and microscopic features
- Affected organ becomes enlarged.
- Intracellular deposits of glycogen in cells of kidneys, liver and muscles.
- Small clear vacuoles seen in distal portion of proximal convoluted tubules, hepatocytes etc.
- It can be stained as bright red by Best's. Carmine and PAS and reddish brown by iodine.

Chapter 7

Necrosis, Gangrene and Post-mortem Changes

NECROSIS

Local death of tissue/ cells in living body is known as necrosis, It is characterized by the followings.
- *Pyknosis* is condensation of chromatin material, nuclei becomes dark, reduced in size and deeply stained
- *Karyorrhexis* is fragmentation of nucleus
- *Karyolysis* is dissolution of nucleus into small fragments, basophilic granules/ fragments.
- *Chromatolysis* is lysis of chromatin material.
- *Necrobiosis* is physiological cell death after completion of its function *e.g.* RBC after 140 days.

Necrosis is further classified into coagulative, caseative, liquifactive and fat necrosis which are different from apoptosis.

COAGULATIVE NECROSIS

Local death of cells/ tissue in living body characterized by loss of cellular details, while tissue architecture remains intact.

Etiology
- Infections
- Ischemia
- Mild irritant *e.g.* toxins/ chemical poisons
- Heat, trauma

Macroscopic and microscopic features
- Organ becomes gray/ white in colour, firm, dense, depressed with surrounding tissue.

- Cellular out line present, which maintains the architecture of tissue/ organ.
- Nucleus absent or pyknotic.
- Cytoplasm becomes acidophilic.

CASEATIVE NECROSIS

Local death of cells/ tissue in living body; the dead cells/ tissue is characterized by presence of firm, dry and cheesy consistency. It occurs due to coagulation of proteins and lipids.

Etiology
- Chronic infections *e.g. Mycobacterium tuberculosis*.
- Systemic fungal infections.

Macroscopic and microscopic features
- Dead tissue looks like milk curd or cottage cheese.
- Tissue dry, firm, agranular, white/ gray/ yellowish in colour
- Disappearance of cells; no cell details/ architecture.
- Purplish granules on H&E staining, blue granules from nucleus fragments, red granules from cytoplasm fragments.

LIQUEFACTIVE NECROSIS

Local death of cells/ tissues in living body characterized by rapid enzymatic dissolution of cells. The intracellular hydrolases and proteolytic enzymes of leucocytes play role in dissolution of cells.

Etiology
- Pyogenic organisms.

Macroscopic and microscopic features
- Liquefactive necrosed tissue present in a cavity "Abscess".
- It contains small/ large amount of cloudy fluid, which is creamy yellow (Pus).
- Areas of liquefactive necrosis stains pink.
- Infiltration of neutrophils

- Sometimes empty spaces but infiltration of neutrophils at periphery.

FAT NECROSIS
Local death of adipose cells in living body.

Etiology
- Trauma
- Increased action of enzymes due to leakage of pancreatic juice.
- Starvation

Macroscopic and microscopic features
- Chalky white mass deposits in organ.
- White opaque firm mass.
- Adipose cell without nucleus.
- Macrophages giant cells contain fat droplets.
- Presence of lime salts in tissues.

Differential features of various types of Necrosis

	Coagulative	Liquifactive	Caseative	Fat
Macroscopic features	1. Organ becomes gray/ white in colour, firm, dense, depressed with surrounding tissue	1. Liquifactive necrosed tissue present in a cavity "Abscess" 2. It contains small/ large amount of cloudy fluid, which is creamy yellow (Pus)	1. Dead tissue looks like milk curd or cottage cheese 2. Tissue dry, firm, agranular, white/ gray/ yellowish in colour	1. Chalky white mass deposits in organ 2. White opaque firm mass
Microscopic features	1. Cellular out line present, which maintains the architecture of tissue/ organ 2. Nucleus absent or pyknotic 3. Cytoplasm becomes acidophilic	1. Areas of liquifactive necrosis stains pink. 2. Infiltration of neutrophils 3. Sometimes empty spaces but infiltration of neutrophils at periphery	1. Disappearance of cells; no cell details/ architecture 2. Purplish granules on H&E staining, blue granules from nucleus fragments, red granules from cytoplasm fragments.	1. Adipose cell without nucleus 2. Macrophages giant cells contain fat droplets. 3. Presence of lime salts in tissues.

APOPTOSIS

Apoptosis is a finely tuned mechanism for the control of cell number in animals; the process is operative during foetal life, tumor regression and in the control of immune response. Apoptosis plays an important role in the development and maintenance of homeostasis and in the maturation of nervous and immune system. It is also a major defense mechanism of the body, removing unwanted and potentially dangerous cells such as self reactive lymphocytes, virus infected cells and tumor cells.

Most cells in animal have the ability to self destruct by activation of an intrinsic cellular suicidal programme when they are no longer needed or are seriously damaged. The dying cell exhibits morphological alterations including shrinkage of cell, membrane blebbing, chromatin condensation and fragmentation of nucleic acid. Cells under going apoptosis often fragment into membrane bound apoptotic bodies that are readily phagocytosed by macrophages or neighbouring cells without generating an inflammatory response. These changes distinguish apoptosis from cell death by necrosis. Necrosis refers to the morphology most often seen when cells die from severe and sudden injury such as ischemia, sustained hyperthermia or physical and chemical trauma. In necrosis, there are early changes in mitochondrial shape and function; cell losses its ability to regulate osmotic pressure, swells and ruptures. The contents of the cell are spilled into surrounding tissue, resulting in generation of a local inflammatory response.

Necrosis is the consequence of a passive and degenerative process while the apoptosis is a consequence of an active process.

Execution of apoptosis requires the coordinated action of aspartate specific cysteine proteases (caspases) which are responsible for cleavage of key enzymes and structural proteins resulting in death of cell. Apoptosis is triggered by a variety of signals which activate the endogenous endonucleases to cause fragment action of nuclear DNA into oligonucleosomal size fragments. Initially, the DNA fragments are large (50-300 Kb) but are later digested to oligonucleosomal size (multimers of 180-200 bp). The formation of this distinct DNA ladder is considered to be a biochemical hallmark of apoptosis.

There is rounding of nucleus with pyknosis and rhexis, chromatin coalesces to form a crescent along the nuclear membrane. Cell fragments to form blebs, which may have one or more organelles. Such changes occurs in apoptotic cells within 20 min of duration.

Apoptosis is generally synonymously used with "programmed cell death" but it differs from programmed cell death as apoptosis cannot be prevented by cycloheximide or actinomycin D, rather these chemicals accelerate the process of apoptosis while programmed cell death is prevented by these chemicals.

GANGRENE

Necrosis of tissue is followed by invasion of saprophytes. Gangrene is mainly divided into three types: Dry, moist and gas gangrene.

DRY GANGRENE

Dry gangrene occurs at extremities like tail, tip of ears, tip of scrotum, hoof etc. due to necrosis and invasion of saprophytes. The evaporation of moisture takes place resulting into dry lesions.

Etiology
- Mycotoxins from fungus *Fusarium equiseti* found on paddy straw in low lying areas with moisture (Degnala disease).

Macroscopic and microscopic features
- Dry, fragmented crusts like lesions on tail, scrotum, ear.
- Hoof becomes detached due to necrosis and gangrene, sloughing, exposing the red raw surface.
- Blackening of the affected area.
- Necrosis and invasion of saprophytes in skin of tail, ear or scrotum.

MOIST GANGRENE

Moist gangrene mostly occurs in internal organs of body like lungs, intestine, stomach etc. It occurs due to necrosis and invasion of saprophytes leading to dissolution of the tissues.

Etiology
- Drenching of milk, medicines etc. *e.g.* Aspiration pneumonia/ Drenching pneumonia.
- Volvulus/ Intussusception or torsion in intestine.

Macroscopic and microscopic features
- Greenish or bluish discoloration of the affected organ.
- Dissolution of affected part into fragments
- Presence of foreign material like milk, fiber, oil, etc.
- Necrosis and invasion of saprophytes
- Presence of foreign material like milk, fibers, oil etc.

GAS GANGRENE

Gas gangrene occurs in muscles particularly of thigh muscles of hind legs in heifers in case of black leg (Black Quarter).

Etiology
- *Clostridium chauvei*
- Gram positive, rod, anaerobe.
- Produces toxins under anaerobic conditions which causes disease.
- Stress, trauma, transportation predisposes animals.

Macroscopic and microscopic features
- Oedema of Muscles in affected part particularly thigh region.
- Blackening of muscles due to production of H_2S by bacteria and its chemical reaction with iron of free hemoglobin producing iron sulphide.
- Presence of gas in the area giving *crepitating sound* on palpation.

- Necrosis of muscles
- Presence of Gram positive rod shaped Clostridia
- Dissolution of muscle fibers due to saprophytes/ toxins of the organism.

Differential features of various types of Gangrene

	Dry	Moist	Gas
Macroscopic features	1. Dry, fragmented crusts like lesions on tail, scrotum, ear 2. Hoof becomes detached due to necrosis and gangrene, sloughing, exposing the red raw surface. 3. Blackening of the affected area.	1. Greenish or bluish discoloration of the affected organ. 2. Dissolution of affected part into fragments 3. Presence of foreign material like milk, fiber, oil, etc.	1. Oedema of Muscles in affected part particularly thigh region. 2. Blackening of muscles due to production of H_2S by bacteria and its chemical reaction with iron of free hemoglobin producing iron sulphide. 3. Presence of gas in the area giving crepitating sound on palpation
Microscopic features	1. Necrosis and invasion of saprophytes in skin of tail, ear or scrotum	1. Necrosis and invasion of saprophytes 2. Presence of foreign material like milk, fibers, oil, etc.	1. Necrosis of muscles 2. Presence of Gram positive rod shaped Clostridia 3. Dissolution of muscle fibers due to saprophytes/ toxins of the organism

POST-MORTEM CHANGES

Alterations in cells/ tissues occur after death of animal. The degree of such alterations and their speed depends upon the environmental temperature, size of animal, species of animal, external insulation and nutritional state of the animal. The postmortem changes occur rapidly in high environmental temperature, large animal, fur/ wool bearing and fatty animals.

Autolysis: Autolysis is the digestion of tissue by its own enzymes and is characterized by uniform destruction of cells without any inflammatory reaction. After death, a state of hypoxia occurs leading to decreased ATP. The cell organelles degenerate and the membrane of lysosomes dissolved which releases the lysosomal enzymes in the cell responsible for digestion of cells/ tissues. These enzymes cause disintegration of cell components into small granules in the cell. Microscopically, autolysis is characterized by uniform dead cells without any circulatory changes and inflammatory reaction.

Putrefaction: Putrefaction is decomposition of tissue after death by saprophytes leading to production of foul odour. After autolysis the saprophytes invade from external environment into the body, multiply and eventually digest the tissues with their enzymes. The tissue becomes frazile and produces foul odour.

Pseudomelanosis: Pseudomelanosis is greenish or bluish discolouration of tissues/ organs after death. Saprophytes causing putrefaction also produce hydrogen sulfide which chemically reacts with iron portion of hemoglobin to produce iron sulfide. Iron sulfide is a black pigment and produces green, gray or black shades on combination with other tissue pigments.

Rigor mortis: Rigor mortis is the contraction and shortening of muscles after death of animal leading to stiffening and immobilization of body. It occurs 2-4 hrs after death and remains till putrefaction sets in. Rigor mortis begins in cardiac muscles first and then in skeletal muscles of head and neck with a progression towards extremities. It is enhanced by high temperature and increased metabolic activity before death; while it is delayed by starvation, cold and cachexia. Rigor appears quickly in case animal is died due to strychnine poisoning as a result of depletion of energy source ATP. Muscle fibers shorten due to contraction and remain in contraction in the absence of oxygen, ATP and creatine phosphate. Rigor mortis remains till 20-30 hrs of death, the duration depends on autolysis and putrefaction. It disappears in same order as it appeared from head, neck to extremities. It can be used to determine the length of time after the death of animal.

Algor mortis: Algor mortis is cooling of body. As there is no circulation of blood after death, which maintains the body temperature, body becomes cool after death. However, it takes

2-4 hrs depending on the species, environmental temperature and type of animal.

Livor mortis: Livor mortis is the staining of tissues with hemoglobin after death of animals. It gives pinkish discolouration to the tissues.

Hypostatic congestion: Due to gravitational force, the blood is accumulated in dependent ventral parts of body. It is helpful in establishment of the state of the body at the time of death.

Post-mortem emphysema: It occurs due to decomposition by gas producing organisms including saprophytes. The gas is mainly accumulated in gastrointestinal tract causing rupture of the organ.

Post-mortem clot: It is clotting of blood after death of animal mainly due to excessive release of thrombokinase from dying leucocytes and endothelial cells. It is smooth in consistency and glistening surface with red or yellow in colour. Post-mortem clot is uniform in structure and it does not attach on wall of blood vessel as thrombus does. In anthrax, postmortem clot does not appear. Post-mortem clot in formed in two types: Red or current jelly clot forms when the components of blood are evenly distributed throughout the clot. It occurs due to rapid clotting of blood. The yellow or chicken fat clot occurs when the components of blood are not distributed evenly. The ventral position is red and upper position in yellow due to WBC fibrin and serum. It occurs due to prolonged coagulation time of blood leading to sediment of red blood cells.

Displacement of organs: Displacement of internal organs due to rolling of dead animal. Mainly intestine/ stomach and uterus are affected with displacement which can be differentiated from antemortem by absence of passive hyperemia.

Imbibition of bile: Cholebilirubin present in the gall bladder diffuses to the surrounding tissues/ organs and stains them with yellow/ greenish pigmentation.

Chapter 8

Disturbances in Calcification and Pigment Metabolism

CALCIFICATION

Calcification is the deposition of calcium phosphates and calcium carbonates in soft tissues other than bones and teeth. It may be classified as dystrophic and metastatic calcification.

DYSTROPHIC CALCIFICATION

Dystrophic calcification is characterized by the deposits of calcium salts in necrosed tissue of any organ.

Etiology/ Occurrence
- Necrosis
- Parasitic infections
- **Tuberculous lesions**

Macroscopic and microscopic features
- Organ becomes hard, nodular.
- Gray/ white deposits in necrosed tissue looking like honey comb.
- Gritty sound on cutting.
- Irregular deposits of calcium salts in necrosed tissue.
- Calcium takes black/ purplish colour on H & E staining.

METASTATIC CALCIFICATION

Metastatic calcification is characterized by deposition of calcium salts in soft tissue as a result of hypercalcemia.

Etiology
- Hyperparathyroidism
- Renal failure
- Excess of vitamin-D
- Increased calcium intake.

Macroscopic and microscopic features
- Organ becomes hard
- Wall of arteries becomes hard due to calcium deposits.
- Deposition of calcium in soft organs like myocardium, arteries, muscles, etc.
- Purplish/ black colour calcium surrounded by comparatively normal tissue.

MELANOSIS

Melanosis is the deposition of melanin, a brown/ black pigment in various tissues/ organs specially in lung, blood vessels and brain.

Etiology
- Hyperadrenalism
- Melanosarcoma
- Melanoma

Macroscopic and microscopic features
- Organ/ tissue involved becomes black in colour.
- Discolouration may be focal or diffused.
- Brown/ black colour pigment is seen in cells.
- The size, shape and amount of pigment vary.

HEMOSIDEROSIS

Hemosiderosis is characterized by deposition of hemosiderin pigment in spleen and other organs. Hemosiderin is a blood pigment with a shiny golden yellow colour and is usually found within the macrophages.

Etiology/ Occurrence
- Extensive lysis of erythrocytes
- Haemorrhage
- Hemolytic anemia

Macroscopic and microscopic features
- Colour of organ becomes brownish
- Brown induration of lungs
- Presence of golden yellow/ golden brown pigment in red pulp of spleen, lungs, liver and kidneys.
- In most of the cases, the pigment is found intracellularly in macrophages.

BILE PIGMENTS

Bile pigments are derived from the breakdown of erythrocytes such as bilirubin and biliverdin. The icterus is hyperbilirubinemia as a result of either excessive lysis of erythrocytes or due to damage in liver or obstruction in the bile duct. The haemolysis resulted into iron, globin and porphyin; the latter being converted into biliverdin. Biliverdin is reduced to produce bilirubin, an orange yellow pigment and bound to albumin and transported by RE cells to liver. In hepatic cells, it is separated from albumin and conjugated with glucuronic acid and excreted in bile as bilirubin diglucuronide. In intestine, it is further reduced by bacteria to urobilinogen, which is reabsorbed into circulation and carried to liver for reexcretion in bile while small amount enters in circulation and excreted through urine. The unabsorbed urobilinogen is oxidized in lower intestine to form urobilin and stercobilin, which gives normal pigment to faeces.

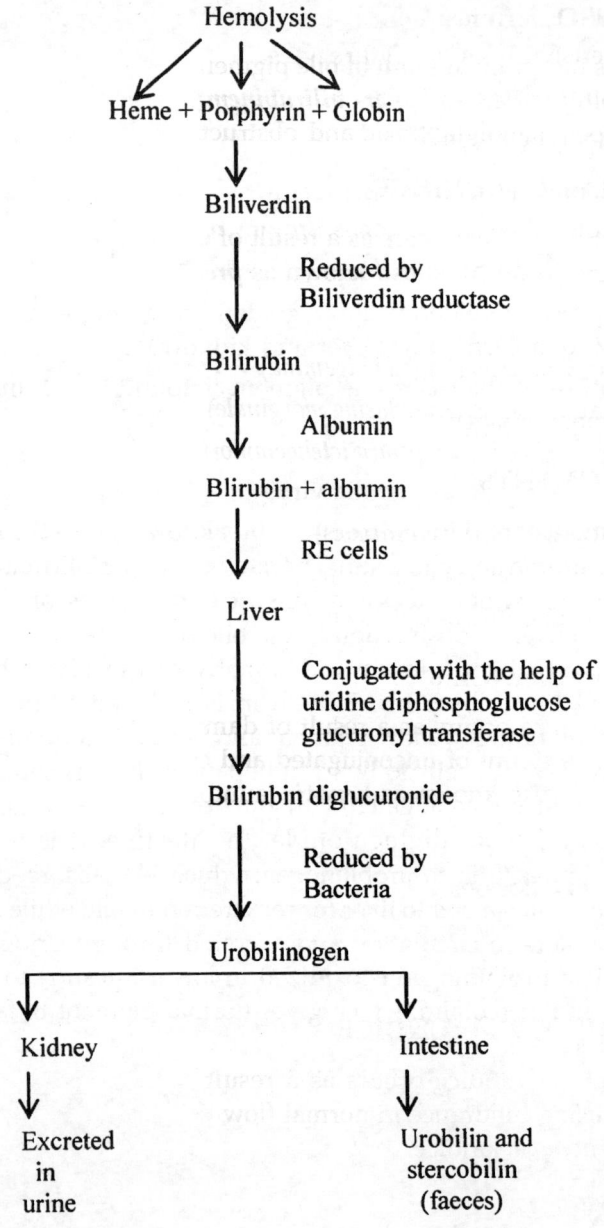

ICTERUS

Icterus is increased amount of bile pigments in blood circulation and is often called as *hyper- bilirubinemia* or *jaundice*. It is of three types hemolytic, toxic and obstructive jaundice.

HEMOLYTIC JAUNDICE

Hemolytic jaundice occurs as a result of excessive hemolysis in circulating blood. It is also known as *prehepatic* jaundice.

Etiology
- Piroplasmosis (*Babesia bigemina*)
- Anaplasmosis (*Anaplasma marginale*)
- Leptospirosis(*Leptospira ictehaemmorrhagae*)
- Equine infectious anemia virus
- Anthrax (*Bacillus anthracis*)
- *Clostriduum hemolyticum*
- β- haemolytic streptococci

TOXIC JAUNDICE

Toxic jaundice occurs as a result of damage in liver leading to increased amount of unconjugated and conjugated bilirubin in blood. It is also known as *hepatic* jaundice.

Etiology
- Toxin/ Poisons
- Copper poisoning
- Leptospirosis

OBSTRUCTIVE JAUNDICE

Obstructive jaundice occurs as a result of obstruction in bile duct causing hindrance in normal flow of bile. It is also known as *post hepatic* jundice.

Etiology
- Blocking of bile canaliculi by swollen hepatocytes

- Obstruction in bile duct (Liver flukes, tapeworms and ascaris)
- Biliary cirrhosis, Cholangitis and Cholelithiasis
- Pressure on bile duct due to abscess, neoplasm.
- Inflammation and swelling at duct opening in duodenum.

Macroscopic features
- Mucous membrane yellow in colour.
- Omentum, mesentry, fat become yellow.
- Increased yellow colour in urine.
- Conjunctiva becomes yellow.
- Brownish pigment in tubules of kidney
- Bile pigments in spleen
- Hemolysis, erythrophagocytosis
- Hepatitis

Differential features of various types of Jaundice

	Hemolytic (Prehepatic)	Toxic (Hepatic)	Obstructive (Post hepatic)
Etiology	1. Piroplasmosis (*Babesia bigemina*) 2. Anaplasmosis (*Anaplasma marginale*) 3. Leptospirosis (*Leptospira ictehaemmorrhagae*) 4. Equine infectious anemia virus 5. Anthrax (*Bacillus anthracis*) 6. *Clostridium hemolyticum* 7. β- haemolytic streptococci	1. Toxin/ Poisons 2. Copper poisoning 3. Leptospirosis	1. Blocking of bile canaliculi by swollen hepatocytes 2. Obstruction in bile duct (Liver flukes, tapeworms and ascaris) 3. Biliary cirrhosis, Cholangitis and Cholelithiasis 4. Pressure on bile duct due to abscess, neoplasm. 5. Inflammation and swelling at duct opening in duodenum.
Vanden Berg's reaction Direct Indirect	Negative Positive	Positive Positive	Positive Negative

Disturbances in Calcification and Pigment Metabolism

Diagnosis
- Van-den-Bergh reaction
- Direct reaction detects bilirubin diglucuronide (Obstructive jaundice)
- Indirect reaction detects hemobilirubin (Hemolytic jaundice)
- Both reaction (Toxic jaundice)

Vanden Berg's reaction

	Type of reaction	Type of jaundice	Type of pigment
1.	Direct reaction (+)	Obstructive	Cholibilirubin
2.	Indirect reaction (+)	Hemolytic	Hemobilirubin
3.	Biphasic reaction (+)	Toxic/ Hepatocellular	Both present

PNEUMOCONIASIS

Pneumoconiasis is the deposition of dust/ carbon particles in lungs through air inhalation. It is also known as anthracosis (carbon), silicosis (silica) or asbestosis (asbestos).

Etiology/ Occurrence
- Dusty air containing carbon/ silica/ asbestos
- Near factory/ coal mines.

Macroscopic and microscopic features
- Hard nodules in lungs
- Nodules my have black/ brown/ gray colour
- Nodules may produce cracking sounds on cut
- Presence of carbon/ other exogenous pigment in intercellular spaces or in cytoplasm of alveolar cells and macrophages.
- Formation of granuloma around the foreign particles including the infiltration of macrophages, lymphocytes, giant cells and fibrous tissue proliferation.

CRYSTALS

Deposition of different kinds of crystals in tissues like uric acid, sulfonamides and oxalates etc. The uric acid and urates when deposits in tissues it is known as *gout*.

GOUT

Gout is a disease condition in which urates and uric acid deposited in tissues characterized by intense pain and acute inflammation.

Etiology
- Common in poultry due to deficiency of uricase enzyme.
- Deficiency of vitamin-A
- Absence or inadequate amount of uricase

Macroscopic and microscopic features
- White chalky mass of urates and uric acid.
- Deposition of urates/ uric acid on pericardium, kidneys etc.
- Dialation of ureter due to excessive accumulation of urates.
- Presence of sharp crystals in tissue
- Crystals are surrounded by inflammatory cells including macrophages, giant cells and lymphocytes

Chapter 9
Inflammation and Healing

INFLAMMATION

Inflammation is a complex process of vascular and cellular alterations occurs in body in response to injury. The term inflammation has been derived from a Latin word inflammare, means to set on fire. The inflammation is considered as an important event in body for implementation of existing defence mechanisms in circulating blood to dilute, naturalize or kill the irritant/ causative agent. Thus, it is said that the immunity is the resistance of body, while inflammation is the implementation of that immunity. It is beneficial to body except chronic persistent and immune origin. Inflammation starts with sublethal injury and ends with healing.

Etiology
- Any irritant/ injury
- Bacteria, virus, parasite, fungus etc.
- Trauma
- Physical or chemical injury

Macroscopic and microscopic features
- Inflammation is characterized by 5 cardinal signs
- Redness
- Swelling.
- Heat
- Pain
- Loss of function
- Acute inflammation is characterized by more intense vascular changes like congestion, oedema, hemorrhages, leak-

age of fibrinogen and leucocytes.
- Chronic inflammation is characterized by more proliferative and/or regenerative changes such as proliferation of fibroblasts and regeneration of epithelium alongwith infiltration of leucocytes.

TERMINOLOGY IN INFLAMMATION

Inflammation may occur in each and every organ/ tissue depending upon the type of injury and irritant. The inflamed organ is called most often with a suffix as "itis"; the detail nomenclature is as under for different organs/ tissues.

Abomasum	–	Abomasitis
Artery	–	Arteritis
Bileduct	–	Cholangitis
Bone & bone marrow	–	Osteomyelitis
Bone	–	Osteitis
Brain	–	Encephalitis
Bronchi	–	Bronchitis
Bursa	–	Bursitis
Caecum	–	Typhlitis
Cervix	–	Cervicitis
Colon	–	Colonitis
Conjunctiva	–	Conjunctivitis
Connective tissue	–	Cellulitis
Cornea	–	Keratitis
Crop	–	Ingluvitis
Durameter	–	Pachymeningitis
Ear	–	Otitis
Endocardium	–	Endocarditis
Eosophagus	–	Esophagitis
Epididymis	–	Epididymitis
Eustachian tube	–	Eustachitis
External ear	–	Otitis externa
Eyelid	–	Blepheritis

Inflammation and Healing

Eyes	–	Ophthalmitis
Fascia	–	Fascitis
Fat	–	Steatitis
Gall bladder	–	Cholecystitis
Gizzard	–	Ventriculitis
Glans penis	–	Balanitis
Gums	–	Gingivitis
Heart	–	Carditis
Inner part of uterus	–	Endometritis
Internal ear	–	Otitis interna
Intestine	–	Enteritis
Iris	–	Iritis
Joints	–	Arthritis
Kidney & pelvis	–	Pyelonephritis
Kidney	–	Nephritis
Lacrimal gland	–	Dacryadenitis
Larynx	–	Laryngitis
Ligament	–	Desmitis
Lip	–	Cheilitis
Liver	–	Hepatitis
Lungs	–	Pneumonitis/ Pneumonia
Lymph nodes	–	Lymphadenitis
Lymph vessels	–	Lymphangitis
Meninges	–	Meningitis
Middle ear	–	Otitis media
Mouth cavity	–	Stomatitis
Muscle	–	Myositis
Myocardium	–	Myocarditis
Nasal passage	–	Rhinitis
Nerve	–	Neuritis
Omasum	–	Omasitis

Ovary	–	Oophoritis
Oviduct	–	Salpingitis
Palates	–	Lampas/ palatitis
Pancreas	–	Pancreatitis
Pericardium	–	Pericarditis
Peritoneum	–	Peritonitis
Pharynx	–	Pharyngitis
Piameter	–	Leptomeningitis
Pleura	–	Pleuritis
Prepuce	–	Posthitis
Rectum	–	Proctitis
Reticulm	–	Reticulitis
Retina	–	Retinitis
Rumen	–	Rumenitis
Salivary glands	–	Sialadenitis
Sinuses	–	Sinusitis
Skin	–	Dermatitis
Spermatic cord	–	Funiculitis
Spinal cord	–	Myelitis
Spleen	–	Splenitis
Stomach	–	Gastritis
Synovial membrane of joints	–	Sinovitis
Tendon	–	Tendinitis
Testes	–	Orchitis
Tongue	–	Glossitis
Trachea	–	Tracheitis
Ureter	–	Ureteritis
Urethra	–	Urethritis
Urinary bladder	–	Cystitis
Uterus	–	Metritis
Vagina	–	Vaginitis
Vein	–	Phlebitis

Vertebra   -   Spondylitis
Vessel   -   Vasculitis
Vulva   -   Vulvitis

PATHOGENESIS OF INFLAMMATION

Inflammation starts with sublethal injury and ends with healing; in between there are many events take place which are described as under:

Transient vasoconstriction

The blood vessels of the affected part becomes constricted for a movement as a result of action of irritant.

Vasodialation and Increase in permeability

The blood vessels become dialated. Endothelium becomes more permeable and releases procoagulant factors and prostaglandins. Fluid and proteins come out due to leakage in endothelium. Fluid contain water, immunoglobulins, complement component, biochemical factors of coagulation and mediators of inflammation.

Blood flow decrease

Due to stasis of blood in blood vessel, there is increase in leakage of fluids/ cells out side the blood vessels. It gives rise to congestion/ hyperemia. There is margination of leucocytes also known as *pavementation.*

Cells in perivascular spaces

Due to pseudopodia movement, leucocytes come out from the dialated blood vessels through intact and swollen endothelium and this process is known as *"diapedesis"*. Cells also come out through break in blood vessel and this process is called as *"rhexis"*.

Leucocytes degranulate in perivascular tissue spaces.

Leucocytes when reaches in tissue spaces, they release chemical mediators of inflammation, antimicrobial factors in tissues such as cationic proteins, hydrogen peroxide, hydrolytic enzymes, lysozymes, proteases, kinins, histamine, serotonin, heparin, cytokines, and complement.

Irritant is removed and damaged tissue healed

By the process of inflammation irritant is neutralized/ removed or killed. Fluids are absorbed through lymphatics and debris is removed by phagocytosis. Blood vessel becomes normal.

If the irritant is strong and not normally removed by the inflammatory process, it remains at the site and covered by inflammatory cells and after some time by fibrous cells in order to localize the irritant. *e.g.* Granuloma.

VASCULAR CHANGES

In inflammation, there is transient vasoconstriction followed by vasodialation increased capillary permeability and decrease in blood flow. Circulatory changes are more pronounced in acute inflammation.

Etiology
- Any irritant/ injury causing inflammation

Macroscopic and microscopic features
- Congestion of the affected organ/ tissue
- Edema
- Haemorrhage
- Congestion of blood vessels
- Edema, presence of fibrin net work
- Infiltration of leucocytes such as neutrophils, lymphocytes, macrophages, eosinophils etc.

CELLULAR CHANGES

In inflammation, there is infiltration of leucocytes in the inflammed area in order to provide defense to the body and to kill or neutralize the etiological factors.

Etiology
- Any irritant/ injury causing inflammation

Macroscopic and microscopic features
- Formation of pus/ abscess if there is increased number of neutrophils in the inflammed area.
- Area becomes hard, painful, swelling/ nodule
- Presence of leucocytes in the inflammation area.
- Presence of the type of cell may also determine the type of inflammation.

Cells of inflammation are polymorphonuclear cells, lymphocytes, macrophages, eosinophils, mast cells, plasma cells, giant cells, etc.

Polymorphonuclear cells

They are also known as neutrophils (mammals) and heterophils (birds). Size of these cells vary from 10m-20m. They are attracted by certain chemotactic factors like bacterial proteins, C_3a, C_5a, fibrinolysin and kinins. These cells are produced in bone marrow and are short lived only for 2-3 days. Mature cells have multilobed nucleus and two types granules. Primary granules are the azurophilic granules present in lysosomes containing acid hydrolases, myeloperoxidases and neuraminidases. Secondary or specific granules are having lactoferin and lysozymes. These cells degranulate through Fc receptor binding with non-specific immune complexes or opsonins.

Lymphocytes

Lymphocytes are produced in primary lymphoid organs like thymus, bursa of Fabricious and bone marrow and their maturation takes place in secondary lymphoid organs like spleen, lymphnodes, tonsils, and mucosa associated lymphoid tissue etc. These cells may survive for years and in some cases for whole life of an animal. There are two types of lymphocytes seen on light microscopy i.e. small and large. Small lymphocytes are mainly T-helper or T-cytotoxic cells having nuclear cytoplasm ratio (N:C) high. The larger lymphocytes are having N:C ratio low and are mainly B cells and NK Cells. There are large numbers of molecules present on cell surface of lymphocytes which are used to distinguish the type of cells. These are known as markers and are identified by a set of monoclonal antibodies and are termed as Cluster of Differentiation (CD system of classification) e.g. CD_4 T- helper cells, CD_8 T-Cytotoxic cell, CD_2 and CD_5 Pan - cell marker and CD_7 NK cells.

B–lymphocytes are characterized on the basis of presence of mature immunoglobulins (IgG, IgA, IgM, IgE, IgD) on their surface. They comprise only 5-15% of total peripheral blood lymphocytes. The B – cells having IgM, IgG, IgD are present in blood while IgA bearing B-lymphocytes are present in large numbers on mucosal surfaces. The B-lymphocytes can be further divided into B_1 and B_2; B_1 are present predominantly in peritoneal cavity and are predisposed for autoantibody production while B_2-cells are conventional antibody producing cells.

Natural Killer (N.K. cells) are also present in 10-15% of total peripheral blood lymphocytes. These are defined as the lymphocytes which do not have any conventional surface antigen receptor i.e. TCR or immunoglobulin. In other words, they are neither T nor B cells. The NK cells do not have CD_3 molecule but CD_{16} and CD_{56} are present on their surface. These may kill tumor cells, virus containing cells and targets coated by IgG non specifically. They excret gamma interferon interleukin 1 and GM- CSF.

Macrophages

The mononuclear macrophages are the main phagocytic and antigen presenting cells which develop from bone marrow stem cells and may survive in body till life. The professional phagocytic cells destroy the particulate material while antigen presenting cells (APC) present the processed antigen to the lymphocytes. They are having horse shoe shape nucleus and azurophilic granules. They have a well developed Golgi apparatus and many intra cytoplasmic lysosomes which contain peroxidases and hydrolases for intracellular killing of microorganism. Macrophages have a tendency to adhere on glass or plastic surface and are able to phagocyte the bacteria and tumor cells through specialized receptors. These cells are also having CD_{14} receptors for lipopolysacharide (LPS) binding protein normally present in serum and may coat on Gram negative bacteria. There are CD_{64} receptor for binding of Fc portion of IgG responsible for opsonization, extracellular killing and phagocytosis. Antigen presenting cells (APC) are associated with immunostimulation, induction of T-helper cell activity and communication with other leucocytes. Some endothelial and epithelial cells may under certain circumstances also acquire the properties of APC when stimulated by cytokines. They are found in skin, lymphnodes, spleen and thymus.

Eosinophils

Eosinophils comprise 2-5% of total leucocyte count in peripheral blood. They are responsible for killing of large objects which can not be phagocytosed such as parasites. However, they may also act as phagocytic cells for killing the bacteria but it is not their primary function. These cells are having bilobed nucleus and eosinophilic granules. The granules are membrane bound with crystalloid core. These granules are rich in major basic protein which also releases histaminase and aryl sulfatase and leucocyte migration inhibition factor.

Mast cells/ Basophils

There are 0.2% basophils in peripheral blood which are having deep violet blue coloured granules. The tissue basophils are known as mast cells. They are of two types, mucosal mast cells and connective tissue mast cells. Basophilic granules present in these cells are rich in heparin, SRS-A and ECF-A. When any antigen or allergen comes in contact with cells, it cross links with IgE bound on the surface of mast cells and stimulate the cells to degranulate and release histamine which plays an active role in allergy.

Platelets

Platelets are derived from bone marrow and contains granules. These cells help in clotting of blood and are involved in inflammation. When endothelial surface gets damaged, platelets adhere and aggregate on damaged endothelium and release substances to increase permeability, attract leucocytes and activate complement.

Plasma cells

The plasma cells are modified B-lymphocytes meant for production of immunoglobulins. Plasma cells have smooth spherical or elliptical shape with increased cytoplasm and eccentrically placed cart wheel shaped nucleus. The cytoplasm stains slightly basophilic and gives a magenta shade of purplish red. In the cytoplasm, there is a distinct hyaline homogenous mass called **Russell body** which lies on the cisternae of the endoplasmic reticulum. This* is the accumulation of immunoglobulin produced by these cells. Such cells are present in almost all types of inflammation.

Epithelioid cells

They are the activated macrophages mostly present in granuloma when macrophages become large and foamy due to accumulation of phagocytosed material (bacteria) and degenerated tissue debris. These cells are considered as *hallmark of granulomatous inflammation.* They are elongated with marginal nucleus looking like a columnar epithelial cells and hence their name "Epithelioid" cells.

Giant cells

The giant cells are multinucleated macrophages fused together to kill the microorganisms. They are formed by the fusion of many macrophages to phagocytose larger particles such as yeast fungi and mycobacteria. They are having many usually more than one nucleus and abundant cytoplasm. Such cells are formed when macrophages fails to phagocytose the particulate material. They are of several types as listed blow.

Foreign body giant cells: They are having many nuclei upto 100 which are uniform in size and shape and resemble the macrophage nucleus. The nuclei are scattered in the cytoplasm. Such cells are seen in chronic infectious granulomas of tuberculosis.

Langhans giant cells: They are horse shoe shaped giant cells having many nuclei and are of characteristically present in tubercle. The nuclei resemble with that of macrophages and epithelioid cells. The nuclei are mostly arranged at periphery giving horse shoe shape.

Touton giant cells: They are multinucleated cells having vacuolation in the cytoplasm due to increased lipid content. They mostly occurs in xanthoma.

Tumor giant cells: These are larger, pleomorphic and hyperchromatic cells having numerous nuclei with different size and shape. Nuclei of such cells do not resemble with that of macrophages or epithelioid cells. They are not true giant cells and not formed from macrophages but are found in cancers as a result of fast division of nuclei in comparison to cytoplasm.

Fibroblasts

Fibroblast proliferates to replace its own tissue and others which are not able to regenerate. The new fibroblasts originate from fibrocyte as well as from the fibroblasts through mitotic division. Collagen fibers begin to appear on 6th day as an amorphous ground substance or matrix. They are characteristic of chronic inflammation and repair. Fibroblasts are elongated cells having long nuclei sometimes looking like the smooth muscle fibers. The proliferation of fibroblasts is extremely active in neonates and slow and delayed in old animals. The fibroplasia can be enhanced by removal of necrosed tissue debris and by fever.

CHEMICAL CHANGES

There is a long list of chemical mediators responsible for acute inflammation. These are endogenous biochemical compounds, which can increase the vascular permeability, vasodilation, chemotaxis, fever, pain and cause tissue damage. Such chemical mediators are released by cells, plasma or damaged tissue and are broadly classified as: cell and plasma derived chemical mediators of inflammation.

CELL DERIVED MEDIATORS

Vasoactive amines

Histamine: Histamine is found in basophilic granules of mast cells or basophils and in platelets. It is released through stimuli due to heat, cold, irradiation, trauma, irritant, chemical and immunological reactions and anaphylotoxins C3a, C5a and C4a. Histamine is also released due to action of histamine releasing factors from neutrophils, monocytes and platelets. It acts on blood vessels and causes vasodilation, increased vascular permeability, itching, and pain.

Serotonin (5-Hydroxy-tryptamine): It is present in tissues of gastrointestinal tract, spleen, nervous tissue, mast cells and platelets. It is also acting on blood vessels to cause vasodilation and increased permeability but its action is mild in comparison to histamine.

Arachidonic acid metabolites

Arachidonic acid is a fatty acid, which either comes directly from the diet or through conversion of linoleic acid to arachidonic acid. Arachidonic acid is activated by C5a to form its metabolites through either cyclo-oxygenase or lipo-oxygenase pathways. Cyclo-oxygenase is a fatty acid enzyme which acts on arachidonic acid to form prostaglandin endoperoxidase (PGG) which is further transformed into prostaglandins like PGD_2, PGE_2, PGF_2, thromboxane A_2 (Tx A_2) and prostacyclin (PGI_2). Prostaglandins act on blood vessels to cause vasodilation, increased permeability bronchodilation except PGF_2a, which is responsible for vasodilation and bronchoconstriction. Thromboxane A_2 is a vasoconstrictor, bronchoconstrictor, and causes aggregation of platelets leading of increased function of inflammatory cells. Prostacylin is found to be responsible for vasodilation, bronchodilation and inhibitory action on platelet aggregation. Lipo-oxygnese acts on arachidonic acid to form hydroperoxy eico-satetraenoic acid (5HPETE) which is further converted into 5 HETE a chemotactic agent for neutrophils and leucotrienes (LT) or slow reacting substance of anaphylaxis (SRS-A). The leucotrienes include an unstable form leucotriene A (LTA), which is soon converted into leucotriene B (LTB), a chemotactic and adherence factor for phagocytic cells, and leucotriene C, D and E (LTC, LTD, LTE) causing contraction of smooth muscles leading to vasoconstriction, bronchoconstriction and increased vascular permeability.

Lysosomal components

Lysosomal granules are released by neutrophils and macrophages to cause degradation of bacterial and extracellular components, chemotaxis and increased vascular permeability. These lysosomal granules are rich in acid proteases, collagenases, elastases and plasminogen activator.

Platelet activating factor (PAF)

Platelet activating factor (PAF) is released from IgE sensitized mast cells, endothelial cells and platelets. It acts on platelets for their aggregation and release, chemotaxis, bronchoconstriction, adherance of leucocytes and increased vascular permeability. In low amount PAF causes vasodilation while in high concentration it leads to vasoconstriction.

Cytokines

Cytokines are hormone like substances produced by activated lymphocytes (*Lymphokines*) and monocytes (*Monokines*). These are glycoprotein in nature with low molecular weight (8-75KD) and composed of single chain. They differ from hormones which are specifically produced by endocrine glands to maintain homeostasis through endocrine action while cytokines are produced by many different cell types and acts on different cells of body with very high functional activity. They cause autocrine, paracrine and endocrine action leading to tissue repair and resistance to infection. Cytokines are broadly classified as interleukins, interferon, cytotoxins and growth factors.

Interleukins (IL)

Interleukins are cytokines required for cell to cell interaction among immune cells. They are numbered serially in order to their discovery; however, their actions are different and not related with each other.

Sl. No.	Type of interleukin	Size MW (KD)	Source	Target/ Action
1.	Interleukin-1 (IL-1α, IL-1β and IL-1RA)	17	Macrophages, Langerhans cells, T-cells, B-Cells, Vascular endothelium, Fibroblasts, Keratinocytes	T-cells, B-cells, Neutrophils, Eosinophils, Dendritic cells, Fibroblasts, Endothelial cells, Hepatocytes, Macrophages.
2.	Interleukin-2 (IL –2)	15	T- helper-1 cells (Th-1)	T-cells, B-cells, NK Cells.
3.	Interleukin-3 (IL-3)	25	Activated T-cells, Th-1 cells, Th-2 cells, Eosinophils, Mast cells.	Stimulates growth and maturation of bone marrow stem cells, Eosinophilia, Neutrophilia Monocytosis, Increases phagocytosis, Promotes immuno-globulin secretion by B- cells.
4.	Interleukin-4 (IL – 4)	20	Activated Th-2 cells.	B-Cells, T-cells, Macrophages, Endothelial cells, Fibroblasts, Mast cells, IgE Production in allergy, Down regulate IL1, IL6, and TNF-α.

5.	Interleukin-5 (IL-5)	18	Th-2 cells, Mast cells, Eosinophils	Eosinophils, Increases T-Cell, cytotoxicity
6.	Interleukin-6 (IL-6)	26	Macrophages, T-cells, B-cells, Bone marrow stromal cells, Vascular endothelial cells, Fibroblasts, Keratinocytes, Mesangial cells.	T-cells, B-cells, Hepatocytes, Bone marrow stromal cells, Stimulates acute phase protein synthesis, Acts as pyrogen.
7.	Interleukin-7 (IL-7)	25	Bone marrow, Spleen cells, Thymic stromal cells.	Thymocytes, T-cells, B-cells, Monocytes, Lymphoid stem cells, Generates cytotoxic T-cells.
8.	Interleukin-8 (IL-8)	8	Macrophages	T-Cells, Neutrophils.
9.	Interleukin-9 (IL-9)	39	Th-2 cells	Growth of Th-cells, Stimulates B-cell, Thymocytes, Mast cells.
10.	Interleukin-10 (IL-10)	19	Th cells, B-cells, Macrophages, Keratinocytes, Th-2 cells	Th-1 cells, NK cells, Stimulates B cells, Thymocytes, Mast cells.
11.	Interleukin-11 (IL-11)	24	Bone marrow stromal cells, Fibroblasts	Growth of B-cells, Megakaryocyte colony formation, Promotes the production of acute phase proteins.
12.	Interleukin-12 (IL-12)	75	Activated macrophages	Th-1 cells activity, T-cell proliferation and cytotoxicity, NK cell proliferation and cytotoxicity Suppresses IgE production, Enhances B-cell immunoglobulin production.

13.	Interleukin-13 (IL-13)	10	Th-2 cells	B-Cells, Macrophages, Neutrophils, Inhibits macrophage activity, Stimulates B-cell proliferation, Stimulates neutrophils.
14.	Interleukin 14 (IL-14)	53.	T-cells, Malignant B-cells	Enhances B-cell proliferation, Inhibits immunoglobulin secretion.
15.	Interleukin-15 (IL-15)	15	Activated macrophages, Epithelial cells, Fibroblasts.	T-cells, NK cells, Proliferation of both cytotoxic and helper T-cells, Generates LAK cells
16.	Interleukin-16 (IL-16)	13	T-cells (CD_8 cells)	T cells, CD_4 cells, Chemotactic for lymphocytes
17.	Interleukin-17 (IL-17)	17	CD_4 cells	Promotes the production of IL-6, IL-8.
18.	Interleukin-18 (IL-18)		Macrophage	Induces γ-interferon production
19.	Interleukin-19 (IL-19)		Macrophage	Inhibit inflammatory and immune responses, suppress activities of T_h1 and T_h2 cells
20.	Interleukin-20 (IL-20)		Activated keratinocytes	Proliferation of keratinocytes and their differentiation, modulate skin inflammation

21. Interleukin–21 (IL-21)	Activated T-cells	Regulation of haematopoiesis and immune responses, promotes production of T-cells, fast growth and maturation of NK cells and B-cells population
22. Interleukin–22 (IL-22)	Activated T-cells	Induction of acute phase responses and proinflammatory role
23. Interleukin–23 (IL-23)	Monocytes, activated dendritic cells	Induces γ interferon production and T_h1 lymphocyte differentiation
24. Interleukin–24 (IL-24)	T_h2 cells	Tumor suppression
25. Interleukin–25 (IL-18)	T_h2 cells	Stimulates release of IL-4, IL-5 and IL-13 from non lymphoid accessory cells
26. Interleukin–26 (IL-26)	T- cells	Proinflammatory role, cutaneous and mucosal immunity
27. Interleukin–27 (IL-27)	CD_4 cells	Rapid clonal expansion of naïve T-cells and CD_4 cells, induces proliferative response and cytokines production by Ag specific effector/ memory T_h1 cells
28. Interleukin–28 (IL-28)	Virus induced peripheral blood mononuclear cells	Immunity to viral infection (antiviral activity)
29. Interleukin–29 (IL-29)	Virus induced peripheral blood mononuclear cells	Immunity to viral infection (antiviral activity)

Interferons

Interferons are glycoproteins having antiviral action and inhibit the virus replication in cells. These are of 5 types like alpha (α), beta (β), gamma (γ), omega (ω), and tau (ι).

Sl. No.	Interferon	Source	Action
1.	Interferon alpha (IFN-α)	Lymphocytes, Monocytes, Macrophages	Inhibit viral growth, activate macrophages
2.	Interferon beta (IFN-β)	Fibroblasts	Inhibit viral growth, Activates macrophages
3.	Interferon Gamma (IFN-γ)	Th-1 cells, Cytotoxic T-cells, NK cells, Macrophages	Stimulates B-cells, Production, Enhances NK Cells activity Activates macrophages and phagocytosis. Promotes antibody dependent and cell mediated cytotoxicity.
4.	Interferon Omega (IFN-ω)	Lymphocytes, Monocytes Trophoblasts	Virus infected cells to check viral growth Activate Macrophages
5.	Interferon tau (IFN-ι)	Trophoblasts	Virus growth, Immunity to fetus through placenta.

Tumor necrosis factor or cytotoxins

Tumor necrosis factor or cytotoxins are produced by macrophages and T-cells and are associated with apoptosis in tumors. Tumor necrosis factor beta (TNF-β) is produced by T-helper 1 cells and activates CD_8^+ T-cells, neutrophils, macrophages, endothelial cells and B-lymphocytes. Tumor necrosis factor alpha (TFN-a) is produced by macrophages, T-cells, B-cells and fibroblasts and it activates macrophages and enhances immunity and inflammatory reaction.

Chemokines

Chemokines are small proteins divided into two a and b subfamilies. Alpha- chemokines include IL-8, which is produced by fibroblasts, macrophages endothelial cells, lymphocytes, granulocytes, hepatocytes and keratinocytes. It acts as chemotactic agent for basophils, neutrophils, and T-cells. The neutrophils get activated and release their granules and leucotrienes. There is increased respiratory burst. Besides, it also acts on basophils and lymphocytes. Macrophage inflammatory protein MIP-1 of b-chemokines are produced by macrophages, T and B-lymphocytes, mast cell and neutrophils. It acts on monocytes, eosinophils, B and T-lymphocytes. Beta-chemokines includes macrophage inflammatory protein (MIP-1), monocyte chemoattractant protein (MCP) and RANTES protein. The MCP is produced by macrophages, T-cells, fibroblasts, keratinocytes and endothelial cells and activates the monocytes and stimulating them for respiratory burst and lysosomal enzyme release. RANTES is released by T-lymphocytes and macrophages and it acts as chemotactic agent for monocytes, eosinophils, basophils and some T-cells.

Growth factors

Many cytokines are also known as growth factors which act on cells and stimulate them to proliferate thus they play very important role in inflammation and healing. These are glycoprotein in nature, which controls the proliferation and maturation of several blood cells. The growth factors also include interleukin 3,7,11, and 15. The granulocyte colony stimulating factor (G-CSF) is produced by fibroblasts, endothelial cells and macrophages. It acts on granulocyte progenitors and regulate their maturation and production of superoxide. Macrophage colony stimulating factors (M-CSF) are the glycoproteins released by lymphocytes, macrophages, fibroblasts, epithelial cells and endothelial cells. They act on monocyte progenitors for their proliferation and differentiation and promotes their killing activity. Granulocyte macrophage colony stimulating factor (GM-CSF) is released from macrophages, T-lymphocytes, endothelial cells and fibroblasts and facilitates phagocytosis, antibody dependent cell cytotoxicity (ADCC) and superoxide production. It activates eosinophils to enhance superoxide production and macrophages for increased phagocytosis and tumoricidal activity. Transforming growth factor (TGF) are five related proteins (TGF-B_1, B_2, B_3 in mammals; B_4 and B_5 in poultry) released from neutrophils, macrophages, T-and B-lymphocytes and they inhibit the proliferation of macrophages, T- and B-lymphocytes and stimulates the proliferation of fibroblasts.

PLASMA DERIVED MEDIATORS

Plasma derived mediators of inflammation are kinins, clotting, fibrinolytic and complement systems; each of them has initiators and accelerators in plasma depending upon their need through feed back mechanism. During inflammation Hagman factor (Factor XII) is activated through leakage in endothelial gaps in increased permeability of blood vessels. The activated factor XII acts on kinin, clotting and fibrinolytic systems and end product of these systems activate complement to generate C3a and C5a, which are potent mediators of inflammation.

Kinin system: Through activation of factor XII, kinin system generate the bradykinin which causes contraction of smooth muscles. The activated factor XII (XIIa) acts on prekallikrein activator which in turn converts the plasma prekallikrein into kallikrein.

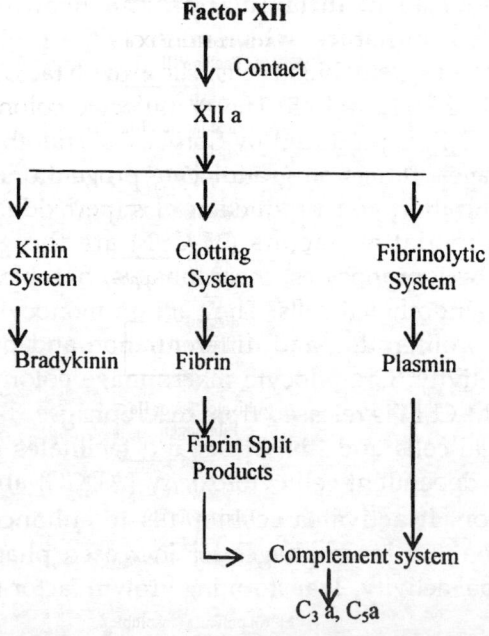

Inflammation and Healing

The bradykinin is formed from kininogen through the action of kallikrein. The bradykinin acts on smooth muscles leading to their contraction. Bradykinin is also found to be responsible for vasodilation, increased vascular permeability and pain.

Clotting mechanism: The activated Hagman factor (XIIa) initiates the cascade of clotting system and activates factor XI into XIa which is along with factor VIIa changes factor X into Xa. Factor Xa along with factor Va converts prothrombin into thrombin which acts on fibrinogen to form fibrin responsible for clotting of blood.

Clotting system

(a) Extrinsic mechanism

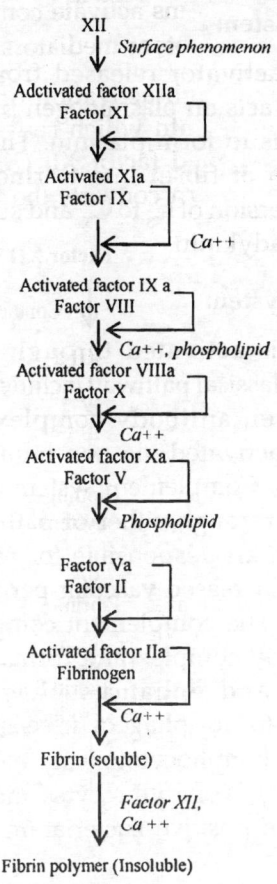

105

(b) Intrisic mechanism

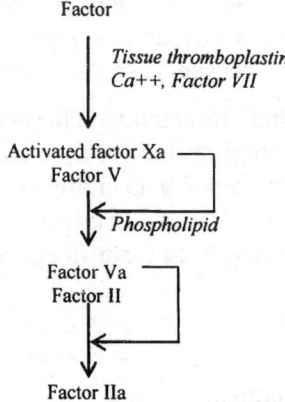

Fibrinolytic system

Plasminogen activator released from endothelial cells and leucocytes and acts on plasminogen present as a component of plasma proteins to form plasmin. The plasmin is responsible for breakdown of fibrin into fibrinopeptides or fibrin split products, conversion of C_3 to C_{3a} and stimulates the kinin system to generate bradykinin.

Complement system

Complement is activated through classical and alternate pathways; the classical pathway include activation of complement through antigen-antibody complexes while the alternate pathway gets activated via non immunologic agents such as bacterial toxins. Complement system on activation generates 3 anaphylotoxin-through either of pathway including C3a, C5a and C4a which are responsible for release of histamine from the mast cells, increased vascular permeability and chemotaxis for leucocytes. The complement components are activated by antigen antibody complex and forms AAC1423 which causes opsonization and enhances phagocyosis. C567 acts as chemotactic factor for phagocytic cells. AAC_{1-7} renders the cell susceptible for lymphocytotoxicity by T-cell. The complement AAC_{1-9} causes lysis of erythrocytes and Gram negative bacteria. However, Gram positive bacteria are resistant to complement lysis.

Inflammation and Healing

Antigen- antibody complex (AA)
On cell surface

$\downarrow C_1$

AAC_1

$\downarrow C_4 \longrightarrow C_4a$

AAC_{14}

$\downarrow C_2 \longrightarrow C_2x$
Kinin like product

AAC_{142}

$\downarrow C_3 \longrightarrow C_3a$
Anaphylotoxin

AAC_{1423}

$\downarrow C_5 \longrightarrow C_5a$
$ C_6 $ *Anaphylotoxin*

AAC_{142356}

$\downarrow C_7 \longrightarrow C567$
Chemotactic factor

$AAC_{1423567}$

$\downarrow C_8$

AAC_{1-8}

$\downarrow C_9$

AAC_{1-9}

$\downarrow$

Cell lysis

PHAGOCYTOSIS

Phagocytosis is the process of engulfment and digestion of particulate matter by certain cells of body (Phagocytes; Phagocytic cells). Mainly there are two types of the cells which perform the phagocytosis including polymorphonuclear neutrophils (PMN) or microphages and monocytes or tissue mononuclear cells also known as macrophages. The process of phagocytosis is almost similar by these micro and macrophages and involves 4 stages.

I. Chemotaxis

The phagocytic cells, neutrophils and monocytes, are present in circulating blood while there are several tissue macrophages found in inflammation. Vasodilation and decreased blood flow leads to disturbances in blood stream resulting in margination of leucocytes. At that time endothelial cells of blood vessels express certain proteins known as *selectins* and *integrins* that bind with neutrophils. Since they are attracted by certain chemical mediators, these cells are directed to migrate towards the chemical mediators, this directed migration of phagocytic cells is known as chemotaxis. Various chemotactic agents for different phgocytic cells are as under:

Chemotactic agents	Phagocytic cells
C_{3a}, C_{5a}, C_{567}, Leucotriene B_4, Bacterial proteins, LPS.	Neutrophils
C_{3a}, C_{5a}, C_{567}, Bacterial products Neutrophilic cationic protein Cytokines, Kinins	Macrophages/ monocytes
ECF-A, Parasitic proteins, Complement C_{3a}, C_{5a}.	Eosinophils

The chemotactic agents diffuse at the site of tissue damage to attract the phagocytic cells. However, large dose of chemotactic molecules may make the phagocytic cells insensitive to chemoattraction and such non-responsive cells may migrate from the damaged area after completion of phagocytosis.

II. Adherence and opsonization

The phagocytic cells and foreign particle like bacteria both are suspended in body fluid with negative charge that repel each other. The negative charge on foreign particle is neutralized by coating of positively charged protein and such proteins are immunoglobulins (IgG) and $C_{3b,}$ the complement component. Thus, the particle coated with (IgG or C_{3b}) reduced its surface charge and it is attracted towards phagocytic cells. The molecules (IgG or C_{3b}) coating on particulate matter to facilitate phagocytosis are known as *opsonins* and this process is termed as *opsonization*. This opsonin word is derived from Greek language means *sauce*, implying that it makes the particles more tastier to phagocytic cells. The phagocytic cells are also having receptors for Fc portion of IgG and C_3b protein that facilitates the adherence of the particles on the surface of the cells. Another mechanism is trapping of particulate material through pseudopodia movement of the phagocytic cells.

III. Ingestion

The phagocytic cell forms pseudopodia around the particles to cover it from outside. The particle is bound to the surface of cells through opsonization and is drawn inside the cytoplasm through engulfment. The phagocytic cell forms vacuole through enveloping the particle which is known as *phagocytic vacuole*. The plasma membrane covering phagocytic vacuole breaks and the ingested particle lies free in cytoplasm of phagocytic cell. The lysosome present in cell cytoplasm binds with phagocytic vacuoles to form *phagolysosome* or *phagosome*.

There is degranulation on the particle and liberation of hydrolytic enzymes and antibacterial substances to kill the ingested particle.

IV. Digestion

The ingested particles are destroyed by the phagocytic cells through two separate mechanisms, the respiratory burst and by action of lysosomal enzymes

Respiratory Burst

Soon after the ingestion of particulate material phagocytic cell increases its oxygen consumption nearly 100 fold and also activates the cell surface enzyme NADPH-oxidase. This activated enzyme converts NADPH to $NADP^+$ with release of electrons.

$$NADPH + O_2 \xrightarrow{NADPH-Oxidase} NADP^+ + 2O + H^+$$

One molecule of oxygen accepts a single donated electron, leading to the generation of one molecule of superoxide anion. $NADP^+$ increases the hexose monophosphate shunt and converts sucrose to a pentose, carbon dioxide and energy for utilization of the cellular functions. Two molecules of superoxide anions interact to generate one molecule of hydrogen peroxide under the influence of enzyme superoxide dismutase.

$$2(2O^-) + 2H^+ \xrightarrow{Superoxide\ dismutase} H_2O_2 + O_2$$

Superoxide anions do not accumulate in the cell because under the influence of dismutase enzyme they rapidly convert into hydrogen peroxide. However, there is accumulation of hydrogen peroxide in the cells which is also converted into bactericidal compounds the hypohalids through the action of myeloperoxidase.

$$H_2O_2 + Cl^- \xrightarrow{Myeloperoxidase} H_2O_2 + OCl^- (Hypochloride)$$

Hypochloride kills bacteria by oxidizing their proteins and enhancing the bactericidal activities of the lysosomal enzymes.

Lysosomal enzymes

Once the phagolysosomes are formed, the lysosomal enzymes are released in the particulate matter, that can kill the bacteria. Many Gram positive and Gram negative bacteria are destroyed by the lysosomal enzymes. However, there are certain bacteria like Brucella, Listeria which are so resistant that they even grow inside the cell and may become fatal to the cell. Dying neutrophils release elastases and collagenase which act as chemotactic factors for macrophages. The macrophages destroy the particulate material/ bacteria by both oxidative and non oxidative mechanisms. In cattle, macrophages after activation synthesize the nitric oxide synthatase. This enzyme acts on L-arginine by using oxygen and NADPH to produce nitric oxide and citrulline. Nitric oxide is not highly toxic but it reacts with superoxide anions released during respiratory burst to produce very toxic derivatives such as NO_2, N_2O_3 ONOO and NO_3 which can kill the ingested bacteria and cause severe tissue damage. Macrophages are also used by the body as scavenger cells to remove the dead or dying cells.

When the foreign particulate material persists for longer period, macrophages accumulate in large number around it to kill and remove from the system. The phagocytosed particles are so potent that they kill the macrophages also. Then after destruction of macrophages it is rephagocytosed. This continuing destruction of macrophages leads to excessive release of lysosomal enzymes and reactive oxygen and nitric oxide metabolites resulting in chronic tissue damage and chronic inflammation. In such situation, macrophages become elongated looking like epithelial cells and such cells are termed as *epithelioid cells*. If these cells are also unable to destroy the ingested material then they combine/ fuse together to form multinucleated giant cells.

TYPES OF INFLAMMATION

Inflammation is classified according to the duration in acute, subacute and chronic form. The acute inflammation is characterized by the presence of more vascular alterations while chronic inflammation is identified on the basis of presence of more proliferative changes, fibrosis and less vascular alterations.

Sl. No.	Changes	Acute	Subacute	Chronic
1.	Vascular changes	+++	++	+
2.	Proliferative changes	+	++	+++

On the basis of the presence of exudate, the inflammation is divided into catarrhal, serus, fibrinous, suppurative, eosinophilic, lymphocytic, haemorrhagic, granulomatous etc., described as under:

CATARRHAL INFLAMMATION

Catarrhal inflammation occurs on mucus surfaces and is characterized by the presence of increased amount of mucin as principal constituent of exudates *e.g. Catarrhal enteritis, catarrhal rhinitis.*

Etiology
- Mild irritant on mucous membrane *e.g.* Rotavirus infection in calves.
- Cold exposure causes excessive mucous discharges from nasal mucosa.

Macroscopic and microscopic features
- Congestion
- Presence of increased amount of slimy, stringy mucin along with stool.
- Mucus nasal discharge, if respiratory mucosa is involved
- Mucous vaginal discharges, in uterine disorders or as physiological phenomenon.
- Increased number of goblet cells on mucous surface.
- Increased amount of mucin, which takes basic stain.
- Hyperplasia of epithelial cells on mucous surface.
- Infiltration of neutrophils, lymphocytes and macrophages.

SEROUS INFLAMMATION

Serous inflammation occurs due to any mild irritant and is characterized by the presence of serum/ plasma as main constituent of the exudates.

Etiology
- Mild irritants *e.g.* Chemicals
- Physical trauma

- Infection
- Virus *e.g.* Pox, FMD
- Bacteria *e.g. Pasteurlla multocida*

Macroscopic and microscopic features
- Congestion
- Watery exudate in cavity/ vesicle/ in intercellular spaces
- On rupture of vesicle clear fluid comes out
- Congestion
- Presence of serus exudate-acidophilic in tissue.
- Infiltration of neutrophils/ lymphocytes/ mononuclear cells.

FIBRINOUS INFLAMMATION

Fibrinous inflammation is characterized by the presence of fibrin as main constituent of the exudates.

Etiology
- Chemicals
- Thermal injury
- Bacteria *e.g. Corynebacterium diphtheriae*
- Viruses *e.g.* Herpes virus, influenza virus

Macroscopic and microscopic features
- Organ becomes firm and tense.
- Surface of organ lost its shine.
- Produces adhesions in between two layers or two organs.
- Congestion
- Presence of fibrin network (thread like) on the surface or in the organ.
- Infiltration of inflammatory cells like neutrophils, lymphocytes and macrophages.

False membrane/ crupous membrane present, which can be removed easily *e.g.* fibrinous membrane over heart and liver due to colisepticemia in birds.

SUPPURATIVE INFLAMMATION

Suppurative inflammation is characterized by the presence of neutrophils (polymorphonuclear cells) as principal constituent of the exudates.

Etiology
- Bacterial infection *e.g.* Staphylococci.
- Chemicals *e.g.* Turpentine.

Macroscopic and microscopic features
- Presence of pus in lesion
- Pus is white yellow/ greenish, thin, watery or viscid/ material.
- When pus present in a cavity it is known as *abscess*. While the presence of pus diffusely scattered throughout the subcutaneous tissue is known as *Phlegmon* or *cellulitis*.
- Congestion
- Presence of neutrophils as main constituent of the exudate.
- Liquifactive necrosis of the cells/ tissue.

HEMORRHAGIC INFLAMMATION

Hemorrhagic inflammation is characterized by the presence of erythrocyte as principal constituent of the exudate.

Etiology
- Extremely injurious chemicals *e.g.* phenol.
- Bacterial infection *e.g.* Anthrax, H.S.
- Viral infection *e.g.* R.P., Blue tongue

Macroscopic and microscopic features
- Colour of organ/ tissue becomes red/ cyanotic.
- Exudate contains clot of blood.
- Petechial, echymotic haemorrhages on the surfaces of organs.
- Mucous membranes become pale/ anemic.
- Presence of erythrocytes out side the blood vessels in extracellular spaces along with neutrophils/ lymphocytes/ macrophage.

- Serous/ serofibrinous exudates.

LYMPHOCYTIC INFLAMMATION

Lymphocytic inflammation is characterized by the presence of lymphocytes as principal constituent of the exudate.

Etiology
- Viral/ Bacterial infections
- Toxic conditions

Macroscopic and microscopic features
- No characteristic gross lesion; sometimes there is formation of small modules on serosa of the affected organ.
- Enlargement of lymphnodes
- Congestion
- Presence of white/ gray lymphoid nodules in organ.
- Presence of lymphocytes in abundant number as principal constituent of the exudate.
- Congestion.
- Accumulation of lymphocytes around the blood vessels, "Perivascular cuffing"
- Aggregation of lymphocytes leading to lymphofollicular reaction.

GRANULOMATOUS INFLAMMATION

Granulomatous inflammation is a chronic condition, characterized by the presence of granuloma in the organs. The granuloma consists of central caseative necrosis surrounded by lymphocytes, macrophages, epithelioid cells, giant cells and fibrous connective tissue.

Etiology
- Chronic bacterial infection *e.g.* Tuberculosis.
- Fungal infections *e.g.* Blastomycosis.

Macroscopic and microscopic features
- Presence of hard, tiny, nodules in the organ.
- Lungs become hard, patchy.

- Lymphnodes become hard and fibrus.
- Later the affected organ calcified and gives cracking sound on cut.
- Presence of granuloma in the tissue/ organ.
- Central caseative necrosis, surrounded by epithelioid cells, macrophages, lymphocytes, giant cells and covered by fibrous connective tissue capsule.
- Caseative area contains causative organisms also, which can be demonstrated by special staining *e.g.* Tuberculous organisms by Acid-fast staining.
- Calcification of necrosed area at later stage looking black/ violet colour on H & E stain.

EOSINOPHILIC INFLAMMATION

It is characterized by the presence of eosinophils as the main constituents of the exudates.

Etiology
- Allergy/ Hypersensitivity
- Parasitic diseases

Macroscopic and microscopic features
- Congestion
- No characteristic gross lesion
- Presence of eosinophils in abundant numbers
- Congestion
- Accumulation of eosinophils around the parasites and/or blood vessels.

HEALING

Healing is characterized by the body response to injury in order to restore normal structure and function of the damaged organ/ tissue. It is of two types.

Regeneration

Healing is by proliferation of parenchymatous cells leading to complete restoration of the original tissue

Differential features of various types of inflammation

	Catarrhal	Serous	Fibrinous	Suppurative	Hemorrhagic	Lymphocytic	Granulomatous	Eosinophilic
Macroscopic features	1. Congestion 2. Presence of increased amount of slimy, stringy mucin along with stool. 3. Mucus nasal discharge, if respiratory mucosa is involved 4. Mucous vaginal discharges, in uterine disorders or as physiological phenomenon.	1. Congestion 2. Watery exudate in cavity/ vesicle/ in intercellular spaces 3. On rupture of vesicle clear fluid comes out	1. Organ becomes firm and tense. 2. Surface of organ lost its shine. 3. Produces adhesions in between two layers or two organs. 4. False membrane/ crupous membrane present, which can be removed easily e.g. fibrinous membrane over heart and liver due to colisepticemia in birds.	1. Presence of pus in lesion 2. Pus is white yellow/ greenish, thin, watery or viscid/ material. 3. When pus present in a cavity it is known as abscess. While the presence of pus diffusely scattered throughout the subcutaneous tissue is known as Phlegmon or cellulitis.	1. Colour of organ/ tissue becomes red/ cyanotic. 2. Exudate contains clot of blood. 3. Petechial, echymotic haemorrhages on the surfaces of organs. 4. Mucous membranes become pale/ anemic.	1. No characteristic gross lesion; sometimes there is formation of small modules on serosa of the affected organ. 2. Enlargement of lymphnodes 3. Presence of white/ gray lymphoid nodules in organ.	1. Presence of hard, tiny, nodules in the organ. 2. Lungs become hard, patchy. 3. Lymphnodes become hard and fibrous. 4. Later the affected organ calcified and gives cracking sound on cut.	1. Congestion 2. No characteristic gross lesion

	Catarrhal	Serous	Fibrinous	Suppurative	Hemorrhagic	Lymphocytic	Granulomatous	Eosinophilic
Microscopic features	1. Increased number of goblet cells on mucous surface. 2. Increased amount of mucin, which takes basic stain. 3. Hyperplasia of epithelial cells on mucous surface. 4. Infiltration of neutrophils, lymphocytes and macrophages.	1. Congestion 2. Presence of serus exudate- acidophilic in tissue. 3. Infiltration of neutrophils/ lymphocytes/ mononuclear cells	1. Congestion 2. Presence of fibrin network (thread like) on the surface or in the organ. 3. Infiltration of inflammatory cells like neutrophils, lymphocytes and macrophages.	1. Congestion 2. Presence of neutrophils as main constituent of the exudate. 3. Liquifactive necrosis of the cells/ tissue.	1. Presence of erythrocytes out side the blood vessels in extracellular spaces along with neutrophils/ lymphocytes / macrophage. 2. Serus/ serofibrinous exudates.	1. Presence of lymphocytes in abundant number as principal constituent of the exudate. 2. Accumulation of lymphocytes around the blood vessels, "Peri vascular cuffing" 3. Aggregation of lymphocytes leading to lymphofollicular reaction.	1. Presence of granuloma in the tissue/ organ. 2. Central caseative necrosis, surrounded by epithelioid cells, macrophages, lymphocytes, giant cells and covered by fibrous connective tissue capsule. 3. Caseative area contains causative organisms also, which can be demonstrated by special staining e.g. Tuberculous organisms by Acid-fast staining. 4. Calcification of necrosed area at later stage looking black/ violet colour on H&E stain.	1. Presence of eosinophils in abundant numbers 2. Congestion 3. Accumulation of eosinophils around the parasites and/or blood vessels.

Macroscopic and microscopic features
- No significant gross lesion
- Proliferation of parenchymal cells
- Hyperplasia of the cells

Repair

Repair is the replacement of injured tissue by proliferation of fibrous tissue.

Macroscopic and microscopic features
- Pink/ red granules (granulation tissue) appear on healing part. These are the indication of formation of new blood vessels.
- It can be seen just beneath the scab.
- Formation of granulation tissue *i.e.* fibroblasts, angioblasts, histiocytes, macrophages and parenchymal cells of organ.
- Fibroblasts are elongated fibrillar cells with ovoid hyperchromatic nuclei.
- Mitosis is frequently observed.

Chapter 10
Concretions

CONCRETIONS

Concretions are solid, compact mass of material endogenous or exogenous in origin found in tissues, body cavities, ducts or in hollow organs. Concretions are stone like bodies commonly occur in urinary system, gall bladder and gastrointestinal tract. Concretions of endogenous origin are known as *calculi* while those formed from exogenous material are known as *piliconcretion* (Hair), *phytoconcretion* (plant fibers) and *polyconcretion* (Polythenes).

Calculi

Calculi are formed due to deposition of salts around the nucleus/ nidus consisting of either fibrin, mucus, desquamated epithelial cells or clumps of bacteria. Due to the gradual and repeated precipitation of salts, calculi becomes laminated. In the formation process of calculi the inner structural arrangement gets shrinkage producing a rough superficial surface. Calculi formation is more common in urinary system and in gall bladder of man and animals; however, they may also occur in salivary gland, pancreas and intestines.

URINARY CALCULI

Urinary calculi are formed in renal tubules, pelvis or in urinary bladder which may carried away through urine and may cause obstruction in ureter or urethra. Urinary calculi is also known as urolith and the process of formation of calculi is termed as *urolithiasis*.

Etiology
- Vit A deficiency
- Bacterial infection *e.g.* E.coli, Micrococci, Streptococci.
- Sulfonamide therapy
- Hormonal therapy
- Hyperparathyroidism

Macroscopic and microscopic features
- May vary in size from 1 mm to several mm
- Mostly rounded, pearl like, laminated.
- Brown, grey and yellowish in colour.
- Enlargement and fibrosis of kidneys.
- In kidney sections tiny, laminated bodies of concretion.
- Hydronephrosis
- Chemical composition of urinary calculi may vary in various species of animals.
- *Horse-* Calcium carbonate, calcium phosphate, magnesium carbonate
- *Ruminants-* Calcium phosphate, magnesium phosphate, aluminium phosphate, calcium oxalate.
- *Pigs-* Ammonium phosphate, magnesium phosphate, calcium carbonate, magnesium carbonate, magnesium phosphate, magnesium oxalate.
- *Dogs-* Calcium carbonate, calcium phosphate, sodium urate, ammonium urate.

BILIARY CALCULI

Biliary calculi are formed in gall bladder and bile ducts and are also known as cholelith. These are common in man; however, in cattle and pigs gall stones are also seen. They are semisolids but become hard and brittle on drying.

Etiology
- Bacteria
- Sand particles

- Particles of ingesta/ intestinal contents
- Desquamated epithelium

Macroscopic and microscopic features
- In gall bladder and bile duct
- 1 mm to 3-4 cm in diameter.
- Their number vary from 1 to many
- Obstructive jaundice
- Cholecystitis and cholangitis
- In sections, concentric layers of cholesterin, bilirubin, calcium carbonate and coagulated material.
- Cholecystitis, cholangitis.

SALIVARY CALCULI

Salivary calculi are formed in excretory ducts of the parotid, sublingual and submaxillary salivary glands. Size of such calculi vary upto 25-30 mm diameter. They are made up of salts like calcium carbonate, calcium phosphate, magnesium carbonate, sodium carbonate, calcium carbonate, around the plant fibers. Salivary calculi also known as *sialolith*.

PANCREATIC CALCULI

Pancreatic calculi or pancrealolith are rare in occurrence in animals but may be found in cattle. Pancreatic calculi is gray in colour with size upto few centimeter. They are made up of calcium carbonate, calcium oxalate and calcium phosphate around a nidus of cholesterol or fatty acids.

ENTERIC CALCULI

Enteric calculi or enterolith are common in horses, which occur mostly in large intestine 'colon'. In horse, a nidus is surrounded by wheat and rye bran containing magnesium phoshphate. The nidus may be a piece of metal or sand on which concentric layers are deposited. They may be looking like a ball in round or oval in shape. Colour of enterolith may vary from grayish to dark brown. In dogs, bone in diet may provide a nidus and such concretions are known as *coproliths*.

PILICONCRETIONS

Piliconcretions are hair balls occur due to excessive licking of skin in calves or in adults. Due to licking, animals swallow large amount of hairs taking a shape of ball due to movements of stomach. Mostly, the hair balls are found in stomach or in colon.

PHYTOCONCRETIONS

Phytoconcretions are formed around the food materials and may occur in stomach and intestine of animals and in crop of poultry. They may cause obstruction of bowel. They are also known as *phytobezoars*.

POLYCONCRETIONS

They are made-up of polythenes and excessive deposition of salts around them. They may vary in size from few centimeters to several centimeters and weighed upto kilograms. They cause obstruction leading to death of animals.

Such concretions are observed in cattle wandering on street in cities and in zoo animals. The polythene containing vegetable extra or green leaves and food materials are thrown away on roads, which is easily available to the animals. Polythene is not degraded in stomach and remained there to form a nidus, around which the salts are deposited and takes the shape of calculi leading to obstruction of digestive tract passage.

Chapter 11
Immunity and Immunopathology

IMMUNITY

Immunity is the resistance of body against extraneous etiological factors of disease, which is afforded by the interaction of chemical, humoral and cellular reactions in body. This is an integral part of the body without, which one cannot think of life. During the process of evolution, nature has provided this defence mechanism in body of all living creatures particularly of higher animals and man that protects them from physical, chemical and biological insults. It can be classified as natural or paraspecific and acquired or specific immunity.

Natural/ paraspecific immunity

There are some species resistant for a particular disease due to presence of natural resistance against them *e.g.* Horse, pig, cat are resistant to canine distemper virus; dogs are resistant to feline panleucopenia virus, chickens are resistant to anthrax. Even within species, there is natural resistance that protects some individuals while others are susceptible *e.g.* Indian Deshi cattle Zebu (*Bos indicus*) is quite resistant to piroplasmosis in comparison to *Bos taurus*. Besides, there are the mechanisms or barriers in body provided by nature, which are:

- *Skin and mucous membrane* prevent organisms from gaining entrance in body
- Mucous prevents from infections by trapping and keep them away.
- *Saliva, gastric juice and intestinal enzymes* kill bacteria

- *Tears, nasal and GI tract secretions* are bactericidal due to presence of lysozymes.
- *Phagocytic cells* such as neutrophils kill bacteria through phagocytosis.
- *Macrophages* kill organisms through phagocytosis
- *Natural antibodies* acts as opsonins and helps in phagocytosis.
- *Interferons* have antimicrobial properties. They are host/species specific and arrest the viral replication.
- *Interleukins, cytotoxins and growth factors* stimulate the immune reactions and inflammation
- *Natural killer cells* kill targets coated with IgG.

Acquired/ specific Immunity

Acquired immunity develop in body as a result of prior stimulation through antigen. It is specific to a particular antigen against which it was developed. It can be restimulated on second or subsequent exposure with antigen and thus, it has memory for a particular antigen. It differs from natural immunity in respect of prior stimulation, specificity and memory. It can be classified as humoral and cell mediated immunity.

Humoral Immunity

The immunity present in fluids of body mainly in blood. There are antibodies in serum of blood, which protect body from diseases. It is specific to particular antigen. Antibodies are formed in blood as a result of exposure of the foreign substances including bacteria, virus, parasite and other substances.

Antigen is foreign substance, which is able to stimulate the production of antibodies in body. They may be of high molecular weight protein, polysaccharides, and nucleic acids. Simple chemicals of low molecular weight are not able to induce immunity. However, they may be conjugated with a large molecular weight molecules such as protein then they become antigenic and induce antibody production, such substances are termed as *haptens*.

Antibodies are protein in nature present in serum and produced as a result of antigen. Antibodies are specific to antigen. Most of the microorganisms have several antigenic determinants and antibodies are produced against each antigenic determinant specifically. The antibody response to antigen can be enhanced if the antigen is released slowly in body. There are several substances like oils, waxes, alum, aluminium hydroxide, which may be added with antigen so that it is released slowly in body to increase the antibody production. Such substances are known as *adjuvants*. Antibodies are also known as *immunoglobulins* as they are the part of globulins. They are glycoprotein in nature and are of 5 types IgG, IgA, IgM, IgD and IgE.

Immunoglobulin G (IgG)

It is the main antibody found in high concentration (75%) in serum with a mw 150 KD. It is produced by plasma cells in spleen, lymphnodes and bone marrow. It has two identical light chains and two gamma heavy chains. The light chains may be of kappa or lamda type. IgG is the smallest immunoglobulin which may pass through blood vessels with increased permeability. It has the capacity to quickly bind with foreign substances leading to opsonization. Its binding with antigen may also activate the complement.

Immunoglobulin M (IgM)

This is about 7% of total serum immunoglobulins. It is also produced by plasma cells in spleen, lymphnodes and bone marrow. It is pentamer, five molecules of conventional immunoglobulin with mw 900 KD. These five molecules are linked through disulfide bonds in a circular form. A cysteine rich polypetide of 15KD mw binds two of the units to complete circle and is known as 'J' chain. It is produced in body during primary immune response. It is considered to be more active than IgG for complement activation, neutralization of antigen, opsonization and agglutination. IgM molecules are confined to the blood and have no or little effect in tissue fluids, body secretions and in acute inflammation.

Immunoglobulin A (IgA)

It is secreted as dimmer (mw 300 KD) by plasma cells present under body surfaces like intestinal, respiratory and urinary system, mammary gland and skin. Its concentration is very little in blood. IgA produced in body surfaces is either secreted on surface through epithelial cells or diffuse in blood stream. IgA is transported through intestinal epithelial cells having a receptor of 71 KD which binds with the secretary component covalently to form a secretary IgA. This secretary component protects IgA in the intestinal tract from digestion. It cannot activate the complement and cannot perform the opsonization. IgA can neutralize the antigen and agglutinate the particulate antigen. IgA prevents adherence of foreign particles/ antigen on the body surfaces and it can also act inside the cells. It is about 16% of total immunoglobulins present in serum.

Immunoglobulin E (IgE)

It is also present on body surfaces and produced by plasma cells located beneath the body surfaces. It is in very low concentration in serum. It can bind on receptors of mast cells and basophils. When any antigen binds to these molecules, it causes degranulation from mast cells leading to release of chemical mediators to cause acute inflammation. It mediates hypersensitivity type I reaction and is responsible to provide resistance against invading parasitic worms. It is of shortest half life (2-3 days) and thus is unstable and can be readily destroyed by mild heat treatment. It is 0.01% of total immunoglobulin in serum with 190 KD molecular weight.

Immunoglobulin D (IgD)

IgD is absent in most domestic animals. However, it is present in very minute amount in plasma of dog, non human primates and rats. IgD can be detected in plasma. However, it can't be found in serum due to lysis by proteases during clotting. It is only 0.2 % of total immunoglobulin in serum with mw 160 KD.

On the basis of their function, antibodies are classified as:

- *Antitoxins* have the property to bind with toxins and neutralise them.
- *Agglutinins* are those antibodies, which can agglutinate the RBC's and/or particulate material such as bacterial cells.
- *Precipitins* can precipitate the proteins by acting with antigen and inhibit their dissemination and chemical activity.
- *Lysins* can lyse the cells or bacteria through complement.
- *Opsonins* have the property to bind with foreign particles, non specifically leading to opsonization, making the foreign material palatable to phagocytic cells.
- *Complement fixing antibodies* bind with antigen and fix the complement for its lysis.
- *Neutralizing antibodies* are those, which specifically neutralizes/ destroy the target/ antigen; merely binding with antigen can't be considered as neutralizing antibodies.

Immune response

The antigen when enters in body of animal is trapped, processed and eliminated by several cells including macrophages, dendritic cells and B-cells. There are two types of antigen in body i.e. exogenous and endogenous. The exogenous or extra cellular antigens are present freely in circulation and are readily available for antigen processing cells.

The endogenous or intracellular antigens are not free and are always inside the cells such as viruses. But when these viruses synthesize new viral proteins using biosynthetic process of the host cells, these proteins also act as antigen and are termed as endogenous or intracellular antigens.

The processing of antigen by macrophages is comparatively less efficient as most of the antigen is destroyed by the lysosomal proteases. An alternate pathway of antigen processing involves antigen uptake by a specialized population of mononuclear cells known as *dendritic cells* located throughout the body specially in lymphoid organs. Such dendritic cells have many long filamentous cytoplasmic processes called dendrits and lobulated nuclei with clear cytoplasm containing characteristic granules. Antigen presenting cells process the exogenous antigen and convert into fragments to bind with MHC class II molecules. Such processed antigen along with MHC class II molecule and certain cytokines such as IL-1 is presented to antigen recognizing cells (T-helper cells). Macrophages also regulate the dose of antigen to prevent inappropriate development of tolerance and provide a small dose of antigen to T- helper cells. However, if the antigen is presented to T-Cells without MHC class II molecule, the T cells are turned off resulting into tolerance. On an average, an antigen presenting cell possesses about 2×10^5 MHC class II molecules. A T-Cell require activation by 200-300 peptide- MHC class II molecules to trigger an immune response. Thus, it is estimated that an antigen-presenting cell may present several epitopes simultaneously to T-helper cells. A counterpart of T- helper cells also exists and known as suppressor T-cells (T_s cell) which suppresses the immune response. The viral encoded proteins, endogenous antigens are handled in a different manner from exogenous antigens. Such antigens are bound to MHC class Ia molecules and transported to the cell surface. Such antigen and MHC class Ia molecule complex triggers a lymphocytic response *i.e.* T-cytotoxic cells (Tc-cells). These cytotoxic T-cells recognize and destroy virus infected cells. However, there is some cross priming leading to cell mediated immune response by exogenous antigens and humoral immune response by endogenous antigens. Some lymphocytes also function as memory cells to initiate secondary immune response.

On antigen exposure, there is a latent period of about four to six days and only after that serum antibodies are detectable. The peak of antibody titre is estimated around 2 weeks after exposure to antigen and then declines after about 3 weeks. During this primary immune response, majority antibodies are of IgM type where as in secondary immune response, it is always predominated by IgG.

Immunity and Immunopathology

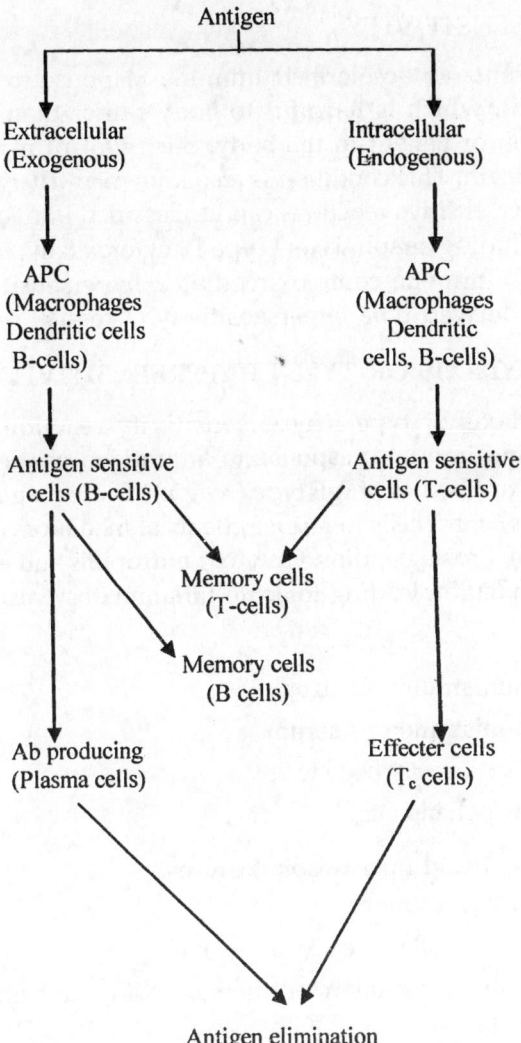

IMMUNOPATHOLOGY

Immunopathology includes the disorders of immune system characterized by increased response or hypersensitivity, response to self antigens (autoimmunity) and decreased responses (Immunodeficiencies).

HYPERSENSITIVITY

It represents an accelerated immune response to an antigen (allergen), which is harmful to body rather than to provide protection or benefit to the body. Such violent reactions may lead to death. This condition is also known as *allergy* or *atopy*. The hypersensitive reactions can be classified into four classical form including anaphylaxis (Type I), cytotoxic hypersensitivity (Type-II), Immune complex mediated hypersensitivity (Type III) and delayed type hypersensitivity (Type-IV) reaction.

ANAPHYLAXIS OR TYPE-I HYPERSENSITIVITY

Anaphylaxis or type I hypersensitivity reaction is rapidly developing immune response to an antigen characterized by humoral antibodies of IgE type *(reagin)*. These reagins sensitize basophils/ mast cells to release chemical mediators (Histamine, Serotonin, Prostaglandins, CFA for neutrophils and eosinophils) of inflammation leading to acute inflammatory reaction.

Etiology
- Administration of drugs
- Administration of serum
- Bite of insects, bee etc.
- Dust, pollens etc.

Macroscopic and microscopic features
- Bronchial asthma.
- Wheel and flare reaction on skin.
- Oedema, congestion, erythema, itching on skin.
- Rhinitis
- Congestion, pulmonary oedema, emphysema, constriction of bronchioles.
- Edema, congestion, haemorrhage on skin

CYTOTOXIC OR TYPE II HYPERSENSITIVITY REACTION

Cytotoxic reactions are characterized by lysis of cells due to antigen- antibody reaction on the surface of cells in the presence of complement.

Etiology/ Occurrence
- Blood transfusion
- Hemolytic anemia
- Infections such as Equine infectious anemia, rickettsia, parasites (trypanosomiosis, babesiosis)
- Thrombocytopenia
- Drugs such as penicillin, phenacetin, quinine cephalosporins.

Macroscopic and microscopic features
- Anemia
- Jaundice
- Haemoglobinuria
- Erythrophagocytosis
- Lysis of erythrocytes/ agglutination of erythrocytes.
- Increased number of hemosiderin laden cells in spleen.

IMMUNE COMPLEX MEDIATED OR TYPE-III HYPERSENSITIVITY REACTION

Type-III hypersensitivity reaction is characterized by the formation of immune complexes as a result of antigen - antibody reaction and their deposition in body tissues leading to inflammatory reaction.

Etiology
- Immunoglobulins
- Tumor antigens, nuclear antigens
- Environmental pollutants *e.g.* pesticides
- Infections such as Leishmaniasis

Macroscopic and microscopic features
- Arthus reaction is focal area of inflammation, necrosis at the site of infection.
- Serum sickness is necrotizing vasculitis, endocarditis and glomerulonephritis.

- Chronic Immune complex disease is renal failure due to glomerulonephritis, vasculitis, chroiomeningitis and arthritis.
- Deposition of immune complexes in wall of blood vessels.
- Deposition of immune complexes in glomeruli.
- Infiltration of inflammatory cells such as neutrophils, macrophages and lymphocytes.
- Lesions of glomerulonephritis, polyarthritis.

DELAYED TYPE HYPERSENSITIVITY (DTH) OR TYPE IV HYPERSENSITIVITY REACTION

DTH reaction is mediated by sensitized T- lymphocytes and is the manifestation of cell- mediated immune response.

Etiology
- Tuberculin reaction
- Graft versus host reactions
- Granulomatous reaction

Macroscopic and microscopic features
- Formation of nodules, which are hard, painful to touch.
- Rejection of transplants/ grafts.
- Heavy infiltrations of mononuclear cells particularly of T-lymphocytes and macrophages.
- Congestion and oedema
- Lymphocytic infiltration is more common around the blood vessels
- Lymphofollicular reaction.

AUTOIMMUNITY

In autoimmunity (auto=self) the immune response is generated against self antigens. It is an aberrant reaction that serves no useful purpose in body. Rather, the immunity developed against self antigens destroys the tissues of body causes inflammation leading to death.

Differential features of various types of Hypersensitivity Reaction

	Anaphylaxis or Type-I Hypersensitivity Reaction	Cytotoxic or Type II Hypersensitivity Reaction	Immune Complex Mediated or Type-III Hypersensitivity Reaction	Delayed Type Hypersensitivity (DTH) or Type IV Hypersensitivity Reaction
Macroscopic features	1. Bronchial asthma. 2. Wheel and flare reaction on skin. 3. Edema, congestion, erythema, itching on skin. 4. Rhinitis	1. Anemia 2. Jaundice 3. Hemoglobinuria	1. Arthus reaction is focal area of inflammation, necrosis at the site of infection. 2. Serum sickness is necrotizing vasculitis, endocarditis and glomerulonephritis. 3. Chronic Immune complex disease is renal failure due to glomerulonephritis, vasculitis, chroiomeningitis and arthritis.	1. Formation of nodules, which are hard, painful to touch. 2. Rejection of transplants/ grafts.
Microscopic features	1. Congestion, pulmonary edema, emphysema, constriction of bronchioles. 2. Edema, congestion, haemorrhage on skin	1. Erythrophagocytosis 2. Lysis of erythrocytes/ agglutination of erythrocytes. 3. Increased number of hemosiderin laden cells in spleen.	1. Deposition of immune complexes in wall of blood vessels. 2. Deposition of immune complexes in glomeruli 3. Infiltration of inflammatory cells such as neutrophils, macrophages and lymphocytes. 4. Lesions of glomerulonephritis, polyarthritis.	1. Heavy infiltrations of mononuclear cells particularly of T-lymphocytes and macrophages. 2. Congestion and oedema 3. Lymphocytic infiltration is more common around the blood vessels 4. Lymphofollicular reaction.

Etiology/ Occurrence
- Hidden antigens *e.g.* spermatozoa
- Alteration of antigens *e.g.* Infections, mutations, chemicals bind with normal body proteins recognized as foreign.
- Cross reaction between antigens of self and foreign
- Forbidden clones of immunocytes

Macroscopic and microscopic features
- Autoimmune hemolytic anemia.
- Anti-glomerular basement membrane (GBM) nephritis
- Lymphocytic thyroditis
- Lupus erythematosus- antinuclear antibodies.
- Hemolytic anemia
- Leukopenia
- Presence of antinuclear antibodies
- Infiltration of lymphocytes/ macrophages (Lymphocytic thryroditis).
- In anti-GBM nephritis, there is immune complex mediated glomerulonephritis.

IMMUNODEFICIENCY

The alterations in immune system, which decrease the effectiveness or destroy the capabilities of the system to respond to various antigens are designated as immunodeficiency. This precarious situation may be attributed to poorly developed immunocompetence or depressed immunity as a result of genetic and environmental factors. Immunodeficiences are thus classified as congenital or primary and acquired or secondary.

Congenital immunodeficiency

In this type of immunodeficiency, the defect in immunity is genetically determined and is present in animals since their birth.

Etiology/ Occurrence
- Defect in basic cellular components *e.g.* stem cells
- Defective genes
- Defect in enzymes
- Defective expression of cell components.

Types
Combined immunodeficiency syndrome (CIS)
- Absence of stem cells of immunocytes
- Agammaglobulinemia
- Absence of T and B cells in blood, leucopenia

Defects in T-lymphocytes
- Thymic hypoplasia
- B-cells are normal and adequate amount of immunoglobulins present in blood
- Absence of T-dependent regions in lymphnodes
- In Danish cattle, exanthema, alopecia, parakeratosis occurs due to T-cell defect with A- 46 lethal trait gene.

Defects in B- lymphocytes
- In equines – equine agammaglobulinemia
- Normal T-cell count, absence of B-cells, absence of all classes of immunoglobulins
- 'X' linked defects in gene occurs in males
- Absence of primary lymphoid follicles in germinal centres in spleen and lymphnodes.
- Selective IgA, IgM and IgG deficiency may also occur.
- Transient hypogammaglobulinemia in new born calves.

Partial T and B cell defects
- Partial presence of T and B-lymphocytes.
- Recurrent infections, eczema, purpura.
- Due to 'X' chromosome linked genetic defect.
- Poor platelet aggregation

Deficiency of complement
- Rare, associated with abnormal regulation of immune responses leading to autoimmunity
- Complement component C_1 C_2 and C_3 are deficient and deficiency is associated with systemic lupus erythematosus, polyarteritis nodosa, glomerulonephritis, rheumatoid arthritis.
- C_5, C_6, C_7 and C_8 deficiency leads to recurrent infections
- Absence or deficiency of C_3 makes animal susceptible to bacterial infections due to lack of opsonization, chemotaxis and phagocytosis

Defects in phagocytosis
- Neutropenia, leucopenia
- Defects in neutrophils, macrophages, platelets, melanocytes and eosinophils
- Defective chemotaxis, phagocytosis and bactericidal activity
- Persistent bacterial infections, pyogenic infections
- Associated with autosomal recessive gene defect and is also known as "Chediak Higashi syndrome"

ACQUIRED OR SECONDARY IMMUNODEFICIENCY

An animal can acquire the suppression of immune system due to drugs, diseases, deficiency of nutrition, neoplasm or environmental pollution which is clinically manifested by increased susceptibility to infections, vaccination failures, recurrent infections and occurrence of new diseases and neoplasms.

Etiology/ Occurrence

Drugs
- Corticosteroids, azathioprines, alkalating agents, cyclophosphamide, cyclosporin A, antibiotics
- Azathioprines used to suppress graft rejection
- Cyclophosphamides and chlorambucil affect the DNA reduplication of T- and B- lymphocytes leading to immuno-

suppression with no affect on macrophages
- Cyclosporin A depresses CMI responses
- Aspirin decreases phagocytosis and lymphocyte functions
- Antibiotics like gentamicin, chloramphenicol, cephalosporin etc. causes decrease in immunity.

Infections

- Bovine herpes virus-1 (BHV-1) decreases CD_4^+ and CD_8^+ cells in blood.
- Equine herpes virus (EHV- 1) causes reduction in T-cell functions
- Marek's disease virus acts as lymphocytolytic agent in lymphoid follicles of spleen, bursa and thymus.
- Bovine viral diarrhoea virus reduces CD_4^+ and CD_8^+ T-lymphocytes, B-lymphocytes, neutrophils and IL- 2 in cattle.
- Respiratory syncytial virus inhibits lymphoproliferative responses in sheep and cattle leading to increased susceptibility to *Pasteurella multocida* infection.
- Blue tongue virus infects CD_4^+ and CD_8^+ lymphocytes and causes their destruction.
- Canine parvovirus causes depletion of lymphoid cells. Canine distemper virus activates the T-suppresser cells (T_s cells) leading to suppression of immunity.
- Infectious bursal disease virus selectively affects B-lymphocytes leading to increased susceptibility of birds
- Infectious laryngotracheitis virus infects macrophages and causes their destruction.
- Feline leukemia virus causes lymphoid depletion, glomerulonephritis, defects in macrophages and complement.
- Feline immunodeficiency virus causes neutropenia, lymphopenia and inhibits the T- and B- cells co-operation.
- Bovine immunodeficiency virus replicates in macrophages and CD_4^+ lymphocytes leading to their destruction and immunosuppression. It also causes lymphadenopathy, lymphocytolysis, reduction in lymphokine production.

Trauma/ surgery
- Trauma or surgical interventions reduces specific immune responses and functional capacity of phagocytic cells.
- Such defects are transient and may reverse after healing of trauma/ surgery.
- Surgical operation/ trauma increases the number of T-suppressor cells (T_s cells), which in turn depresses the immunity.

Environmental pollution
- Pesticides used in agriculture, animal husbandry and public health operations remains in ecosystem and food items for longer period and enters in body of animals and man through food, air, water and affects the immune system leading to its depression and increased susceptibility to infections.
- Heavy metals are common contaminants of pesticides, fertilizers and are inadvertently accumulated in soil, plant, water, which enters directly or indirectly in the animal's body. These heavy metals (lead, mercury, cadmium) may exert their immunotoxic effects leading to immunosuppression.
- Mycotoxins such as aflatoxin, ochratoxin, zearalenone etc also affect the immune system of animals leading to its suppression resulting increased susceptibility to infectious diseases.

Chapter 12
Pathology of Cutaneous System

DEVELOPMENTAL ANOMALIES

Congenital icthyosis

Congenital icthyosis is scaly epidermis which resembles with skin of fish and occurs due to a simple autosomal recessive homozygous gene in calves. This condition is characterized by scaly, horny, thick epidermis divided into plates by deep fissures. Microscopically, there is thick keratin layer over the epidermis.

Epitheliogenesis imperfecta

Epitheliogenesis imperfecta is a congenital defect characterized by discontinuity of epithelium on skin leaving patches without squamous epithelium mostly at feet, claws and oral mucosa. Such defect may occur in calves which succumb to infection after birth or such foetus may abort. This disease condition is inherited as an autosomal recessive trait.

Congenital alopecia

Alopecia or hairlessness on the skin with complete lack of hair follicles has been observed in dog and other animals. Such hair less sites may follow a regular pattern or occurs in patches. This is a hereditary defect recognized in certain breeds.

Congenital albinism

Albinism is absence of melanin pigmentation due to deficiency of tyrosinase. This congenital abnormality is encountered sporadically due to a recessive trait in most species. The melanocytes are present but there is lack of melanin synthesis due to tyrosinase deficiency.

Congenital cutaneous asthenia

The collagen fibers are irregular in size and orientation and become fragmented due to disorganization of fibrils within the fibers. This condition occurs due to a deficiency in procollagen peptidase responsible for formation of collagen. This condition leads to hyperelasticity and fragility of skin and hypermotility of joints in cattle, sheep and dogs.

ACANTHOSIS NIGRICANS

This is increased amount of melanin in skin along with hyperkeratosis. This condition commonly occurs in dogs, at ventral abdomen and medial surface of legs.

Etiology
- Hormonal imbalance
- Tumors of testicles and pituitary gland

Macroscopic and microscopic features
- Colour of skin becomes black
- Dry and scaly skin due to hyperkeratosis
- Proliferation of melanocytes and melanoblasts.
- Black/ brown colour pigment intracellular/ extracellular.
- Cells appear as black or brown globular mass.
- Melanin granules are minute, dirty brown in colour and spherical in shape.
- Hyperkeratinization.

DERMATITIS

Dermatitis is the inflammation of skin characterized by hyperemia, erythema, serus exudation and infiltration of neutrophils and mononuclear cells.

Etiology
- Bacteria, Viruses, Chemicals, Allergy, Trauma, Fungi and their toxins.

Macroscopic and microscopic features
- Erythematous patches on skin
- Swelling of skin, itching sensation leads to damage/ scratch due to rubbing.
- Loss of hairs, patches on skin, alopecia.
- Hyperemia
- Serous exudate
- Infiltration of neutrophils and mononuclear cells.
- Presence of fungus in skin scrapings.

VESICULAR DERMATITIS

Vesicular dermatitis is excessive accumulation of clear fluid in dermis and epidermis leading to vesicle/ blisters formation. It is also known as hydropic dermatitis.

Etiology
- Sunburn
- Heat
- Foot and Mouth Disease virus
- Pox virus

Macroscopic and microscopic features
- Oedematous fluid in dermis and epidermis resulting in thickening of skin
- Hyperemia, vesicles.
- Break of vesicles leads to clear fluid discharge.
- Hyperemia
- Accumulation of clear fluid in epidermis and dermis, which is characterized by clear spaces or takes light pink stain of eosin.
- Some cells show hydropic degeneration.

- Infiltration of leucocytes.

PARASITIC DERMATITIS (ACARIASIS)

Acariasis or mange is caused by mites and characterized by hyperkeratosis and inflammation of skin leading to itching, rubbing and scratching.

Etiology
- Mites
- *Sarcoptes scabei*
- *Psoroptic* sp.
- *Demodectic* sp.
- *Chorioptic* sp.

Macroscopic and microscopic features
- Hyperkeratosis of skin, dry and scaly appearance of skin.
- Hemorrhage/ trauma due to rubbing/ scratching as a result of intense itching.
- Absence of hairs on lesions.
- Hyperkeratinization of skin.
- Hyperemia
- Infiltration of neutrophils, lymphocytes, macrophages, eosionophils
- Presence of mites at the site of lesions

ALLERGIC DERMATITIS

This is the inflammation of skin sensitized to certain substances, known as allergens. Such inflammation can be seen as a result of delayed type hypersensitivity (DTH) reaction.

Etiology
- Chemicals (DNCB/ DNFB).
- Tuberculin reaction.
- Allergic reaction
- Soaps, detergents, organic chemicals

- Parasites- fleas

Macroscopic and microscopic features
- Hyperemia, Erythema
- Edematous/ nodular swelling, hard to touch.
- Hot, painful
- Atopy with vesicular rash, pruritus, serus exudate.
- Infiltration of eosinophils and mononuclear cells, macrophages, lymphocytes.
- Hyperemia, Edema, necrosis

GANGRENOUS DERMATITIS

Gangrenous dermatitis is the inflammation of skin alongwith formation of gangrene caused by fungal toxins and characterized by sloughing of skin, dry gangrene with break in epidermis.

Etiology
- *Fusarium* sp. toxins
- Rice straw feeding- Degnala disease

Macroscopic and microscopic features
- Presence of gangrenous inflammation on extremities such as legs, udder, ears, tail, scrotum.
- Sloughing of skin leaving raw surface.
- Sloughing of hoofs with haemorrhage
- Inflammation of skin and invasion by saprophytes causing dissolution of cells/ tissue
- Infiltration of mononuclear cells at the periphery of the lesion.

EQUINE CUTANEOUS GRANULOMA

There is development of chronic, ulcerated and bloody granuloma on limb of horses due to wire cuts or other cutaneous injury.

Etiology
- Skin cuts/ injury
- Habronemiasis
- Phycomycosis
- *Hyphomyces destruens*
- *Entomorphthora coronata*

Macroscopic and microscopic features
- Granulation tissue in wound.
- Presence of yellowish/ white specks.
- Summer sores/ Bursatti.
- Tissue composed of newly formed fibrous tissue, with large number of capillaries, infiltration of eosinophils
- Presence of necrotic masses stains deep red with H&E
- Presence of helminths in section- cutaneous habronemiasis
- Presence of septate hyphae of fungus

MISCELLANEOUS LESIONS OF SKIN

Papule: Focal Hyperplasia of stratum spinosum epithelium leading to hard nodular eruption on skin.

Vesicle: A cavity in epidermis containing fluid and covered by a thin layer of epidermis elevated from the surface.

Pustule: A vesicle filled with pus.

Acanthosis: Thickening of epidermis due to hyperplasia of stratum spinosum/ prickle cell layer.

Hyperkeratosis: Thickening of keratin layer stratum corneum.

Parakeratosis: The retention of nucleus in keratin layer.

Bulla/ bleb: Cavitations in epidermis filled with fluid and larger than vesicle.

Erosion/ Excoriation: Superficial loss of epithelium.

Fissure: Linear defect in epidermis, which may be crusted at mucocutaneous junctions.

Abscess: A circumscribed cavity filled with pus.

Ulcer: A break in the continuity of the epidermis exposing dermis.

Urticaria: A circumscribed area of swelling/ oedema involving dermis

Folliculitis: Inflammation of hair follicles.

Acne: Enlargement of sealed off hair follicles or sebaceous glands and rupture through the epidermis. It leaves a rounded hole in the epidermis and a canal down to the dermis.

Eczema: Eczema is a form of allergic dermatitis of obscure etiology and characterized by erythema, vesicular rash, serus exudate and pruritus.

Chapter 13
Pathology of Musculoskeletal System

PATHOLOGY OF MUSCLES

EQUINE RHABDOMYOLYSIS

It is also known as ***Azoturia*** or ***Monday Morning Disease***. The disease occurs in well fed horse after a gap of holiday. Suddenly after walking few steps, the horse is unable to move further and feels pain with intense sweating and hardening of muscles.

Etiology
- Accumulation of lactic acid in muscles
- High glycogen storage
- Lack of oxygen supply

Macroscopic and microscopic features
- Hardening of muscle just like wood
- **Urine is dark brown with myoglobin-***myoglobinuria*
- Tonic spasms in muscles
- Atrophy of affected muscles in chronic cases
- Necrosis of muscle fibers
- Edema
- Hyaline degeneration.
- Invasion of sarcolemma by macrophages and lymphocytes
- Degeneration and necrosis of tubular epithelium in kidneys.

WHITE MUSCLE DISEASE

Extensive coagulative necrosis of muscles is observed in calves possibly due to deficiency of vitamin E during 6 month of age.

Etiology
- Vitamin E deficiency
- Selenium deficiency
- Stress

Macroscopic and microscopic features
- Colour of muscle becomes pale pink, yellowish red, grey or white.
- Muscle becomes dry, inelastic and firm.
- Urine is brown/ red or chocolate brown in colour because of myoglobin.
- Coagulative necrosis of muscles.
- In some muscle cells, cloudy swelling can be observed.
- Neutrophils, macrophages, lymphocytes and eosinophils may present.
- Calcium may be deposited in necrosed areas.

ACUTE MYOSITIS

Acute myositis is the acute inflammation of skeletal muscles characterized by the presence of serous, fibrinous or haemorrhagic exudates.

Etiology
- Trauma
- Vitamin E/ Selenium deficiency
- *Clostridium chauvoei*, the cause of black leg in cattle

Macroscopic and microscopic features
- Muscles become extremely moist.
- Colour becomes red, consistency is firm and tense.
- Swelling and accumulation of gas in muscles, crepitating sound on palpation.

- Muscle dark red/ black with gas mixed exudates.
- Presence of serous, fibrinous and/or haemorrhagic exudate.
- Infiltration of neutrophils, macrophages, lymphocytes, etc.
- Degenerative and necrotic changes in muscles.
- Presence of Gram positive rods in exudate.

HEMORRHAGIC MYOSITIS

Haemorrhagic myositis is characterized by the presence of large amount of blood and inflammation in muscles. It may occur due to trauma and muscle rupture.

Etiology
- Trauma
- Clostridial infections

Macroscopic and microscopic features
- Area becomes red/ cyanotic.
- On cut, large amount of blood comes out from muscles.
- On touch, the affected area is hard and painful to touch.
- Regional lymphnodes may become enlarged and swollen.
- Extravasation of blood in between the myofibrils.
- Infiltration of neutrophils, macrophages and lymphocytes in connective tissue between the muscle cells.

CHRONIC MYOSITIS

Chronic inflammation of muscle is characterized by necrosis, calcification and proliferation of fibrous connective tissue. In case of tuberculosis and pseudotuberculosis, there are multiple, focal nodules containing caseation and fibrous capsule.

Etiology
- *Mycobacterium tuberculosis*
- *Corynebacterium pseudotuberculosis*
- *Trichinella* spp. infection
- *Sarcosporidia* spp. infection

Macroscopic features
- Muscles become hard to touch
- Nodules can be seen.
- On cut the lesions of caseation and calcification observed.
- Caseative necrosis, infiltration of macrophages, lymphocytes and proliferation of fibrous tissue.
- Calcification can also be observed.
- In cases of pseudotuberculosis infiltration of neutrophils is seen.
- Extensive infiltration of eosinophils in sarcoporidia infection.

PATHOLOGY OF BONES

FIBROUS OSTEODYSTROPHY

Fibrous osteodystrophy occurs as excessive action of parathyroid hormone on bones and characterized by bone resorption with replacement by fibrous tissue, increased osteoid formation which does not get sufficient minerals for deposition and formation of cysts.

Etiology
- Hyperparathyroidism
- Dietary deficiency of calcium or excess of phosphorus
- Vitamin-D deficiency
- Excessive bran feeding (Disease in horses of flour millers).

Macroscopic and microscopic features
- Lack of calcification in bone
- Resorption of calcium from bone, fibrosis
- Bone becomes shoft, flexible and deformed
- Rubbery jaw due to involvement of facial bones
- Fibrous tissue hyperplasia in bones.
- Enlargement of Haversian canals.

- Boney tissue is replaced by fibroblasts, with osteoclastic giant cells lining the remaining bone tissue.

RICKETS

Rickets is failure of adequate deposition of calcium in bones of growing animals caused by deficiency of calcium and vitamin-D and characterized by bending of limbs, enlargement of ends of long bones and skeletal deformities.

Etiology
- Vitamin D deficiency
- Calcium deficiency
- Deficiency of phosphorus

Macroscopic and microscopic features
- Bending of legs, bow legs
- Pot belly
- Enlarged costochondral articulation
- Softening of bones
- Increase in proliferating cartilage adjacent to the area of ossification and its disorderly arrangement.
- Disorderly penetration of cartilage by blood vessels
- Increased area of uncalcified osteoid tissue
- Fibrosis of marrow

OSTEOMALACIA

Osteomalacia is also known as *adult rickets*. It occurs in bone of adults caused by deficiency of vitamin D and calcium and characterized by softening of bones.

Etiology
- Vitamin-D deficiency
- Calcium-phosphorus ratio disturbance

Macroscopic and microscopic features
- Softening of bones
- Irregular diffuse thickening of bones

- Bone deformities
- Increase in osteoid tissue with failure of calcification
- Increase in osteoclastic activity

OSTEOPOROSIS

Osteoporosis is atrophy of bones caused by possibly hormonal imbalance and characterized by inadequate deposition of calcium, brittleness of bones due to its increased porosity.

Etiology
- Hormonal imbalance
- Vitamin C deficiency
- Copper deficiency

Macroscopic and microscopic features
- Inadequate calcium deposition
- Bone becomes brittle and porous
- Increased fragility of bones
- Widening of Haversian canals
- Increased activity of osteoclasts
- Decrease in zona compacta and thickness of bone trabeculae

OSTEOPETROSIS

Osteopetrosis is enlargement of bone caused by fluorosis or avian leukosis virus and characterized by increase in bony tissue. It is also known as *marble bone disease*.

Etiology
- Avian leukosis virus of retroviridae family
- Fluorosis

Macroscopic and microscopic features
- Enlargement of bone towards outside and inside.
- Reduced marrow cavity
- Bone becomes brittle, marbelling of bones.
- Cartilage is also calcified, surrounded by osteoid tissue.

OSTEOMYELITIS

Osteomyelitis is the inflammation of bone with bone marrow caused by trauma and pyogenic bacteria and characterized by destruction, replacement and excessive growth of new bone adjacent to the infected part.

Etiology
- Hematogenous infection
- Direct infection through trauma/ fracture
- *Actinomyces pyogenes, A. bovis*
- *Staphylococcus aureus*
- *Pseudomonas aeruginosa*

Macroscopic and microscopic features
- Metastatic abscess in bone marrow
- Excessive growth of bone in adjacent area.
- Exostosis or endostosis.
- Infiltration of neutrophils
- Proliferation of osteoid tissue
- Demonstration of bacteria in pus

BONE FRACTURE AND REPAIR

Fracture is the break in the continuity of bone due to trauma. A fracture may be simple or compound depending on the severity of trauma. Healing of fracture occurs by reunion of the broken ends of bone through development and proliferation of fibroblasts, angioblasts, osteoid tissue and infiltration of calcium salts.

Etiology
- Trauma
- Accidents-automobile accidents.

Macroscopic and microscopic features
- Fracture can be identified by break in bones.
- Healing of fracture is characterized by development of callus at the site of reunion of break ends of bone.

- Callus may be soft or hard.
- Proliferation of fibroblasts, angioblasts and metaplasia of connective tissue to osteoid tissue.
- Areas of calcification in osteoid tissue

PULMONARY OSTEOARTHROPATHY

Pulmonary osteoarthropathy is a rare disease of dog, sheep, cat, horse, and lion caused by prolonged anoxia and characterized by cough, dyspnea, respiratory disturbances and formation of new bone leading to thickening and deformity of limbs.

Etiology
- Prolonged anoxia
- Toxaemia

Macroscopic and microscopic features
- Pneumonia
- New bone formation just beneath the periosteum in long bones.
- The proliferation of bone is irregular leading to rough surface.
- Bone becomes enlarged twice to its normal size.
- Heart worms in case of dogs.
- Bronchogenic carcinoma
- Granulomatous lesions of tuberculosis
- Chronic bronchiectasis
- Hyperplasia of osteoid tissue with no indication of any kind of neoplastic growth in bones.

SPONDYLITIS

Spondylitis is the inflammation of vertebrae caused by bacteria/fungi and characterized by caseation, intraosseous abscess formation granulomatous lesions and fibrosis.

Etiology
- *Brucella abortus, Br. ovis, Br. meletensis*
- *Actinomyces bovis*
- *Coccidioidomyces* sp.

Macroscopic and microscopic features
- Intraosseous abscess
- Granuloma encapsulated by fibrous tissue involving one or two adjacent vertebrae.
- Local enlargement of bone.
- Granulomatous lesions with caseation
- Proliferation of osteoid tissue
- Infiteration of neutrophils in intraoseous abscess.

PATHOLOGY OF JOINTS

ARTHRITIS

Arthritis is the inflammation of joint caused by bacteria, virus, chlamydia, mycoplasma and immune complexes and characterized by serus, fibrinous, purulent or ankylosing lesions in joints.

Etiology
- Bacteria- *E. coli, Erysipelas rhusiopathae, Streptococus* sp., *Shigella* sp. *Corynebacterium ovis, Brucella* sp.
- Mycoplasma- *Mycoplasma mycoides, Mycoplasma sinoviae*
- Virus- Reovirus (Tenosynovitis in birds)
- Antigen antibody complexes
- Trauma

Macroscopic and microscopic features
- Swelling of joints with increase in synovial fluid.
- Difficulty in movement
- In chronic cases fusion of two bony processes leaving no joint (ankylosing)

- Synovial fluid diminishes, becomes dirty, thick in chronic illness
- Presence of increased number of leucocytes in synovial fluid.
- Serous, fibrinous or purulent exudate in joints.
- Thickening of synovial membrane
- Presence of plasma cells and immune complexes in synovial fluid.

Chapter 14
Pathology of Cardiovascular System

DEVELOPMENTAL ANOMALIES

Persistent right aortic arch

This is a developmental anomaly of aorta in which the aorta develops from right arch present on right side of trachea and oesophagus. The ductus arteriosus forms a ring around trachea and esophagus by connecting aorta and pulmonary artery. This ring causes partial obstruction of trachea and/or esophagus.

Patent ductus arteriosus

The ductus arteriosus is a short blood vessel which connects pulmonary artery to aorta in foetal life for diversion of blood. Normally soon after birth this duct is sealed and remains in the form of a ligamentum arteriosum. But sometimes this ductus arteriosus remains open and blood is continuously shunted between aorta and pulmonary artery and may led to congestive heart failure, pulmonary hypertension and cyanosis due to mixing of venous and arterial blood.

Interventricular septal defects

In foetal life, there is no partition in ventricles and there is only one chamber which is divided into two right and left by inter ventricular septum. But when interventricular septum does not develop completely and due to defect in formation of complete partition, there is mixing of blood from both chambers. It is responsible for thickening of myocardium, roughening of endocardium and cyanosis.

Transposition of aorta

When there is a shift in position of aorta and pulmonary artery i.e. the aorta arises from right ventricle and pulmonary artery from left ventricle. This results in arterial blood in right and venous blood in left side and has no clinical significance. However, it may create problems when aorta arises from venous ventricle and pulmonary artery from arterial side.

Tetrad of Fallot

Tetrad of Fallot includes 4 developmental defects of cardiovascular system and is also known as *tetralogy of Fallot*.
i. Inter ventricular septal defect
ii. Pulmonary stenosis is characterized by narrowing of lumen of pulmonary artery at its origin due to fibrous tissue causing 'jet' effect.
iii. Hypertrophy of right ventricle
iv. Transposition of aorta.
v. Ectopia cardis

When heart lies outside the thorax under the subcutaneous tissue of lower cervical region.

Interatrial septal defect

There is a developmental defect in inter atrial septa and remains as incomplete partition of atrium. It produces continuous overload on the right side of heart leading to pulmonary hypertension and hypertrophy of right side myocardium. However, a small defect in septum may persist throughout the life of animal without causing any clinical illness.

CARDIAC FAILURE

Cardiac failure is the inability of heart to maintain adequate blood supply leading to death. It can be divided into two types: Acute and chronic heart failure.

Acute cardiac failure

Acute cardiac failure is sudden failure of contraction of heart leading to death within minutes.

Etiology
- Anoxia
- Drugs/ poisons
- Shock
- Cardiac temponade
- Myocardial necrosis
- Sudden occlusion of aorta and/or pulmonary artery.

Macroscopic and microscopic features
- Cardiac temponade
- Occlusive thrombus
- Pulmonary congestion
- Dialation of heart particularly of right ventricle
- Myocardial necrosis
- Centrilobular necrosis in liver "nut meg liver"
- In prolonged cases, congestion and oedema in visceral organs.

CHRONIC CARDIAC FAILURE

Chronic cardiac failure is the inability of heart to maintain balance between its output and venous return of blood. It can be further divided into two left and right sided heart failure.

LEFT SIDED HEART FAILURE

Left sided heart failure is caused by myocardial damage and characterized by congestion and oedema in lungs with hypertrophy of alveolar lining cells.

Etiology
- Myocardial degeneration/ necrosis
- Aortic and mitral valve disease
- Hypertension

Macroscopic and microscopic features

- Congestion and oedema in lungs
- Chronic dialation of heart
- Congestion of alveolar vessels
- Edema in lungs
- Hypertrophy of alveolar lining cells
- Alveolar macrophages contain hemosiderin pigment also called "heart failure cells"

RIGHT SIDED HEART FAILURE

Right-sided heart failure is caused by a disease of lungs or pulmonary vasculature and mostly occurs after a left sided heart failure.

Etiology
- Left sided heart failure
- Pulmonary lesions, congestion

Macroscopic and microscopic features
- Congestion of visceral organs
- Subcutis oedema and ascites
- Pulse in jugular vein
- "Nutmeg appearance" in liver due to centrilobular necrosis.
- Atrophy, necrosis and fibrosis in liver
- Congestion in visceral organs.

PERICARDITIS

Pericarditis is the inflammation of pericardium, the upper layer of heart. It may be serus, fibrinous or suppurative depending on the type of exudate.

Etiology/ Occurrence
- Pasteurellosis
- Salmonellosis in poultry.
- Hydropericardium syndrome in poultry
- Gout in poultry

- Trauma/ Foreign body *e.g.* Traumatic reticulo pericarditis (TRP).

Macroscopic and microscopic features
- Deposition of fibrin in between pericardium and heart gives an appearance of "bread and butter".
- In chronic cases, pericardium becomes thick due to excessive fibrosis.
- Accumulation of fluid (clear, serus) in pericardial sac is termed as *Hydropericardium*.
- Presence of blood in pericardial sac is known as *hemopericardium* and the excessive accumulation of blood leading to heart failure is termed as *cardiac temponade*.
- Accumulation of pus in pericardial sac is called as *pyopericardium*.
- Presence of gas in pericardial sac in termed as *pneumopericardium*.
- Hyperemia and haemorrhage in pericardium
- Deposition of fibrin, formation of fibrin network, infiltration of neutrophils, macrophages and lymphocytes.

MYOCARDITIS

Myocarditis is the inflammation of myocardium, the middle layer of heart. It may be suppurative, eosinophlic or lymphocytic depending on the type of the exudates.

Etiology
- Toxins/ Poisons
- Bacteria/ Virus
- Parasites
- Drugs/ Chemicals

Macroscopic and microscopic features
- Colour of myocardium may become dark red or cyanotic due to accumulation of blood.
- In suppurative myocarditis, one can find abscesses in myo-

cardium from where yellow/ green pus oozes out.
- Yellowish white streaks of necrosis in myocardium.
- Presence of cyst encapsulated by fibroplasia due to cysticercosis.
- Hyperemia and haemorrhages in myocardium.
- Infiltration of neutrophils, eosinophils or lymphocytes.
- Coagulative necrosis of muscle fibers.
- In chronic cases, proliferation of fibrous connective tissue.

ENDOCARDITIS

Endocarditis is the inflammation of the endocardium, the inner layer of heart.

Etiology/ Occurrence
- Chronic septicemic diseases like caused by *Actinomyces pyogenes, Erysipelothrix rhusiopathe*
- Staphylococci
- Streptococci
- *Pseudomonas aeruginosa*
- Clostridial infections.

Macroscopic and microscopic features
- Lesions in heart valves or wall of atrium/ ventricles.
- Presence of thrombi on endocardium.
- Vegetative/ cauliflower like growth on endocardium either in valves (*Valvular vegetative endocarditis e.g.* Swine erysepalas) or in wall (*Mural vegetative endocarditis*).
- Dilation of heart chambers.
- Infiltration of thrombocytes, neutophils, macrophages and lymphocytes.
- Masses of bacterial organisms can be seen.
- Underlying endocardium and myocardium shows the presence of fibrin network and infiltration of RBC, neutrophils and macrophages.

BRISKET DISEASE/ HIGH ALTITUDE DISEASE

Brisket disease is a condition of slow cardiac failure, which occurs at 2500 meters sea level or above where pressure of air is low.

Etiology
- Low oxygen in environment
- Decreased atmospheric pressure of air
- In native cattle morbidity rate is only 2% and in imported cattle at hills it is upto 40%.

Macroscopic and microscopic features
- Dilation of heart
- Hypertrophy of ventricular wall
- Chronic passive congestion in visceral organs
- Edema in sternal region in between forelegs.
- Nut meg liver due to chronic passive congestion
- Polycythemia
- Hypertrophy of muscle fibers in myocardium.

MULBERRY HEART DISEASE

It is characterized by firm contraction of heart and petechial hemorrhage on pericardium giving the appearance of mulberry.

Etiology
- Not known
- May be enterotoxaemia/ poisoning

Macroscopic and microscopic features
- Contraction of heart with petechial haemorrhage on pericardium looking like mulberry "Mulbery heart disease"
- Hydropericardium, hydroperitoneum and pulmonary oedema
- Edema fluid has high protein content resulting in clot formation
- Congestion of fundic portion of stomach.
- Congestion on serosa of visceral organs.

ARTERIOSCLEROSIS

Arteriosclerosis is hardening of arteries causing 3 types of diseases in arteries depending on their size and etiological factors viz., Atherosclerosis, medial sclerosis and arteriolosclerosis.

ATHEROSCLEROSIS

Atherosclerosis is characterized by hardening and thickening of intimal layer of large arteries and aorta due to proliferation of connective tissue, hyaline degeneration, infiltration of fat/ lipids and calcification. These intimal changes may lead to loss of elasticity of artery (*Athere* means mushy substance).

Etiology
- Exact cause is not clear
- Hypercholesterolemia and hyperlipidemia
- Hypertension

Macroscopic and microscopic features
- Fatty streaks running parallel in the direction of the artery.
- Intimal layer of aorta/ coronary arteries is elevated due to plaques which are white/ yellow, fibrous and occluding the lumen of vessel.
- Occlusion of artery may lead to ischemia and infarction.
- Macrophages are filled with lipid droplets including cholesterol, fatty acids, triglycerides and phospholipids.
- Fragmented internal elastic lamina in the intimal layer of artery
- Proliferation of altered smooth muscles may become metaplastic to macrophages.
- Deposition of mucoid ground substance and collagen fibers
- Hyalinization of connective tissue "Fibrous plaques".
- Presence of some fat droplets in between the lesion

MEDIAL SCLEROSIS

Medial sclerosis involve medium sized muscular arteries and

characterized by fatty degeneration and hyalinization of muscular tissue of medial arteries leading to necrosis. This is also known as *Monckeberg medial sclerosis.*

Etiology
- Old age
- Excessive administration of epinephrine (adrenaline).
- Nicotine
- Vitamin D toxicity.
- Hyperparathyroidism

Macroscopic and microscopic features
- Hardening of medium sized arteries
- Hyaline, fatty changes and calcification of arterial wall
- Fatty changes, hyalinization of muscular layer of medium sized arteries.
- Necrosis of myofibrils
- Calcification

ARTERIOLOSCLEROSIS

Arteriolosclerosis affects arterioles in kidneys, spleen and pancreas and is characterized by hyperplasia of intimal cells of arterioles producing concentric lamellations occluding their lumen.

Etiology
- Hypertension

Macroscopic and microscopic features
- No characteristic macroscopic lesion.
- Atrophy of organ, hardening.
- Proliferation of cells present in intima of blood vessels
- Swelling and necrosis of cells in medial layer leading to occlusion of lumen
- Calcification in chronic cases.

ARTERITIS

Arteritis is the inflammation of arteries characterized by infiltration of neutrophils, lymphocytes and macrophages in the media and intima of arterial wall.

Etiology
- Chemicals
- Thermal
- Virus *e.g.* Equine viral arteritis
- Pyogenic bacteria.
- Parasite *e.g. Strongylus vulgaris*

Macroscopic and microscopic features
- Hyperemia
- Conjunctivitis, oedema of eye
- Presence of thrombi in artery
- Presence of thrombi in artery involving intimal layer.
- Equine viral arteritis virus causes infiltration of lymphocytes and macrophages in media.
- Occlusion of lumen of arteries due to thickening of wall.
- In parasitic arteritis, parasitic thrombi may present along with inflammatory reaction in intimal layer.

ANEURYSM

Aneurysm is dilation of an artery or cardiac chamber leading to formation of sac.

Etiology
- Aflatoxin
- Infectious emboli
- Weak vessel wall due to rupture.
- Fracture or necrosis of medial layer of large blood vessel.
- Arteriolosclerosis

Macroscopic and microscopic features
- Fracture or necrosis of medial layer of large blood vessels permitting parallel blood circulation till the next division of blood vessel is called as *Dissecting aneurysm* or *false aneurysm*.
- Formation of sac in artery due to dilation, also known as *True aneurysm*.
- Rough intimal layer
- Wall of blood vessel damaged with inflammatory exudate.

PHLEBITIS

Phlebitis is the inflammation of veins characterized by presence of inflammatory exudate, thickening of the wall and dilation of the lumen.

Etiology/ Occurrence
- Naval infection in calves
- Uterine infections
- In jugular vein due to improper intravenous infection.
- *Varicose veins* are dilated and elongated veins following irregular and tortuous course
- *Telangiectasis* is marked dilation of veins particularly of sinusoidal capillaries in one or more lobules in liver.
- Macroscopic feature
- Wall of vein is thickened.
- Vein contain large thick necrotic material
- Lumen dialated
- Inner surface of vein is rough and hyperemic.
- Infiltration of neutrophils in the wall of veins
- Sometimes calcification may also present.
- Wall of vein becomes thick due to inflammatory cells and/or proliferation of fibrous tissue.

LYMPHANGITIS

Lymphangitis is the inflammation of lymph vessels characterized by aggregation of lymphocytes around lymphatics, oedema of dependent parts and distension of lymphatics.

Etiology/ Occurrence
- *Corynebacterium ovis* causes caseous lymphangitis and lymphadenitis
- Equine epizootic lymphangitis

Macroscopic and microscopic features
- Distension of subcutaneous lymph vessels, nodules of lymphoid aggregates
- Edema due to failure of lymphatic drainage.
- Lymhoid aggregation around lymphatics.
- Lymphatics distended
- Edema of dependent tissue.

Chapter 15
Pathology Respiratory System

PATHOLOGY OF UPPER RESPIRATORY TRACT

In many infectious diseases, there is inflammation of mucosa of upper respiratory passage leading to nasal discharge which is catarrhal, purulent or fibrinous depending on the type of infection. The infection may extend to lower parts of respiratory tract and reach in lungs causing pathological alterations. *Rhinitis* is the inflammation of nasal mucosa. *Sinusitis* is the inflammation of sinuses *e.g.* Frontal sinusitis in dehorned cattle. The larvae of botfly *Oestrus ovis* enters in nasal passage and migrate upto frontal sinuses and turbinate bones and cause mucopurulent inflammation. Similarly leeches (*Dinobdella ferox*) is known to cause nasal cavity inflammation in domestic animals and suck blood. Rhinitis caused by *Bordetella bronchiseptica* in pigs and characterized by mucopurulent exudate, disappearance of nasal septum, retarded growth of snout and plugging of passage by solidified exudate and dead tissue. This condition is known as *porcine atrophic rhinitis*. *Epistaxis* is bleeding from nasal passage due to trauma, neoplasm and ulcerative lesions as a result of infections. *Pharyngitis* is the inflammation of pharynix while *laryngitis* is the inflammation of larynx.

NASAL POLYPS

Nasal polyps are the inflammatory condition of respiratory mucosa resembling neoplastic growth caused by fungus and characterized by formation of new growth simulating benign neoplasm in nasal passage.

Etiology
- *Rhinosporidium sceberi*, a fungus most commonly prevalent in southern India.

Macroscopic and microscopic features
- Formation of a single polyp in respiratory mucosa, pedunculated, elongated, fills nasal cavity.
- Cauliflower like growth may cause bleeding.
- Fibrous covering by mucous membrane and heavily infilterated by neutrophils, lymphocytes, eosinophils, macrophages around fungus.

NASAL GRANULOMA

Nasal granuloma is the gramlomatous inflammation of respiratory mucosa in nasal cavity caused by blood flukes and characterized by the presence of granulomatous growth filling the nasal passage causing obstruction.

Etiology
- *Schistosoma nasalis,* a blood fluke.
- Type II hypersensitivity reaction of nasal mucosa to plant pollens, fungi, mites etc.

Macroscopic and microscopic features
- Nasal pruritus
- Small tiny nodules on nasal mucosa later becomes cauliflower like growth filling the cavity and causing obstruction.
- Edema in lamina propria
- Infiltration of eosinophils, mast cells, lymphocytes and plasma cells and absence of epithelioid cells.
- Proliferation of fibroblasts.
- The lesion is covered by squamous epithelium.
- Mucous glands may have metaplastic pseudostratified columnar epithelium.

TRACHEITIS

Tracheitis is the inflammation of trachea. In canines, it is tracheobronchitis while in poultry it is manifested by laryngotracheitis.

Etiology
- Canine tracheobronchitis caused by adenovirus, influenza virus and herpes virus.
- Avian infectious laryngotracheitis (ILT) is caused by herpes virus.

Macroscopic and microscopic features
- Canine tracheobronchitis or *kennel cough* includes congestion of trachea and presence of catarrhal exudate.
- In poultry, haemorrhage in trachea and caseous plug in trachea towards larynx causing obstruction.
- Inclusion bodies in tracheal and bronchial epithelium in canines
- Haemorrhagic tracheitis, presence of intra nuclear basophilic inclusions in tracheal epithelial cells in infectious laryngotracheitis.

BRONCHITIS

Bronchitis is the inflammation of bronchi, characterized by catarrhal, suppurative, fibrinous or haemorrhagic exudate.

Etiology
- Bacteria *e.g.* Pasteurella
- Virus *e.g.* Infectious bronchitis in poultry
- Parasites
- Allergy/ Inhalation of pollens etc.

Macroscopic and microscopic features
- Coughing, dyspnoea
- Mucous exudate in lumen
- Congestion and/or haemorrhages in bronchi
- Presence of caseaous plugs at the point where bronchi enters in lungs in infectious bronchitis of poultry.
- Mucous exudate alongwith inflammatory cells in the lumen of bronchi.

- Hyperplasia and/or necrosis of bronchiolar epithelium
- Accumulation of mononuclear cells in the bronchial mucosa and in peribronchiolar area.

PATHOLOGY OF LUNGS

ATELECTASIS

Atelectasis is the failure of alveoli to open or the alveoli are collapsed and thus do not have air.

Etiology

- Obstruction in bronchi/ bronchiole
- Pleuritis
- Atelectasis neonatorum in new born animals. In the absence of respiration, lung alveoli remain closed and thus sink in water indicating still birth.

Macroscopic and microscopic features

- Dull red in colour, hard area of lung like liver in consistency
- Atelectic lung sinks in water.
- Compressed alveoli.
- Absence of air spaces
- Collapsed bronchioles
- In inflammatory condition, exudate compresses alveoli

EMPHYSEMA

Emphysema is the increase in amount of air in lungs characterized by dilation of the alveoli. It may be acute or chronic and focal or generalized.

Etiology

- Bronchitis
- Atelectasis in adjoining area of lung
- Pneumonia
- Allergy to dust, Pollens etc

- Pulmonary adenomatosis

Macroscopic and microscopic features
- Lungs are enlarged and flabby
- Imprints of ribs can be seen. Colour of lungs becomes pale.
- Cut surface is smooth and dry.
- Alveoli are distended.
- Some alveoli may rupture and form giant alveoli.
- Alveolar wall becomes thin due to stretching.
- Mild bronchitis.
- Hyperplasia of lymphoid tissue.

PULMONARY EDEMA

In pulmonary edema, there is accumulation of serous fluid in alveoli of lungs.

Etiology
- Bacteria
- Virus
- Allergy

Macroscopic and microscopic features
- Lungs become enlarged
- Weight of lungs increases
- Cut surface releases fluid and frothy exudate in trachea and/or bronchi.
- Serous fluid accumulation in alveoli of lungs
- Fluid may also be seen in some bronchi/ bronchioles.
- Infiltration of inflammatory cells.
- Congestion of lungs.

PNEUMONIA

Pneumonia is the inflammation of lungs characterized by congestion and consolidation of lungs. The pathological lesions in lungs are produced in a similar way irrespective of the type of etiological agent and includes various stages like congestion, red hepatization, grey hepatization and resolution.

Stage of congestion: This stage of lung is characterized by active hyperemia and pulmonary oedema. The capillaries are distended with engorged blood and alveoli are filled with watery serous exudate. This requires 2 minutes to few hours to initiate the congestion.

Stage of red hepatization: This stage of lung is characterized by the consolidation of lungs due to accumulation of blood in blood vessels (congestion). The consolidated lungs are firm and looking like liver and hence the name "red hepatization". Such affected lung always sinks in water. Alveoli are filled with serous or serofibrinous exudate giving hardness to lungs. In inflammatory condition, the neutrophils, macrophages and lymphocytes along with erythrocytes infilterate the affected area of lungs. This stage of red hepatization takes 2 days for development of firmness of lung.

Stage of grey hepatization: The lung remains hard but due to lysis and removal of erythrocytes, it becomes grey or less red in colour. Firmness/ hardness of lung remains same and thus, the name grey hepatization. There is increase in infiltration of inflammatory cells like macrophages, lymphocytes, epithelioid cells depending on the virulence of etiological agents.

Stage of resolution: After a week, the recovery starts in the form of resorption of fluid; autolized cells and debris is removed by phagocytic cells. The causative organism is neutralized or removed from the lungs through immunity of body. After few days the lung parenchyma becomes normal and starts functioning. If the causative agent is more virulent, it may cause death of animal due to respiratory failure or may cause permanent lesions like formation of scar, carnification, granuloma etc. There are various types of pneumonia caused by bacteria, virus, fungi, parasites, allergens, chemicals and all such affections of lungs are classified as under.

BRONCHOPNEUMONIA

Bronchopneumonia is the inflammation of lungs involving bronchi or bronchioles along with alveoli. It is thought to be spread through bronchogenous route and is the common type of pneumonia in animals.

Etiology
- Virus
- Bacteria
- Chemicals
- Mycoplasma
- Chlamydia
- Parasites
- Fungus
- Mainly through bronchogenous route

Macroscopic and microscopic features
- Congestion and consolidation of anterior and ventral parts of lungs (Lobular pneumonia).
- Patchy lesions on one or several lobes and adjacent area shows emphysema.
- Mediastinal lymphnodes are swollen.
- Congestion, oedema or haemorrhage in lung.
- Infiltration of neutrophils, mononuclear cells in and around bronchioles/ bronchi.
- Catarrhal inflammation of bronchi.
- Proliferation of bronchiolar epithelium

INTERSTITIAL PNEUMONIA

Interstitial pneumonia is the inflammation of the lungs characterized by thickening of alveolar septa due to serous/ fibrinous exudate alongwith infiltration of neutrophils and/or mononuclear cells and proliferation of fibroblasts. It is also known as lobar pneumonia.

Etiology
- Bacteria
- Virus

- Chlamydia
- Parasites
- Mainly through hematogenous route

Macroscopic and microscopic features
- Lungs are pale or dark red in colour.
- Edema, dripping of fluid from cut surface
- Alveoli may have serous or fibrinous exudate.
- Thickening of alveolar septa due to accumulation of exudate, inflammatory cells and in chronic cases, proliferation of fibrous tissue.
- Infiltration of mononuclear cells in alveolar septa.

FIBRINOUS PNEUMONIA

Fibrinous pneumonia is the inflammation of lungs characterized by the presence of fibrin in alveoli or bronchioles and may give rise to hyaline membrane formation over the surface of alveoli or bronchiole.

Etiology
- Bacteria
- Virus
- Parasites
- Toxin/ Poisons

Macroscopic and microscopic features
- Antero-ventral portion of lung is congested and consolidation.
- Colour of lungs become deep red due to congestion
- Surface of lungs is covered by fibrin sheet.
- Interlobular septa are prominent due to accumulation of plasma and fibrin.
- Principal exudate is fibrin, fills alveoli, bronchioles and bronchi.
- Congestion and/or haemorrhages

- Infiltration of neutrophils, macrophages and giant cells
- Formation of eosinophilic false membrane of fibrin over the surface of alveoli and bronchiole and then known as *"hyaline membrane pneumonia"*.

VERMINOUS PNEUMONIA

Verminous pneumonia is caused by parasites and characterized by the presence of lesions of broncho-pneumonia along with parasites or their larva.

Etiology
- *Metastrongylus apri* in pig.
- *Dictyocaulus filariae* in sheep and goat.
- *D. viviparus* in cattle and buffaloes.
- *Capillaria aerophila* in dogs and cats.
- *D. arnfieldi* in horse and donkeys.

Macroscopic and microscopic features
- Multiple petechial haemorrhage in lungs at the site of parasite penetration.
- Mature worms in alveoli, bronchioles and bronchi.
- Mucopurulent exudate in alveoli/ bronchi.
- Pulmonary oedema, emphysema.
- Dilation of bronchiole/ bronchi
- Lesions of chronic suppurative bronchiolitis
- Focal areas of inflammation in the vicinity of parasites and around bronchioles.
- Hyperplasia of bronchiolar epithelium.
- Infiltration of eosinophils and lymphocytes.

ASPIRATION PNEUMONIA

Aspiration pneumonia is caused by faulty medication through drenching which reaches in lungs instead of target place (digestive track) and characterized by necrosis and gangrene of lung paranchyma.

Etiology
- Drugs, food, foreign body and oil drench which reaches in lungs through trachea.
- Paresis of throat predisposes the animal for aspiration pneumonia.

Macroscopic and microscopic features
- Congestion and consolidation of anterior and ventral portion of lung.
- Affected part becomes green/ black in colour, moist gangrene.
- Affected lungs are often foul smelling.
- Presence of foreign body like heads of wheats, parts of corn, oil, milk etc.
- Thrombosis of blood vessels.
- Necrosis in lungs.
- Presence of saprophytes, leucocytes and bacteria cause liquefaction and gangrene.
- Gangrenous lesions surrounded by intense inflammation.
- Congestion

MYCOTIC PNEUMONIA

Mycotic pneumonia is caused by a variety of fungi and characterized by the presence of chronic granulomatous lesions in lungs.

Etiology
- *Aspergillus fumigatus*
- *Blastomyces* sp.
- *Cryptococcus* sp.
- *Coccidioidomyces immitis*

Macroscopic and microscopic features
- Nodules in lungs
- On cut, cheese like caseative mass comes out from nod-

ules.
- Caseation involves both bronchiole and alveoli.
- Such lesions may also present in trachea, bronchi and air sacs.
- Presence of granulomatus lesions *i.e.* caseative necrosis, macrophages, epithelioid cells, lymphocytes, giant cells, fibroblasts etc.
- Presence of branched hyphae of fungi in the necrosed area.

TUBERCULOUS PNEUMONIA

Tuberculous pneumonia is caused by *Mycobacterium* sp. and characterized by the presence of chronic granulomatous lesions in the lungs.

Etiology
- *Mycobacterium tuberculosis*
- *M. bovis*

Macroscopic features
- Grey, white or light yellowish nodules in lungs.
- Nodules are hard, painful and/or calcified.
- Animal carcass is cachectic, weak or emaciated.
- On cut, the cheesy material comes out from the nodules.
- Presence of tubercle/ granuloma in lungs which comprises a central necrosed area surrounded by macrophages, epithelioid cells, lymphocytes, Langhan's giant cells and covered by fibrous covering.
- Acid-fast rod shaped bacteria may present in necrosed area.
- Central area may be calcified.

OVINE PULMONARY CARCINOMA (PREVIOUSLY PULMONARY ADENOMATOSIS)

Pulmonary adenomatosis is a slow viral disease of sheep and characterized by metaplasia of alveolar squamous epithelium to cuboidal and/or columnar epithelium leading to glandular appearance of alveoli.

Differential features of various types of Pneumonia

	Bronchopneumonia	Interstitial	Fibrinous	Verminous	Aspiration	Mycotic	Tuberculous
Macroscopic features	1. Congestion and consolidation of anterior and ventral parts of lungs (Lobular pneumonia). 2. Patchy lesions on one or several lobes and adjacent area shows emphysema. 3. Mediastinal lymphnodes are swollen.	1. Lungs are pale or dark red in colour. 2. Edema, dripping of fluid from cut surface	1. Antero-ventral portion of lung is congested and consolidated. 2. Colour of lungs become deep red due to congestion 3. Surface of lungs is covered by fibrin sheet. 4. Interlobular septa are prominent due to accumulation of plasma and fibrin.	1. Multiple petechial haemorrhage in lungs at the site of parasite penetration. 2. Mature worms in alveoli, bronchioles and bronchi. 3. Mucopurulent exudate in alveoli/bronchi. 4. Pulmonary oedema, emphysema.	1. Congestion and consolidation of anterior and ventral portion of lung. 2. Affected part becomes green/black in colour, moist gangrene. 3. Affected lungs are often foul smelling. 4. Presence of foreign body like heads of wheats, parts of corn, oil, milk etc.	1. Nodules in lungs 2. On cut, cheese like caseative mass comes out from nodules. 3. Caseation involves both bronchiole and alveoli. 4. Such lesions may also present in trachea, bronchi and air sacs.	1. Grey, white or light yellowish nodules in lungs. 2. Nodules are hard, painful and/or calcified. 3. Animal carcass is cachectic, weak or emaciated. 4. On cut, the cheesy material comes out from the nodules.

Pathology Respiratory System

Microscopic features	1. Congestion, Edema or haemorrhage in lung. 2. Infiltration of neutrophils, mononuclear cells in and around bronchioles/ bronchi. 3. Catarrhal inflammation of bronchi. 4. Proliferation of bronchiolar epithelium	1. Alveoli may have serous or fibrinous exudate. 2. Thickening of alveolar septa due to accumulation of exudate, inflammatory cells and in chronic cases, proliferation of fibrous tissue. 3. Infiltration of mononuclear cells in alveolar septa.	1. Principal exudate is fibrin, fills alveoli, bronchioles and bronchi. 2. Congestion and/or haemorrhages 3. Infiltration of neutrophils, macrophages and giant cells 4. Formation of eosinophilic false membrane of fibrin over the surface of alveoli and bronchiole and then known as "hyaline membrane pneumonia".	1. Dilation of bronchiole/ bronchi 2. Lesions of chronic suppurative bronchiolitis 3. Focal areas of inflammation in the vicinity of parasites and around bronchioles. 4. Hyperplasia of bronchiolar epithelium. 5. Infiltration of eosinophils and lymphocytes.	1. Thrombosis of blood vessels. 2. Necrosis in lungs. 3. Presence of saprophytes, leucocytes and bacteria cause liquefaction and gangrene. 4. Gangrenous lesions surrounded by intense inflammation 5. Congestion	1. Presence of granulomatus lesions i.e. caseative necrosis, macrophages, epithelioid cells, lymphocytes, giant cells, fibroblasts etc. 2. Presence of branched hyphae of fungi in the necrosed area.	1. Presence of tubercle/ granuloma in lungs which comprises a central necrosed area surrounded by macrophages, epithelioid cells, lymphocytes, Langhan's giant cells and covered by fibrous covering. 2. Acid-fast rod shaped bacteria may present in necrosed area. 3. Central area may be calcified.

Etiology
- Retrovirus
- Pulmonary adenomatosis virus

Macroscopic and microscopic features
- Multiple focal areas of consolidation in lungs.
- Imprint of ribs on lungs.
- Congestion and hardening of mediastinal lymphnodes.
- Metaplasia of alveolar epithelium leading to formation of glandular structures in alveoli.
- Metaplasia of simple squamous epithelium to cuboidal or columnar epithelium which gives alveoli a gland like look.
- Mild inflammatory reaction.
- Proliferation of fibrous tissue.

HYPERSENSITIVITY PNEUMONITIS

Hypersensitivity pneumonitis is the inflammation of lung caused by an allergic reaction of antigen (allergen) and characterized by interstitial pneumonia, emphysema, hyaline membrane formation and hyperplasia of alveolar epithelium.

Etiology
- Allergens
- Parasites – *Dictyocaulus viviparous*
- Moldy hay
- Fungus- *Aspergillus* sp.

Macroscopic and microscopic features
- Lobes may contain small grey foci
- Presence of yellow and dense mucus in lumen of bronchi
- Excessive accumulation of air in lungs due to emphysema
- Presence of worms/ larvae.
- Extensive infiltration of lymphocytes, monocytes and eosinophils around the bronchi and bronchioles.
- Accumulation of catarrhal exudate in bronchi/ bronchiole.

- Emphysema as a result of widening of alveoli.
- Hyperplasia of bronchiolar musculature.
- Inflammatory cells in interalveolar septa may form small granulomas.
- Formation of hyaline membrane over alveolar and bronchiolar epithelium.

PNEUMOCONIOSIS

Pneumoconiosis is the granulomatous inflammation of lungs caused by aerogenous dust particles of sand, silica, beryllium, carbon or asbestos. It is also known as anthracosis.

Etiology
- Silica
- Asbestos
- Beryllium
- Bauxite
- Graphite
- Carbon
- Bronchogenous/ aerogenous administration of particles inhaled with air, mostly around mines/ factories.
- Generator smoke.

Macroscopic and microscopic features
- Dense fibrous nodules in lungs.
- Presence of carbon particles in trachea/ bronchi mixed with mucous exudate.
- Granuloma formation around the particles of silica/ asbestos infilterated by macrophages, lymphocytes and giant cells
- Silica produces cellular reaction *'Silicosis'*.
- *Beryllium granuloma* looks like tubercule without caseation.
- *Asbestosis* is characterized by the presence of club shaped filaments bearing cells in lesion.

PATHOLOGY OF AIR SACS

AIR SACCULITIS

Air sacculitis is inflammation of air sacs caused by *E.coli*, Mycoplasma, reovirus etc. and characterized by thickening of the wall of air sacs and presence of cheesy exudates.

Etiology
- *Escherichia coli*
- *Mycoplasma gallisepticum*
- Avian reovirus

Macroscopic and microscopic features
- Thickening of the air sac wall, which becomes dirty and cloudy.
- Presence of cheesy exudate in air sacs, congestion of lungs.
- Fibrinous pericarditis
- Liver is covered with thin fibrinous membrane.
- Oedema and infiltration of neutrophils and lymphocytes in air sacs
- Caseous exudate in lungs and air sacs.

PATHOLOGY OF PLEURA

PLEURITIS

Pleuritis is the inflammation of pleura characterized by serous, fibrinous or purulent exudate. It is also known as *pleurisy*.

Etiology
- *Mycobacterium tuberculosis*
- *Mycoplasma mycoides*
- *Haemophilus suis*
- Organisms responsible for pneumonia/ traumatic pericarditis may also cause pleuritis.

Macroscopic and microscopic features
- Congestion of pleura

- Serous, fibrinous or purulent exudate.
- Accumulation of clear fluid in pleura/ thoracic cavity is called as *hydrothorax*.
- Presence of blood in thoracic cavity is known as *Hemothorax*.
- Suppurative exudate in thoracic cavity is known as *pyothorax*.
- Presence of air in pleural cavity is termed as *pneumothorax*, while presence of lymph in pleural cavity is called as *chylothorax*.
- Tuberculous pleuritis is characterized by small nodules on pleura and is known as *"pearly disease"*.
- In chronic cases, development of fibrous tissue causes adhesions and is known as *adhesive pleuritis*.
- Congestion of blood vessels
- Infiltration of neutrophils and lymphocytes.
- Thickening of pleura due to oedema
- Proliferation of fibroblasts producing adhesive lesions.

Chapter 16
Pathology of Digestive System

DEVELOPMENTAL ANOMALIES

Epitheliogenesis imperfecta of tongue

Abnormal smooth surface of tongue due to small filiform papillae. It occurs as a defect in autosomal recessive gene and occurs in Holstein-Friesian cattle. This is also known as smooth tongue.

Cleft palate

This is most common congenital abnormality occurs due to failure of oral-nasal cavity to divide leaving cleft. It may also extend towards lips producing 'hare lip' condition.

Mega colon

There is distention of colon which abruptly terminate in rectum due to mutant gene in dogs.

Duplication of colon

In dog, the colon is duplicated from caecum to rectum and this defect is associated with malformation in the body of vertebrae T_4 and T_5.

Atresia coli

In calf, the absence of colon occurs and the intestine terminates in blind caecum.

Atresia ani

This is absence of anal opening.

PATHOLOGY OF MOUTH CAVITY

STOMATITIS

Stomatitis in the inflammation of mucosa of oral cavity. It includes:

Gingivitis: Inflammation of gums

Glossitis: Inflammation of tongue

Cheilitis: Inflammation of lips

Tonsilitis: Inflammation of tonsil

Palatitis/ Lampas: Inflammation of palates

Etiology
- Trauma due to nails, wire, or any sharp object like needle
- Physical due to hot milk, medicines etc.
- Chemical- Alkali/ acids
- Microorganisms- Bacteria, virus, fungi

Macroscopic and microscopic features
- Catarrhal stomatitis: Mucous exudation in oral cavity.
- Vesicular stomatitis: Vesicles in oral mucosal *e.g.* FMD
- Erosive stomatitis: Erosions in oral mucosa *e.g.* Rinderpest
- Fibrinous stomatitis: False membrane in oral mucosa.
- Ulcerative stomatitis: Presence of ulcers in oral mucosa *e.g.* mucosal disease.
- Congestion of oral mucosa
- Presence of erosions, vesicles or ulcers
- Infiltration of neutrophils, lymphocytes and macrophages
- Presence of fibrinous exudate in the form of diphtheritic membrane.

PATHOLOGY OF ESOPHAGUS AND CROP CHOKE

Choke is complete or partial obstruction of esophagus either due to any foreign material or pressure from adjoining areas.

Etiology
- Beets, turnip, carrots, bone
- Abscess tumor of neck area

Macroscopic and microscopic features
- Tympany
- Gangrene, sapremia and toxaemia
- Sac like dialatation "Esophageal diverticulum"
- Perforation due to sharp bone ends
- Necrosis gangrene at a point of obstruction
- Congestion haemorrhage in perforated cases

ESOPHAGITIS

Esophagitis is the inflammation of esophagus caused by trauma, parasites etc. and characterized by catarrhal inflammation, ulceration or stenosis due to fibrosis.

Etiology
- Trauma due to foreign bodies
- Chemicals- Acids, alkalies
- Infection- Mucosal disease virus
- Parasite- *Spirocerca lupi*
- Nutritional- Vit. A deficiency

Macroscopic and microscopic features
- Congestion
- Ulcer formation.
- Red streaks of catarrhal inflammation.
- Stenosis due to fibrous nodules or inflammatory exudate.
- Enlargement of glands.
- Congestion, haemorrhage
- Ulceration
- Infiltration of neutrophils, lymphocytes
- Sub-epithelial fibrosis/ nodules by *Spirocerea lupi*.

INGLUVITIS

Ingluvitis is the inflammation of crop caused by fungi and characterized by ulcerative or diphtheritic lesions.

Etiology
- *Candida albicans*
- *Monilia albicans*

Macroscopic and microscopic features
- Turkis towl like appearance in crop mucosa.
- Round and raised ulcers.
- In moniliasis, formation of diphtheritic membrane
- Necrotic and ulcerative lesions
- Fibrinous inflammation with infiltration of mononuclear cells

PATHOLOGY OF STOMACH

TYMPANY

Tympany is accumulation of gases in rumen due to failure of eructation as a result of obstruction or due to excessive production of gases characterized by distended rumen and dyspnoea. It is also known as *bloat*.

Etiology
- Choke of esophagus
- Sudden change in animal feed with high content of legumes.
- Excessive lush green fodder

Macroscopic and microscopic features
- Rumen is distended due to excessive accumulation of gases (CO_2, H_2S, CO)
- Distended rumen compresses diaphragm to hinder respiration.
- Tarry colour blood, pale liver and rupture of diaphragm.
- On rupture of rumen gas comes out (dry tympany).

- The gas is trapped in small bubbles in the ruminal fluid forming foams and is not easily removed. This is known as *"frothy bloat"*, which is produced by saponin and water soluble proteins and due to reduction in surface tension in the absence of fatty acids that favours froth formation.
- Haemorrhage in lungs, pericardium, trachea and lymphnodes
- Atelectasis in lungs.

RUMENITIS

Rumenitis is the inflammation of rumen in ruminant animals caused by change in diet, chemicals or drugs and characterized by seropurulent exudate or ulcer formation with or without parakeratosis.

Etiology
- Change in diet, corn or alfa-alfa hay.
- Chemicals/ drugs *e.g.* potassium antimony tarterate.
- *Spherophorus necrophorus* infection

Macroscopic and microscopic features
- Ulcers
- Spherical white nodules of 1-2 cm diameter size.
- Sloughing of mucosa.
- Seropurulent exudate
- Ulcers
- Infiltration of lymphocytes and neutrophils
- Fibrous nodules due to hyperplasia of fibroblasts
- Parakeratosis

RETICULITIS

Reticulitis is the inflammation of reticulum in ruminant animals caused by trauma/ perforation by foreign body including sharp object like needles, wires, etc. and characterized by abscess formation, adhesions, peritonitis and pericarditis.

Etiology
- Foreign body- sharp objects like needles, wires etc.

Macroscopic and microscopic features
- Perforation of reticulum by foreign body.
- Abscessation/ suppuration
- Peritonitis, adhesions of reticulum with diaphragm
- Pericarditis due to foreign body (traumatic reticulo pericarditis).
- Infiltration of neutrophils, macrophages, lymphocytes
- Proliferation of fibroblasts producing adhesions.
- Liquefactive necrosis.

OMASITIS

Omasitis is the inflammation of omasum in ruminant animals caused by *Actinobacillus* sp. and characterized by granulomatous inflammatory reaction.

Etiology
- *Actinobacillus ligneiresi*

Macroscopic and microscopic features
- Granulomatous nodules in omasum
- Typical granuloma formation
- Sulfur granules of Actinobacillus in the centre of lesion.

ABOMASITIS

Abomasitis is the inflammation of abomasum in ruminants caused by chemicals/ drugs, bacteria, virus or parasites and characterized by congestion, edema and/or haemorrhagic ulcers.

Etiology
- Chemicals/ drugs
- Bacteria *e.g. Clostridium septicum* cause of Braxy
- Virus *e.g.* Hog cholera, Mucosal disease
- Parasites *e.g. Theileria* sp.

Macroscopic and microscopic features
- Presence of ulcers (button ulcers in Hog cholera).
- Congestion, oedema of abomasal folds, haemorrhage in braxy.
- Catarrhal, haemorrhagic abomasits
- Presence of gram positive rods in case of braxy.
- Neutrophilic and lymphocytic infiltration.
- Congestion and haemorrhages.
- Ulceration with lymphocytic infiltration.

IMPACTION OF RUMEN AND RETICULUM

Impaction of rumen and reticulum is common in cattle and buffaloes caused by heavy carbohydrate diet and characterized by atony of rumen, indigestion, acidosis and haemorrhage on serous membranes.

Etiology
- Overfeeding of carbohydrate feed.
- Lack of water.
- Defective teeth or damaged tongue.
- Paralysis of rumen.

Macroscopic and microscopic features
- Atony of rumen due to lactic acid production.
- Rumen is filled with hard, caked undigested food with foul odour.
- Hemoconcentration, anuria, blood becomes dark in colour.
- Hemorrhage in lungs.
- Desquamation of ruminal epithelium.
- Lesions of acidosis/ toxicosis.

GASTRITIS

Gastritis is the inflammation of stomach in non-ruminant animals having simple stomach caused by chemicals/ drugs, bacteria, virus, parasite and characterized by congestion, edema, hemorrhage and ulceration. Inflammation of proventriculus in poultry is termed as proventriculitis.

Etiology
- Physical- overfeeding, trauma,
- Chemicals- Acid/ alkali
- Microorganisms such as bacteria, virus, fungi,
- Parasites *e.g. Trichostrongyles* sp., *Hemonchus* sp.
- Uremia

Macroscopic and microscopic features
- Congestion, oedema and haemorrhage of mucosal surface
- Thick mucous exudate in stomach
- Presence of vesicles/ ulcers on gastric mucosa
- Congestion and haemorrhage of gastric mucosa.
- Presence of ulcers/ necrosis.
- Infiltration of mononuclear cells.
- Lymphoid hyperplasia.

PATHOLOGY OF INTESTINES

CATARRHAL ENTERITIS

Catarrhal enteritis is characterized by increased number of goblet cells, congestion and infiltration of neutrophils and mononuclear cells in mucosa of intestine.

Etiology
- Physical- Foreign bodies and corase feed
- Chemical- drugs
- Microorganisms-*E.coli, Salmonella* sp., viruses
- Parasites- Coccidia

Macroscopic and microscopic features
- Presence of catarrhal exudate in lumen of intestine and congestion.
- Thickening of the wall of intestine.

- Diarrhoea.
- Presence of parasites in lumen of intestine.
- Increased number of goblet cells in intestinal villi, reduced length of villi.
- Congestion.
- Infiltration of polymorphonuclear and mononuclear cells.

HEMORRHAGIC ENTERITIS

Haemorrhagic enteritis is characterized by inflammation of the intestines along with haemorrhagic exudates.

Etiology
- Bacteria- *E. coli, Bacillus anthracis, Salmonella* sp.
- Virus- Coronavirus, BVD, MD, RP
- Parasites- Coccidia

Macroscopic and microscopic features
- Hemorrhagic exudate in intestines; blood mixed intestinal contents.
- Petechial or echymotic haemorrhage in mucosa and sub-mucosa of intestine.
- Presence of erosions/ ulcers in mucosa.
- Hemorrhage in the mucosa of intestine
- Infiltration of neutrophils and mononuclear cells.
- Erosion or ulcers in intestinal mucosa
- Presence of coccidia in the mucosa

CHRONIC ENTERITIS

Chronic enteritis is the chronic inflammation of intestine characterized by proliferative changes like proliferation of fibrous tissue, infiltration of mononuclear cells and plasma cells in lamina propria leading to hardening of intestinal wall.

Etiology
- *Mycobacterium paratuberculosis* in bovines

- Intestinal helminths
- *E. coli* in poultry (Hjarre's disease)

Macroscopic and microscopic features
- Thickening of the wall of intestine (Corrugations in Johne's disease).
- Thick mucous cover over mucosa of intestine
- Transverse corrugations in the large intestine.
- Granulomatous nodules in duodenum.
- Small, round, raised necrotic foci on serosal surface of intestine covering whole length of intestine.
- Proliferation of fibrous tissue in lamina propria.
- Infiltration of macrophages, lymphocytes, plasma cells.
- Atrophy of intestinal glands.

NECROTIC ENTERITIS

Necrotic enteritis is characterized by necrosis of mucosal epithelium of intestine leading to erosions/ ulcer formation and exposition of underlying tissues.

Etiology
- Salmonella
- Rinderpest, rotavirus, cornovirus, Hog cholera virus.
- Coccidia, Histoplasma
- Niacin deficiency
- *Clostridium* sp. after coccidial infection in birds.

Macroscopic and microscopic features
- Necrotic patches in intestines.
- Fibrinous deposits over necrotic patches like bran deposits
- Swelling of mesenteric lymphnodes
- Ulcers in intestine.
- Congestion and infiltration of mononuclear cells.

- Necrosis and desquamation of intestinal villous epithelium, leading to exposed underlying tissue.
- Ulcers in mucosa.
- Proliferation of crypt epithelium, presence of abnormal epithelium over villous surface.

PARASITIC ENTERITIS

Parasitic enteritis is caused by parasites and characterized by catarrhal and/or hemorrhagic exudate in intestine, presence of ova/ adult parasite and thickening of the wall of intestine.

Etiology
- Helminths
- Roundworms
- Tapeworms
- Protozoa
- Coccidia
- Histoplasma

Macroscopic and microscopic features
- Presence of parasite helminths in the lumen of intestine.
- Thickening of the wall of intestine.
- Catarrhal or haemorrhagic exudate in intestine.
- Presence of large number of goblet cells in mucosa of intestine.
- Congestion and/or hemorrhage.
- Presence of parasite/ ova in the intestinal lumen
- Infiltration of eosinophils in mucosa and submucosa of the intestines.
- Coccidia can be seen on mucosal scrapings under microscope.

FIBRINOUS ENTERITIS

Fibrinous enteritis is the fibrinous inflammation of intestine characterized by presence of fibrinous exudate comprising of pseudomembrane in the mucosa of intestine.

Etiology
- *Salmonella choleraesuis*
- *Spherophorus necrophorus*

Macroscopic and microscopic features
- Presence of diphtheritic membrane over mucosa of intestine.
- Button ulcers
- Sometimes, diphtheritic membrane covers the faeces.
- Congestion and haemorrhage in intestine.
- Thickening of intestinal wall due to fibrinous exudate.
- Fibrin network in mucosa.

GRANULOMATOUS ENTERITIS

Granulomatous enteritis is caused by bacteria or fungi and characterized by granuloma formation in the intestines.

Etiology
- *Mycobacterium tuberculosis*
- Coli granuloma- *E. coli* in poultry (Hjarre's disease)
- Coccidioiodomycosis/ candidiasis.

Macroscopic and microscopic features
- Granulomatous about one cm diameter elevated/ raised areas on the serous surface of intestine.
- Thickening of the wall of intestine.
- Small, tiny, white necrotic nodules on serosa.
- Granuloma formation consisting of central necrosed area covered by lymphocytes, macrophages, epithelioid cells, giant cells and fibrous connective tissue
- Extensive proliferation of fibrus tissue.
- Presence of bacteria/ fungus in the lesion.

Differential features of various types of Enteritis

	Catarrhal	Hemorrhagic	Chronic	Necrotic	Parasitic	Fibrinous	Granulomatous
Macroscopic features	1. Presence of catarrhal exudate in lumen of intestine and congestion. 2. Thickening of the wall of intestine. 3. Presence of parasites in lumen of intestine.	1. Hemorrhagic exudate in intestines; blood mixed intestinal contents. 2. Petechial or echymotic hemorrhage in mucosa and submucosa of intestine. 3. Presence of erosions/ulcers in mucosa.	1. Thickening of the wall of intestine (Corrugations in Johne's disease). 2. Thick mucous cover over mucosa of intestine. 3. Transverse corrugations in the large intestine. 4. Granulomatous nodules in duodenum. 5. Small, round, raised necrotic foci on serosal surface of intestine covering whole length of intestine.	1. Necrotic patches in intestines. 2. Fibrinous deposits over necrotic patches like bran deposits. 3. Swelling of mesenteric lymphnodes. 4. Ulcers in intestine.	1. Presence of parasite helminths in the lumen of intestine. 2. Thickening of the wall of intestine. 3. Catarrhal or haemorrhagic exudate in intestine.	1. Presence of diphtheritic membrane over mucosa of intestine. 2. Button ulcers. 3. Sometimes, diphtheritic membrane covers the faeces.	1. Granulomatous about one cm diameter elevated/raised areas on the serus surface of intestine. 2. Thickening of the wall of intestine. 3. Small, tiny, white necrotic nodules on serosa.

| Microscopic features | 1. Increased number of goblet cells in intestinal villi, reduced length of villi. 2. Congestion. 3. Infiltration of polymorphonuclear and mononuclear cells. | 1. Haemorrhage in the mucosa of intestine 2. Infiltration of neutrophils and mononuclear cells. 3. Erosion or ulcers in intestinal mucosa | 1. Proliferation of fibrous tissue in lamina propria. 2. Infiltration of macrophages, lymphocytes, plasma cells. 3. Atrophy of intestinal glands. | 1. Congestion and infiltration of mononuclear cells. 2. Necrosis and desquamation of intestinal villous epithelium, leading to exposed underlying tissue. 3. Ulcers in mucosa. 4. Proliferation of crypt epithelium, presence of abnormal epithelium over villous surface. | 1. Presence of large number of goblet cells in mucosa of intestine. 2. Congestion and/or haemorrhage. 3. Presence of parasite/ova in the intestinal lumen 4. Infiltration of eosinophils in mucosa and submucosa of the intestines. 5. Coccidia can be seen on mucosal scrapings under microscope. | 1. Congestion and hemorrhage in intestine. 2. Thickening of intestinal wall due to fibrinous exudate. 3. Fibrin network in mucosa. | 1. Granuloma formation consisting of central necrosed area covered by lymphocytes, macrophages, epithelioid cells, giant cells and fibrous connective tissue 2. Extensive proliferation of fibrous tissue. 3. Presence of bacteria/fungus in the lesion. |

INTESTINAL OBSTRUCTION

Obstruction of intestines may occur as a result of foreign body, enterolith, piliconcretions, phytobezoars, polybezoars or due to hypermotility of intestines leading to intussusception, volvulus or torsion.

Piliconcretions: Piliconcretions are hair balls mostly found in stomach/ intestines of those animals having habit of licking. This vice is more common in suckling calves and in animals with pica related to phosphorus deficiency. The hairs are accumulated in stomach which becomes in rounded shape due to movements of stomach and look like balls. Such hair balls are not degradable in gastrointestinal tract and may cause obstruction.

Phytobezoars/ Polybezoars: Concretions formed in gastrointestinal tract as a result of deposition of salts around a nidus of undigested plants or polythenes. They may cause obstruction in gastrointestinal tract.

Foreign bodies: Foreign bodies like rubber balls, nuts, bones, stones, plastic and rubber materials, polythenes may obstruct the intestinal tract as they are not degradable in the gastrointestinal tract.

Hernia: Hernia is presence of intestinal loop in umbilical area, scrotum or inguinal cavity which causes passive congestion, oedema and obstruction in intestines.

Intussusception: Intussusception is telescoping of intestine means a portion of intestine enters in caudal segment due to violent peristaltic movement. It causes obstruction, passive congestion and oedema.

Volvulus: In volvulus, the loop of intestine passes through a tear in mesentry. It causes obstruction at both ends of loop.

Torsion: Torsion is twisting of intestine upon itself causing obstruction.

Enterolith: Concretions in intestines particularly in horses are responsible for obstruction of intestinal tract and are responsible for "colic in horse" and enterocolitis.

TYPHLITIS

Typhlitis is the inflammation of caecum. It is particularly important in poultry caused by protozoan parasites and characterized by haemorrhage, thickening of the wall, presence of cheesy exudates and/or necrotic ulcers.

Etiology
- *Eimeria tennella*
- *Histomonas meleagridis*

Macroscopic and microscopic features
- Haemorrhage in caecum, blood mixed contents.
- Thickening of the wall, with congestion and cheesy exudates.
- Presence of necrotic ulcers in caecum in case of histomoniasis which is further supported by round, depressed, yellowish green areas of necrosis in liver.
- Congestion, haemorrhage, necrosis
- Presence of protozoan parasites
- Necrotic hepatic lesions.

HEPATITIS

Hepatitis is the inflammation of liver. It may be acute or chronic. Acute hepatitis is characterized by the presence of degeneration and necrosis of hepatocytes and infiltration of neutrophils and mononuclear cells alongwith hyperemia and/or haemorrhage.

Etiology
- Bacteria- Necrobacillosis, *Salmonella, E. coli*
- Virus- ICH
- Chemicals- Carbon tetrachloride
- Parasites- *Fasciola gigantica, Fasciola hepatica*

Macroscopic and microscopic features
- Enlargement of liver.
- Congestion and/or haemorrhage.

- Presence of necrotic patches in liver.
- Presence of fibrinous diphtheritic membrane on liver.
- Cloudy swelling and/or fatty changes in liver.
- Congestion in blood vessels and in sinusoidal area.
- Infiltration of neutrophils, macrophages and lymphocytes.
- Necrosis of hepatic parenchyma.
- In acute toxic hepatitis there is necrosis of hepatocytes. According to location it can be classified as under which is helpful in making diagnosis.
- *Diffuse necrosis* covers a considerable area crossing over the lobular boundaries.
- *Focal necrosis* occupying only a part of lobule *e.g.* EHV induced aborted foetal liver.
- *Peripheral necrosis* is characterized by necrosis at the periphery of lobule which occurs due to presence of strong toxins in blood.
- *Midzonal necrosis* have necrosis of cells in midway of periphery and centre of lobule.
- *Centrilobular necrosis* is characterized by necrosis of hepatocytes around the central vein occurs due to stagnation of blood with toxaemia.
- *Paracentral necrosis* is characterized by necrosis of hepatocytes at one side of central vein *e.g.* Rift valley fever.

CIRRHOSIS

Cirrhosis is the chronic inflammation of liver characterized by extensive fibrosis, hepatic degeneration and necrosis.

Etiology
- Bacteria- Salmonella, *Spherophorus necrophorous*
- Virus- Infectious canine hepatitis
- Chemicals- Carbon tetrachloride
- Parasites- *Fasciola hepatica, F. giantica*

- Poisons/ toxins- Aflatoxins
- Once cirrhosis of liver starts, it is not checked even after removal of the cause as the newly formed fibrous tissue itself acts as an irritant to cause further proliferation of fibroblasts.

Macroscopic and microscopic features
- Liver becomes hard and firm.
- Surface of liver becomes uneven and nodular.
- Size of liver becomes reduced due to atrophy.
- Colour becomes yellowish, grey.
- Increase in fibrous tissue within and around lobules.
- Infiltration of macrophages and lymphocytes.
- Central vein is either absent or placed eccentrically.
- Hepatocytes show degenerative and necrotic changes.
- *Biliary cirrhosis* is characterized by proliferation of fibrous tissue around the bile ducts encircling them *e.g. Fasciola giantica*.
- *Glissonian cirrhosis* is mostly confined to areas at a short distance beneath the capsule.
- *Pigment cirrhosis* is associated with yellow discolouration.
- *Central or cardiac cirrhosis* is increase in fibrous tissue around the central vein as a result of chronic passive congestion.
- *Parasitic cirrhosis* occurs due to damage caused by migration of parasites *e.g. Ascaris lumbricoides, Schistosoma* sp.

CHOLECYSTITIS

Cholecystitis is the inflammation of gall bladder characterized by congestion, thickening of wall and infiltration of mononuclear cells. Cholangitis is the inflammation of bile duct.

Etiology
- Parasites- *Fasciola* sp.
- Foreign body- Stones
- Bacteria- *E. coli*.

Macroscopic and microscopic features
- Thickening of the wall of gall bladder.
- On opening of gall bladder, there may be parasites/ stones/ foreign body.
- Contents of gall bladder may be watery or thick oily.
- Congestion
- Proliferation of fibrous tissue in the wall of gall bladder
- Infiltration of mononuclear cells
- Increased number of mucus secreting cells.

PANCREATITIS

Pancreatitis is the inflammation of pancreas characterized by necrosis of pancreatic tissue, infiltration of neutrophils and mononuclear cells and fibrous tissue proliferation.

Etiology
- Bacteria
- Virus- Reovirus in poultry
- Parasites

Macroscopic and microscopic features
- Pancreas becomes pale, swollen, oedematous.
- In chronic cases, atrophy of pancreas
- Pancreas becomes hard, firm, and fibrous.
- Necrosis of pancreatic cells.
- Edema, infiltration of leucocytes, haemorrhage.
- Fibrosis characterized by proliferation of fibroblasts.

PATHOLOGY OF PERITONIUM

Peritonitis is the inflammation of peritoneum characterized by suppurative, serofibrinous or nodular lesions.

Etiology
- Bacteria- Staphylococci, *Mycobacterium* sp.
- Virus
- Neoplasia

- Parasites

Macroscopic and microscopic features
- Serofibrinous, fibrinous, suppurative or granulomatous lesions
- Accumulation of clear fluid is known as *Hydroperitoneum* or *Ascites*.
- Presence of nodules in tuberculosis is also termed as "*Pearly disease*".
- Serofibrinous, suppurative or granulomatous lesions.
- Thickening of peritoneum, adhesions due to fibrosis.

Chapter 17
Pathology of Hemopoitic and Immune System

DEVELOPMENTAL ANOMALIES

Hereditary anemia

Hereditary anemia has been reported in mice due to defects in erythropoiesis or reduced vitality of erythrocytes. Erythropenia along with leucopenia occurs in mouse foetus on 20th day of gestation due to defective autosomal chromosome 4. Sex linked anemia in mouse is hypochromic with deficient bone marrow and occurs in hemizygus males or homozygus females. This anemia occurs due to deficiency of iron as a result of poor absorption from gastrointestinal tract.

Autoimmune hemolytic anemia in foals

It occurs due to incompatible blood group antigens of male and female parents. The mare does not have that blood group antigen but foetus acquires it from father. The foetal blood exposed to dam through placental exchanges that leads to induction of antibody production in mares against foetal blood group antigen. These antibodies accumulate in colustrum and when foal suck the milk from mares, they are readily absorbed through G.I. tract of foals in blood and causes destruction of erythrocytes leading to anemia.

Congenital defects in lymphocytes

Congenital defects in lymphocytes are classified under stem cell aplasia/ agenesis leading to combined immunodeficiency with absence of both T- and B-lymphocytes in Arabian foals. It occurs either due to inherited gene defect or there is differentiation/ maturation defects in lymphocytes. It is characterized by agammaglobulinemia, lymphopenia, hypoplasia of thymus, lymphnodes and spleen.

Chediak Higashi Syndrome

This syndrome is related with defects in phagocytic cells such as defective neutrophils and monocytes. The defects are in chemotaxis, engulfment and killing of bacteria and associated with defective assembly of cytoplasmic microtubules responsible for degranulation and release of lysosomal enzymes, there is depression of superoxide anions leading to persistent bacterial infections.

ANEMIA

Anemia is the decrease in number of erythrocytes or hemoglobin concentration in erythrocytes per unit of blood and is characterized by pale mucus membrane, dyspnoea, cardiac hypertrophy and weakness. Anemia is classified according to morphological characteristics of erythrocytes and on the basis of causative factors. Morphologically, anemia is classified as macrocytic, normocytic and microcytic depending on the size of red blood cells and normochromic and hypochromic based on the presence of quantity of hemoglobin in RBC. *Macrocytic anemia* is characterized by increased size of RBC and occurs due to acute blood loss or hemolysis resulting in excessive production and availability of immature erythrocytes in blood. Such cells also have reduced amount of hemoglobin and termed as hypochromic. *Macrocytic normochromic* anemia is increase size of RBC with normal hemoglobin and has been observed in deficiency of folic acid, niacin and vitamin B_{12}. *Normocytic anemia* are most common in animals occurs due to neoplasia, irradiation and are also known as *aplastic anemia* as a result of aplasia or agenesis of RBC. Normocytic normochromic, normal size of RBC with normal hemoglobin anemia occurs as a result of depression of erythrogenesis. *Microcytic anemia* is reduction in size of erythrocytes with decreased hemoglobin (Microcytic hypochromic) and occurs in deficiency of iron and pyridoxine or chronic blood loss.

In anemia, the size of RBC varies markedly with some large and some small size and is known as *anisocytosis*. The presence of abnormal shape (elongated, angular, ovoid, distorted) of RBC is termed as *poikilocytosis*. In some blood smears, there are nucleated RBC's which are immature due to increased production to meet the demand. Sometimes, the erythrocytes are having minute dark spots known as *basophilic stippling* which occurs in acute blood loss. Some erythrocytes stain unevenly with some dark and light colour spots and are known as *polychromatophilia* which is an indication of active erythrogenesis. The denaturation and precipitation of hemoglobin leads to appearance of purplish granules in RBC near the cytoplasmic membrane which are known as "Heinz bodies". According to etiological factors, the anemia is classified as hemolytic, haemorrhagic or deficiency anemia.

HEMOLYTIC ANEMIA

Hemolytic anemia occurs due to excessive lysis of erythrocytes and characterized by icterus, hemoglobinuria, and presence of nucleated erythrocytes in blood and hemosiderosis in spleen.

Etiology
- Infections *e.g. Anaplasma* spp. *Babesia* spp., Equine infectious anemia virus
- Toxins/ poisons *e.g.* snake venom, chronic lead poisoning.
- Immune mechanisms *e.g.* autoimmunity against erythrocytes.

Macroscopic and microscopic features
- Pale mucous membranes
- Icterus
- Blood is thin, watery.
- **Hemoglobinurea**
- Decreased number of erythrocytes
- Presence of nucleated/ immature RBC in blood
- Hemosiderin laden cells in spleen

HEMORRHAGIC ANEMIA

Hemorrhagic anemia occurs due to severe haemorrhage, extravasation of blood and characterized by pale mucus membrane and hemorrhage in body.

Etiology
- Infections e.g. Acute septicemic diseases
- Toxins/ poisons e.g. Bracken fern poisoning
- Parasites e.g. *Hemonchus contortus*
- **Deficiency e.g. vitamin C deficiency**

Macroscopic and microscopic features
- Petechiae or Echymotic hemorrhage
- **Pale mucous membrane**
- Hematuria
- Hemorrhage in various tissues/ organs
- Macrocytic or normocytic characters of RBC
- Poikilocytosis
- Hyperplasia of bone marrow

DEFICIENCY ANEMIA

Deficiency anemia occurs as a result of deficiency of iron, copper, cobalt and vitamins and characterized by pale mucus membrane, weak and debilitated body and decreased number of erythrocytes with hypochromasia in blood.

Etiology
- Deficiency of iron
- Deficiency of copper
- Deficiency of cobalt
- Deficiency of vitamin B_{12}, Pyridoxine, riboflavin and folic acid.
- Parasitic infestation may lead to deficiency.

Macroscopic and microscopic features
- Pale mucous membrane
- Thin watery blood with light red colour
- Weak and debilitated carcass
- Heavy parasitic load in gastrointestinal tract.
- Microcytic hypochromic erythrocytes.
- **Poikilocytosis**

TOXIC APLASTIC ANEMIA

Toxic aplastic anemia is agenesis or aplasia of hemopoietic tissues in bone marrow and there is lack of erythrocyte production. It is characterized by the absence of developmental stages of erythrocytes viz., normoblasts, megaloblasts etc.

Etiology
- **Radiation *e.g.* X-rays, g rays, or UV rays**
- Sulfonamides
- Bracken fern toxicity
- Uremia
- **Feline panleukopenia**

Macroscopic and microscopic features
- Pale mucuos membrane
- Weak and debilitated animal
- Dyspnoea
- **Bone marrow becomes yellow/ fatty.**
- Absence of developmental stages or RBC such as normoblasts, megaloblasts etc.
- Agranulocytosis i.e. Reduction of WBC in circulating blood.
- Bone marrow becomes fatty.

AUTOIMMUNE HEMOLYTIC ANEMIA

Autoimmune hemolytic anemia occurs as a result of destruction of erythrocytes by immune mechanisms developed against erythrocytes.

Etiology
- Autoimmune hemolytic anemia in foals.
- Antibodies produced against own RBC of an animal.
- Equine infectious anemia
- Anaplasmosis
- Systemic lupus erythematosus

Macroscopic and microscopic features
- Pale mucous membrane
- Enlargement of liver, spleen and lymphnodes
- Hemoglobinuria
- Lameness due to rheumatoid arthritis
- Erythrophagocytosis
- Demonstration of antibodies against own RBC in sera of animals.
- Active erythropoiesis
- Glomerulonephritis

POLYCYTHEMIA

Polycythemia is increase in number of erythrocytes in circulating blood. It may be relative increase as a result of dehydration or decrease in plasma volume or absolute due to anoxia.

Etiology
- Dehydration due to diarrhoea, vomiting and loss of fluid in oedema/ inflammation.
- Anoxia in high altitudes.
- Heart diseases *e.g.* Patent ductus arteriosus
- Severe pulmonary emphysema
- Erythroid leukemia

Macroscopic and microscopic features
- Dehydration, mucous membrane dry, sticky
- Pulmonary emphysema, fibrosis in lungs
- **Increase hemoglobin concentration**

Differential features of various types of Anaemia

	Hemolytic	Hemorrhagic	Deficiency	Toxic/Aplastic	Autoimmune Hemolytic
Macroscopic features	1. Pale mucus membranes 2. Icterus 3. Blood is thin, watery. 4. Hemoglobinurea	1. Petechiae or Echymotic haemorrhage 2. Pale mucus membrane 3. Hematuria	1. Pale mucous membrane 2. Thin watery blood with light red colour 3. Weak and debilitated carcass 4. Heavy parasitic load in gastro-intestinal tract.	1. Pale mucus membrane 2. Weak and debilitated animal 3. Dyspnoea 4. Bone marrow becomes yellow/ fatty	1. Pale mucous membrane 2. Enlargement of liver, spleen and lymphnodes 3. Hemoglobinuria 4. Lameness due to rheumatoid arthritis
Microscopic features	1. Decreased number of erythrocytes 2. Presence of nucleated/ immature RBC in blood 3. Hemosiderin laden cells in spleen	1. Hemorrhage in various tissues/ organs 2. Macrocytic or normocytic characters of RBC 3. Poikilocytosis 4. Hyperplasia of bone marrow	1. Microcytic hypochromic erythrocytes. 2. Poikilocytosis	1. Absence of developmental stages or RBC such as normoblasts, megaloblasts etc. 2. Agranulocytosis i.e. Reduction of WBC in circulating blood. 3. Bone marrow becomes fatty.	1. Erythrophagocytosis 2. Demonstration of antibodies against own RBC in sera of animals. 3. Active erythropoiesis 4. Glomerulonephritis

- Increased number of erythrocytes
- Severe damage in lungs, congestion, emphysema, fibrosis

LEUCOCYTOSIS

Leucocytosis is increase in number of leucocytes in circulating blood caused by various infections. There is also increase in white blood cells in blood due to neoplastic condition and is known as *Leukemia*. As the leucocytes consist of neutrophils, lymphocytes eosinophils, monocytes and basophils; the increase in number of neutrophils is termed as *neutrophilia*, eosinophils as *eosinophilia*, lymphocytes as *lymphocytosis*, basophils as *basophilia* and of monocytes as *monocytosis*.

Etiology
- Infections
- Bacterial infection- neutrophilia
- Viral infections and chronic bacterial infections- lymphocytosis
- Parasites- eosinophilia
- Allergies- basophilia, lymphocytosis

Macroscopic and microscopic features
- No characteristic lesion.
- Reactive lymph node hyperplasia.
- Enlargement of lymphoid organs such as spleen, thymus and bursa.
- Increase in number of total leucocytes in blood
- Increase in absolute lymphocyte, absolute neutrophil, absolute eosinophil counts.
- Heperplastic lesions in lymphoid organs.

LEUCOPENIA

Leucopenia is decrease in number of white blood cells. The leucocytes are neutrophils, lymphocytes monocytes, eosinophils and basophils. If there is decrease in number of all 5 cells of leucocytes, it is known as *panleucopenia*. The decrease in number of neutrophils is termed as *neutropenia* and lymphocytes as *lymphopenia*.

Etiology
- Congenital *e.g.* Chediak Higashi syndrome
- Infections *e.g.* Feline panleucopenia virus, infectious bursal disease virus
- Chemicals *e.g.* Pesticides, heavy metals
- Radiation *e.g.* X-rays

Macroscopic and microscopic features
- Atrophy of lymphoid organs
- Recurrent infections, vaccination failures, pyogenic disorders.
- Edema, hemorrhage in bursa, atrophy of bursa due to fibrosis in IBD infection.
- Decrease in total leucocyte count and absolute neutrophil and absolute lymphocyte counts
- Degeneration and necrosis of lymphoid cells in follicles of lymphoid organ
- Edema, necrosis, proliferation of fibrous tissue in bursa in IBD infection.

PATHOLOGY OF SPLEEN

SPLENITIS

Spleenitis is the inflammation of spleen characterized by enlargement, infiltration of inflammatory cells, proliferation of lymphoid follicles, congestion and oedema followed by proliferation of fibrous tissue.

Etiology
- Infections *e.g.* bacteria, virus
- Deficiency of vitamins and minerals
- **Amyloidosis**
- Immunodeficiency *e.g.* environmental pollution

Macroscopic and microscopic features
- Enlargement of spleen.
- Necrotic patches on spleen.
- In chronic cases or in immunological disorders.
- There is atrophy of spleen due to fibrosis.
- Necrotic patches and congestion leading to mottling.
- Congestion in spleen.
- Proliferation of lymphoid follicles/ cells.
- Edema.
- In atrophied spleen, proliferation of fibrous tissue, depletion of lymphoid cells/ follicles.

PATHOLOGY OF LYMPHNODES

LYMPHADENITIS

Lymphadenitis is the inflammation of lymphnodes characterized by enlargement/ atrophy, congestion proliferation of lymphoid cells/ depletion of lymphoid cells, oedema AND fibrosis of lymphnodes.

Etiology
- Infections *e.g.* Rinderpest
- Immunological disorders *e.g.* immuno-deficiency
- Deficiency *e.g.* Deficiency of protein
- Environmental pollution *e.g.* pesticides, heavy metals
- Tumors/ neoplasm *e.g.* lymphosarcoma

Macroscopic and microscopic features
- Enlargement of lymphnodes
- Congestion
- Edema
- In chronic cases- fibrosis
- Atrophy
- Congestion, edema, proliferation of lymphoid cells.

- In chronic cases, proliferation of fibrous tissue, depletion of lymphoid cells

PATHOLOGY OF THYMUS

THYMOMA/ THYMIC HYPERPLASIA

It is characterized by congestion and hyperplasia of lymphoid cells in thymus. The inflammation of thymus in chronic cases is characterized by atrophy and proliferation of fibrous tissue.

Etiology
- Immunological disorders
- Environmental pollution *e.g.* Pesticide, Heavy metals
- Toxins/ poisons
- Aging *e.g.* in adult poultry thymus regresses

Macroscopic and microscopic features
- Congestion, reddening of thymus
- Edema
- Increase in size
- Atrophy, thinning like thread.
- Congestion, oedema
- Proliferation of lymphoid cells
- Depletion of lymphoid cells
- Proliferation of fibrous tissue

PATHOLOGY OF BURSA

BURSITIS

Bursitis is the inflammation of bursa of Fabricius in poultry characterized by edema, congestion, haemorrhage or atrophy and depletion of lymphoid cells.

Etiology
- Infectious Bursal disease virus (Birnavirus)
- Environmental pollution *e.g.* Pesticides, heavy metals.

Macroscopic and microscopic features
- Enlargement of bursa
- Congestion and/or hemorrhage
- In chronic cases, atrophy and fibrosis
- Edema
- Depletion of lymphoid tissue
- Degeneration and necrosis of lymphoid cells
- Congestion and/or haemorrhage.
- Proliferation fibrous tissue.

Chapter 18
Pathology of Urinary System

DEVELOPMENTAL ANOMALIES

Aplasia

Absence of one or both kidneys. Absence of one kidney is observed in animals with compensatory hypertrophy of another kidney and such animals may survive well.

Hypoplasia

The size of kidneys remain small which don't grow properly due to defect in a single recessive autosomal gene.

Cyst in Kidney

Single or multiple cysts in pig and dog kidney are reported with tinged yellow in colour. They may arise from nephron due to its distension. Presence of multiple cysts is also termed as congenital polycystic kidney.

- *Type-I* cysts are formed due to dilation and hyperplasia of collecting tubules resulting in spongiform kidneys. In such neonates cystic bile ducts are also present.
- *Type-II* polycystic kidney is formed due to absence of collecting tubules and developmental failure of nephron. The cysts are thick walled with dense connective tissue and may involve one or both kidneys.
- *Type-III* cysts in kidneys occur due to multiple abnormalities during development. Cysts develop from tubules or Bowmen's capsule with part of glomeruli in cyst. This condition is bilateral and causes considerable enlargement of kidney due to clear fluid or blood mixed fluid containing cysts.

FUNCTIONAL DISTURBANCES

Proteinuria: Presence of protein particularly albumin in urine. Protein is found as smooth, homogenous, pink staining precipitate also called as 'cast'. The presence of albumin in urine is indicative of damage in glomeruli. It is also characterized by oedema due to protein deficiency.

Hematuria: Presence of blood in urine giving bright red colour. It may occur due to damage in glomeruli, tubule or haemorrhage anywhere from glomeruli to urethra. The most important cause of hematuria is bracken fern toxicity.

Hemoglobinuria: When hemoglobin is present in urine without erythrocytes due to intravascular hemolysis. The urine becomes brownish red in colour. It must be differentiated from hematuria in which intact erythrocytes are present and settle down after some time leaving clear urine as supernatant. Hemoglobinuria is caused by various infections such as *Leptospira* sp., *Babesia* sp. or phosphorus deficiency in animals.

Anuria

Absence of urine is known as anuria which may be due to:
- Absence of urinary secretion due to glomerulonephritis
- Inelastic renal capsule unable to exert sufficient pressure required for glomerular filtration leading to nephrosis.
- Due to Hydronephrosis or calculi urine already secreted puts back pressure to prevent further secretion.
- Low blood pressure
- Dehydration
- Necrosis of tubular epithelium

Polyuria: Increased amount of urine leading to frequent urination caused due to diabetes insipedus, hormonal imbalance and polydypsia. In this condition, waste products are successfully eliminated.

Uremia: The presence of harmful waste products like uric acid, creatinine and urea in blood. Normally such waste products are removed by excretion through kidneys. But due to damage in kidneys or obstruction by inflammation, neoplasm, abscess and most importantly by presence of calculi urine remains in the system and causes uremia. Uremia is characterized by headache, vomiting, hyperirritability, convulsion, ulcers in oral cavity and stomach, normochromic and normocytic anemia, hemosiderosis and thrombocytopenia.

Glycosuria: Presence of glucose in urine. This is also known as diabetes mellitus, a metabolic disorder. It may occur due to insulin deficiency. This condition is not common in animals. However, it may occur in dogs as a result of hypoglycemia. It may occur in sheep due to enterotoxemia caused by *Clostridium welchii* type D.

Pyuria: Presence of pus in urine due to suppurative inflammation in urinary tract.

Ketonuria: Presence of ketone bodies in urine, which is common in diabetes mellitus, acetonemia, pregnancy toxemia and in starvation.

Oligouria: In this condition, there is decreased amount of urine, which occurs due to glomerulonephritis, obstruction in urinary passage, dehydration, low blood pressure and tubular damage.

NEPHROSIS

Nephrosis is the degeneration and necrosis of tubular epithelium without producing inflammatory reaction. It mostly includes acute tubular necrosis as a result of ischemia or toxic injury to kidney. Nephrosis is characterized by necrosis and sloughing of tubular epithelial cells exhibited by uremia, oligouria, anuria.

Etiology
- Hypotension
- Heavy metals
- Mycotoxins *e.g.* Ochratoxin
- Antibiotics *e.g.* Gentamicin

Macroscopic and microscopic features
- Swelling of kidneys
- Capsular surface smooth, pale and translucent.
- Vacuolation in tubular epithelium.
- Coagulative necrosis.
- Sloughing of tubular epithelium

GLOMERULONEPHRITIS

Glomerulonephritis is the inflammation of glomeruli primarily characterized by pale and enlarged kidneys with potential hemorrhage, oedema of glomeruli, congestion and infiltration of inflammatory cells. Due to presence of mesangial proliferation, it is also called as mesangio-proliferative glomerulonephritis (MPGN).

Etiology
- Streptococci infection
- Immune complexes
- Environmental pollutants such as - Organochlorine pesticides

Macroscopic and microscopic features
- Enlarged kidneys
- Edema, pale kidneys
- Petechiae on kidneys
- Proteinuria, uremia, hypercholesterolemia and increased creatinine level in blood.
- Edema of glomeruli leading to increase in size.
- Infiltration of neutrophils, macrophages.
- Compression of blood capillaries and absence of erythrocytes.
- Thrombosis and necrosis of glomerular capillaries.
- Based on type of lesions, it can be divided into 5 subtypes.

1. Type-I MPGN
- Proliferation of mesangial cells.
- Deposition of immune complexes containing IgG, IgM, IgA and C_3.
- Immune complexes penetrate vascular endothelium but not the basement membrane and are deposited in subendothelial region.
- Proliferation and swelling of endothelial cells.
- Immune complexes induce production of transforming growth factor ($TGFB_1$) which increases production of fibronectin, collagen and proteoglycans leading to thickness of basement membrane; this is also known as "wire loop" lesions.

2. Type-II MPGN (Membranous)
- Deposition of immune complexes in basement membrane (lamina densa).
- Due to uncontrolled activation of complement.
- Proliferation of endothelium and mesangial cells.
- Demonstration of C_3 component, no immunoglobulin.

3. Type III MPGN (Acute Proliferative)
- Subepithelial deposits of immune complexes and disruption of basement membrane.
- Swelling of epithelium and its proliferation forming "Epithelial cresent".
- Demonstration of IgG in subepithelial region.
- Congestion and edema of glomeruli.
- Infiltration of neutrophils, macrophages and lymphocytes.

4. Chronic glomerulonephritis
- Proliferation of epithelial and endothelial cells
- Reduplication, thickening and disorganization of glomerular basement membrane.
- Lumen of capillaries occluded.
- Entire glomerulus is replaced by Hyaline connective tissue.

5. Focal embolic glomerulonephritis
- Focal zone of necrosis in glomeruli
- Infiltration of neutrophils
- Proliferation of epithelial cells and formation of crescent.

INTERSTITIAL NEPHRITIS

Interstitial nephritis is the inflammation of kidney characterized by degeneration and necrosis of tubular epithelium, edema and infiltration of inflammatory cells in interstitium.

Etiology
- Ochratoxins and atrinin.
- Leptospira
- Toxins/ poisons *e.g.* Pesticides.
- Herpes virus
- Endogenous toxaemia *e.g.* Ketosis
- Immune complexes

Macroscopic and microscopic features
- Enlargement of kidneys
- Necrosis, congestion and hemorrhage
- Edema, congestion, hemorrhage
- Necrosis and degeneration of tubular epithelium
- Infiltration of inflammatory cells like neutrophils, macrophages and lymphocytes in interstitium.
- Loss of tubules, foci of mononuclear cells, fibrosis in chronic cases
- Immune complexes are deposited in granular form causing degeneration of epithelial cells of tubules and mononuclear cell infiltration.

PYELONEPHRITIS

Pyelonephritis is the inflammation of renal pelvis and parenchyma i.e. tubules characterized by congestion, suppurative inflammation and fibrosis.

Etiology
- *Corynebacterium renale*
- *Staphylococcus aureus*
- *E. coli*
- *Actinomyces pyogenes*
- *Pseudomonas aeruginosa*

Macroscopic and microscopic features
- Congestion, hemorrhage and abscess formation in renal cortex, pelvis and ureters.
- Pyuria- Pus mixed urine in bladder.
- Enlargement of kidneys
- Congestion, hemorrhage
- Suppurative inflammation of pelvis and kidney parenchyma.
- Necrosis of collecting ducts.
- Purulent exudate in pelvis.
- Infiltration of neutrophils, lymphocytes and plasma cells in interstitium.

NEPHROSCLEROSIS

Nephrosclerosis is chronic fibrosis of kidney characterized by loss of glomeruli and tubules and extensive fibrosis.

Etiology
- Glomerulonephritis
- Interstitial nephritis
- Arteriolscleresis

Macroscopic and microscopic features
- Hard, atrophied kidneys.
- Fibrous nodules on kidneys.
- Thickening of capsule.
- Small white firm kidneys.
- Ischemia, tubular atrophy

Differential features of various types of Nephritis

	Glomerulonephritis	Interstitial	Pyelonephritis
Macroscopic features	1. Enlarged kidneys 2. Edema, pale kidneys 3. Petechiae on kidneys 4. Proteinuria, uremia, hypercholesterolemia and increased creatinine level in blood.	1. Enlargement of kidneys 2. Necrosis, congestion and hemorrhage	1. Congestion, hemorrhage and abscess formation in renal cortex, pelvis and ureters. 2. Pyuria- Pus mixed urine in bladder. 3. Enlargement of kidneys
Microscopic features	1. Edema of glomeruli leading to increase in size. 2. Infiltration of neutrophils, macrophages. 3. Compression of blood capillaries and absence of erythrocytes. 4. Thrombosis and necrosis of glomerular capillaries.	1. Edema, congestion, hemorrhage 2. Necrosis and degeneration of tubular epithelium 3. Infiltration of inflammatory cells like neutrophils, macrophages and lymphocytes in interstitium. 4. Loss of tubules, foci of mononuclear cells, fibrosis in chronic cases 5. Immune complexes are deposited in granular form causing degeneration of epithelial cells of tubules and mononuclear cell infiltration.	1. Congestion, hemorrhage 2. Suppurative inflammation of pelvis and kidney parenchyma. 3. Necrosis of collecting ducts. 4. Purulent exudate in pelvis. 5. Infiltration of neutrophils, lymphocytes and plasma cells in interstitium.

- Loss of glomeruli and tubules
- Extensive fibrosis
- Deposition of hyaline mass
- **Infiltration of mononuclear cells.**

UROLITHIASIS

Urolithiasis is the formation of stony precipitates any where in the urinary passage including kidneys, ureter, urinary bladder or urethra.

Etiology
- Bacterial infections
- Metabolic defects
- Vitamin A deficiency
- Hyperparathyroidism
- **Mineral imbalance**

Macroscopic and microscopic features
- Nephrosis, Hydronephrosis
- Distension of ureters
- Distension of ureters and urinary bladder
- **Hard enlarged kidneys**
- **Presence of calculi/ stone in kidney, ureter, bladder or urethra.**
- Presence of crystals/ stone in lumen of tubules.
- Degeneration and necrosis of tubular epithelium.
- Hemorrhage
- Proliferation of fibrous tissue

There are various types of calculi, which differ in size, shape and composition. Some of them are as under:

Oxalate calculi are hard, light yellow, covered with sharp spines found in urinary bladder and formed due to calcium oxalate. It causes damage in urinary bladder leading to haemorrhage.

Uric acid calculi are composed of ammonium and sodium urates and uric acids, yellow to brown in colour, formed in acidic urine, spherical and irregular in shape and they are not radioopaque.

Phosphate calculi are white or grey in colour, chalky in consistency, soft, friable and can be crushed with mild pressure. They are mostly multiple in the form of sand like granules. They are composed of magnesium ammonium phosphate and occur as a result of bacterial infection.

Xanthine calculi are brownish red, concentrically laminated, fragile and irregular in shape. They rarely occur in animals.

Cystine calculi are small, soft with shiny and greasy in appearance, yellow in colour which becomes darker on air exposure. Insoluble amino acid cystine precipitates in bladder to form calculi. Such calculi may cause obstruction of urethra with cystinuria.

PATHOLOGY OF URETER

URETERITIS

Ureteritis is the inflammation of ureter characterized by enlargement, thickening of wall due to accumulation of urates, or calculi, pyonephrosis and pyelonephritis.

Etiology
- Tuberculosis
- Calculi
- Hydronephrosis
- Pyelonephritis
- Pyonephrosis

Macroscopic and microscopic features
- Deposits of whitish/ yellowish urates in ureter in poultry.
- Obstructions of ureter due to calculi leads to its enlargement and formation of diverticulum.
- Thickening of the wall due to congestion and infiltration of inflammatory cells.

- Extensive fibrosis with infiltration of mononuclear cells in chronic cases.

PATHOLOGY OF URINARY BLADDER

CYSTITIS

Cystitis is the inflammation of urinary bladder characterized by congestion and fibrinous, purulent or hemorrhagic exudates.

Etiology
- Urinary calculi
- Tuberculosis
- **Blockage in urethra**
- **Bracken fern poisoning**

Macroscopic and microscopic features
- Congestion, hemorrhage.
- Enlargement of urinary bladder.
- Thickening of the wall.
- Presence of small nodules on wall.
- Thickening of wall due to infiltration of neutrophils and macrophages.
- Granuloma in tuberculosis.
- Fibrosis
- Presence of neoplasm.

PATHOLOGY OF URETHRA

URETHRITIS

Inflammation of urethra is known as urethritis, which occurs as a result of catheter injury and calculi. It is characterized by congestion, obstruction, hydronephrosis and strictures.

Etiology
- Calculi
- Catheter injury

- *Trichomonas foetus* infection
- Picorna virus infection

Macroscopic and microscopic features
- Transient inflammation, congestion and hemorrhage.
- Strictures (male), diverticulum (female)
- Obstruction due to calculi, presence of calculi
- Thickening due to inflammatory exudate.

Chapter 19
Pathology of Genital System

FEMALE GENITAL SYSTEM

DEVELOPMENTAL ANOMALIES

Agenesis

Absence of ovary, uterus, oviduct and cervix in females. It may be unilateral or bilateral.

Hypoplasia

Complete or partial lack of germ cells in ovaries. Hypoplasia of uterus is related with agenesis of gonads. Ovaries of freemartin are also hypoplastic. Hermaphrodite animal has ovary and testicular tissue both in the gonads.

Hermaphroditism

In hermaphrodites, there is presence of organs of both sexes in same individual animal. Both ovarian and testicular tissue occur in one animal leads to sterility in animal (true hermaphrodite) while in pseudohermaphrodite the gonadal tissue of only one sex is present but there is some degree of development of opposite sex organs.

Uterus unicornis

Uterus unicornis is presence of only one horn of uterus instead of two, seen in animals with white heifer disease.

White heifer disease

White heifer disease occurs due to a single sex linked gene defect responsible for white coat colour. In such animals, there are normal ovaries, oviduct but uterus is incomplete and may lack communication with cervix. There is hypoplasia of cervix and vagina.

Uterus didelphys

Uterus didelphys is the occurrence of two cervix with two uterine bodies and single or double vagina. It occurs due to failure of Mullerian ducts to fuse at their distal end. Sometimes failure of fusion may affect only cervix and there is two cervix which is termed as *Cervix bifida*.

CYSTIC OVARIES

Cystic ovaries are defined as an ovary, which contains one or more clear cysts ranging from one to several centimeters in size.

Etiology
- Hormonal imbalance

Macroscopic and microscopic features
- Presence of cysts in ovaries.
- Hormonal imbalance of animal leads to sterility, continuous estrus, nymphomania due to follicular cyst.
- Lutein cysts may cause pyometra leading to pseudopregnancy.
- Follicular cyst
- Ova absent several layers of granulosa or a single layer of epithelium.
- Many follicular cysts are present
- Lutein cyst covered by fat containing granulosa cells.

OOPHORITIS

Oophoritis is the inflammation of ovary caused by trauma, infection and characterized by granulomatous or lymphocytic inflammation of ovary.

Etiology
- *Mycobacterium tuberculosis*
- Herpes virus

Macroscopic and microscopic features
- Hard, nodular lesions in ovary, encapsulated with fibrous tissue.
- Granuloma of tuberculosis through hematogenous infection.
- Infiltration of lymphocytes leading to lymphofollicular reaction in follicles.
- Atrophy or absence of ova.

SALPINGITIS

Salpingitis is the inflammation of oviduct or fallopian tube characterized by congestion, catarrhal or purulent exudate leading to distended lumen.

Etiology
- Mycoplasma
- Streptococci
- Tuberculosis (*Mycobacterium tuberculosis*)
- Trichomoniasis (*Trichomonas foetus*)

Macroscopic and microscopic features
- Congestion, abscess formation
- Distension of oviduct lumen due to accumulation of serous exudate which is known as ***Hydrosalpinx.***
- Accumulation of pus in oviduct is termed as ***Pyosalpinx.***
- Fibrosis, hardness
- Occlusion of lumen due to inflammatory exudate resulting in sterility.
- Inflammatory exudate is toxic to ova as well as sperms leading to sterility.

- Suppurative inflammation
- Infiltration of neutrophils, macrophages and lymphocytes
- Proliferation of fibrous tissue
- Debris of desquamated cells

METRITIS

Metritis is the inflammation of uterus characterized by suppurative exudate, hemorrhage and necrosis of uterus.

Etiology
- Actinomyces pyogenes
- E.coli
- Staphylococci
- Streptococci
- *Trichomonas foetus*
- *Campylobacter foetus*

Macroscopic and microscopic features
- Congestion, catarrhal or purulent exudate
- Hemorrhage
- Enlargement, oedema
- Oozing out of pus from uterus on pressure
- Seropurulent exudate in uterine wall.
- Edema
- Infiltration of macrophages and lymphocytes
- Desquamation of lining epithelium

PYOMETRA

Pyometra is an acute or chronic suppurative inflammation of uterus resulting in accumulation of pus in the uterus.

Etiology
- Occurs under the influence of progesterone.
- *E. coli*

- *Actinomyces pyogenes*
- *Proteus* spp.
- *Staphylococcus aureus*
- *Trichomonas foetus*

Macroscopic and microscopic features
- Discharge of thin cream like pus from vulva soiling the tail and perineal region.
- Pus discharge is more on sitting position of animal.
- Enlargement of abdomen due to distension of uterus.
- Uterus looking like as pregnant uterus as a result of accumulation of pus. This condition is also known as ***Pseudocyesis*** or ***pseudopregnancy.***
- Rention of lutein cyst.
- Congestion, infiltration of neutrophils, lymphocytes and plasma cells.
- Necrosis of mucosal epithelium of uterus.
- Proliferation of endometrial epithelium.
- Edema, glandular hyperplasia.

ENDOMETRITIS

Endometritis is the inflammation of endometrium, the mucosa of uterus. It may be catarrhal or purulent and may occur after metritis.

Etiology
- *Trichomonas foetus*
- *Campylobacter foetus*
- Staphylococci
- Streptococci
- Organism enters in uterus as a result of coitus, artificial insemination or as iatrogenic infection.
- Strong chemicals/ medicines administered in uterus.

Macroscopic and microscopic features
- Catarrhal discharge from uterus containing desquamated cells.
- Sterility due to toxic environment of uterus to sperms.
- Congestion.
- Congestion
- Moderate infiltration of lymphocytes, plasma cells and neutrophils in mucosa.

CERVICITIS

Cervicitis is the inflammation of cervix as a result of either descending infection from uterus or ascending infection from vagina and characterized by catarrhal inflammation.

Etiology
- Etiological agents are similar as in endometritis.

Macroscopic and microscopic features
- Congestion
- Enlargement of cervix.
- Catarrhal inflammation of cervical mucosa.
- Hyperplasia of mucous glands with tall mucin containing epithelial cells.
- Presence of mucin in lumen.

VAGINITIS

Vaginitis is the inflammation of vagina characterized by congestion, granularity as a result of elevations in mucosa. This is also known as *infectious pustular vulvovaginitis* in cattle caused by herpes virus.

Etiology
- *Mycoplasma bovigenitalium*
- Bovine herpes virus-1 (BHV-1)
- Picorna virus
- *Trichomonas foetus*

Macroscopic and microscopic features
- Granular elevation in vaginal mucosa.
- Congestion
- Prolapse due to limitation.
- Accumulation of lymphocytes in sub epithelial region.
- Congestion

ABORTION

Abortion is expulsion of dead embryo or foetus before attaining normal gestation. There are two other terms related to abortion i.e. stillbirth and premature birth. *Stillbirth* is defined as expulsion of dead foetus on its full maturity while *premature birth* is birth of a live foetus before attaining full gestation period.

Etiology
- Brucellosis (*Brucella abortus, B. meletensis, B. ovis*)
- *Campylobacter foetus*
- *Salmonella abortus-equi*- mares
- Equine herpes virus- mares
- Bovine herpes virus-1- cattle
- *Chlamydia psittasci*
- *Trichomonas foetus*
- *Listeria monocytogenes* (*Listeria ivanovii*)
- *Leptospria* spp.
- *Mycobacterium tuberculosis*
- *Toxoplasma gondii*
- *Mycoplasma mycoides*
- Fungi- *Aspergillus* spp., *Coccidioides* spp. *Absidia* spp.
- Toxins/ poisons

Macroscopic and microscopic features
- Expulsion of dead foetus in early stage (3-4 month) of gestation (Trichomoniasis)

- Abortion in middle of gestation (Campylobacteriosis).
- Late abortions (7-9 months) occur due to Brucellosis, BHV-1 infection.
- Liver of foetus has necrotic foci, congestion.
- Stomach contents used for confirmation of **Etiology.**
- In some cases of abortion, there is retention of placenta (*e.g.* Brucellosis)
- Placenta becomes oedematous and necrotic (Placentitis)
- If the foetus becomes dead and not expelled outside the body due to non-opening of cervix, the dead foetus remains in uterus under sterile conditions. Such foetus undergoes autolysis and liquified. Liquid material is absorbed in uterus through lymph or blood and bones/ skin etc. remain in uterine horn sometimes causing irritation or damage to endometrium. Such foetus becomes shrunken with wrinkled skin and dried as mummy and are known as *"Mummified foetus".*
- Necrotic hepatitis with lymphofollicular reaction in foetus (Brucellosis, BHV-1 infection).
- Granulomatous lesions (tuberculosis, fungal infection), lymphofollicular reaction (mycoplasma, chlamydia).
- Demonstration/ isolation of causative organisms in foetal stomach contents.
- Liver of foetus icteric (leptospirosis)
- Endometritis in dam.
- Bronchopneumonia in foetus *e.g.* brucellosis.

RETAINED PLACENTA/ PLACENTITIS

Retention of placenta occurs after abortion or parturition as a result of inflammation characterized by swelling, edema or fibrosis which prevent the separation of chorion from endometrium.

Etiology
- Lack of progesterone

- Infection *e.g.* Brucellosis, Trichomoniasis.

Macroscopic and microscopic features
- Retained placenta undergoes autolysis, putrefaction
- Toxaemia in dam.
- Endometritis, Pyometra
- Placenta is oedematous and congested
- Infiltration of neutrophils, mononuclear cells.
- Proliferation of fibroblasts.

MASTITIS

Mastitis is the inflammation of mammary gland characterized by oedema, haemorrhage and fibrosis of udder. Mastitis is always infectious and is a disease of lactating glands. There is no hematogenous infection and infections enter through teat canal to cause mastitis.

Etiology
- Bacteria *e.g. Streptococcus agalactiae, Streptococcus dysgalactiae, Staphylococcus aureus, Actinomyces pyogenes, Pseudomonas aeruginosa, Brucella abortus, Mycobacterium tuberculosis, E. coli, Pasteurella multocida* and many more.
- Virus *e.g.* FMD virus, pox virus, BHV-1
- Mycoplasma *e.g. Mycoplasma mycoides*
- Fungi *e.g. Candida ablicans, Trichosporon* spp. *Nocardia asteroids, Cryptococcus neoformans.*

Macroscopic and microscopic features
- Edema of udder
- Flakes (coagulated milk proteins) in milk.
- Blood mixed milk
- **Watery dirty grey or dark colour milk in animals, which are in dry period caused by *Actinomyces pyogenes* and is known as *"summer mastitis"*.**
- Terminal atrophy or shrunken quarter
- Gangrene formation

- Congestion, haemorrhage
- Infiltration of neutrophils, macrophages, lymphocytes
- Necrosis of alveolar epithelium, hyperplasia of epithelial lining.
- Proliferation of fibrous tissue
- Increase in WBC count in milk (more than 100/ ml milk).

MALE GENITAL SYSTEM

DEVELOPMENTAL ANOMALIES

Testicular hypoplasia

Testicular hypoplasia occurs in animals with chromosomal abnormality such as XXY chromosomes or Klinefelter's syndrome. Hypoplasia is also seen in hermaphrodites and in animals with cryptorchidism.

Spermatocele

There is failure of development of mesonephric tubules and does not connect with vas deferens resulting into blind tubules filled with spermatozoa. Rupture of tubules may lead to spermatic granuloma.

Cryptorchidism

The testicle fails to descend in scrotum through inguinal canal after birth and remains in abdominal cavity. This permanent retention of testicles in abdominal cavity causes their hypoplasia leading to lack of spermatogenesis. Such testes are more prone for development of neoplastic growth.

Phimosis

Phimosis is the failure of extension of penis from its sheath.

Paraphimosis

Paraphimosis is the failure of withdrawal of extended penis.

Hypospadias

In hypospadias, there is urethral opening in ventral side of the penis.

Epispadias

There is urthral opening on the dorsal side of the penis

Phallocampsis

Phallocampsis is the deviation of penis, which may be spiral (*Cork screw penis*) or ventral deviation (*rainbow penis*).

ORCHITIS

Orchitis is the inflammation of testes characterized by edema, necrosis and infiltration of neutrophils, macrophages, lymphocytes and proliferation of fibrous tissue leading to atrophy in chronic cases.

Etiology

- *Brucella* spp.
- *Campylobactor* spp.
- *Salmonella* spp.
- *Trichomonas* spp.
- *Corynebacterium pseudotuberculosis*
- *Actinomycess pyogenes*
- *Pseudomanas aeruginosa*
- *Actinomyces bovis*

Macroscopic and microscopic features
- Enlargement of testes, oedema.
- Accumulation of serous fluid in scrotal sac/ tunica vaginalis is called as *hydrocele*.
- Enlargement of scrotum.
- Congestion
- Atrophy and hardening in chronic cases.
- Congestion
- Infiltration of neutrophils and mononuclear cells

- Necrosis of germinal cells
- Proliferation of fibrous tissue and infiltration of mononuclear cells.
- Granulomatous lesions in case of actinomycosis and tuberculosis
- Aspermatogenesis

EPIDIDYMITIS

Epididymitis is the inflammation of epididymis characterized by catarrhal or suppurative exudate with necrosis of lining epithelium.

Etiology
- *Brucella ovis* in sheep
- Other organisms that cause orchitis which is preceded by epidiymitis

Macroscopic and microscopic features
- Enlargement of epididymis
- Edema of scrotum
- Accumulation of mucus and/or purulent exudate in epididymis.
- Accumulation of serous exudate in scrotum.
- Necrosis of lining epithelium of epididymis
- Infiltration of neutrophils, macrophages and lymphocytes
- Edema
- Formation of granuloma in chronic cases.

FUNICULITIS

Funiculitis is inflammation of scirrhous cord characterized by enlargement of scrotum due to chronic abscess.

Etiology/ Occurrence
- Botryomycosis
- Actinomycosis
- Castration

- Unsanitary conditions

Macroscopic and microscopic features
- Enlargement of scrotum
- Hard swelling/ chronic abscess
- Chronic hyperplastic/ proliferative changes.
- Fibroplasia
- Infiltration of macrophages, lymphocytes, neutrophils around sulfur granules forming rosette.

SEMINAL VESICULITIS

Seminal vesiculitis is the inflammation of seminal vesicle characterized by metaplasia of the columnar epithelial lining to cornfied stratified squamous epithelium.

Etiology
- *Pseudomonas aeruginosa*
- *Chlamydia psittasci*
- *Mycoplasma bovigenitalium*
- *Actinomyces pyogenes*
- *Corynebacterium renale*
- *Brucella abortus*
- *E. coli*

Macroscopic and microscopic features
- Melanosis in bulbourethral glands.
- Enlargement/ hardness of seminal vesicle
- Metaplasia of columnar epithelium into severely cornified stratified squamous epithelium.
- Proliferation of melanoblasts/ melanocytes.

PROSTATITIS

Prostatitis is the inflammation of prostate gland by formation of painful abscess, atrophy, hyperplasia of epithelial cells, proliferation of fibroblasts and formation of cysts. It occurs in dogs.

Etiology
- Hormonal imbalance
- Pyogenic staphylococci, streptococci

Macroscopic and microscopic features
- Presence of abscess encapsulated by fibrous tissue
- Enlargement of prostate causing obstruction of urethra
- Obstruction in rectal passage
- Hematuria
- Infiltration of neutrophils and liquefied necrosis.
- Chronic inflammation is characterized by hyperplasia of glandular epithelium, fibroblasts and smooth muscle fibers.
- Cystic glandular hyperplasia.
- Infiltration of lymphocytes.

BALANOPOSTHITIS

Balanoposthitis is the inflammation of prepuce and glans penis characterized by phimosis or paraphimosis and pain during copulation. Balanitis is inflammation of glans penis and posthitis is inflammation of prepuce.

Etiology
- *Trichomonas foetus*
- BHV-1 virus
- Vesicular exanthema virus
- *Mycoplasma* spp.
- *Pseudomonas aeruginosa*
- *Actinomyces pyogenes*
- *Corynebacterium renale*

Macroscopic and microscopic features
- Phimosis and paraphimosis due to pain, adhesions
- Congestion
- Fibrinopurulent exudate
- Lymphocytic infiltration, congestion.

Chapter 20
Pathology of Nervous System

Nervous system is composed of brain, spinal cord, and peripheral nerves. The neuron is a basic functional unit of nervous system. Necrosis of neurons in brain is known as *encephalomalacia* while necrosis of neurons in spinal cord is termed as *myelomalacia*. If the necrosis occurs in gray matter it is known as *polioencephalomalacia* while necrosis of neurons in white matter is called as *leukoencephalomalacia*. There are three types of scavenger cells in nervous system known as *microglia, oligodendroglia* and *astrocytes*. Microlial cells surround the necrotic neurons and are known as *satellite cells* and the process is called as *satellitosis*. As the neuron dies, it is engulfed by microglial cell and this process is termed as *neuronophagia*. The necrosis of nerve fibers starts from myelin sheath and this change is called as *demyelination* or *Wallerian degeneration*.

The brain and spinal cord is covered by meninges. The inflammation of meninges is termed as *meningitis*. *Meningoencephalitis* is used for inflammation of both meninges and brain. Inflammation of duramater is known as *pachymeningitis* and of piamater is termed as *leptomeningitis*. *Hydrocephalus* means accumulation of clear fluid in ventricles and in sub arachnoid space due to obstruction in drainage. Hydrocephalus occurs in neonatal calves due to influenza and parainfluenza virus and is termed as *congenital hydrocephalus*.

Some nutritional deficiency like vitamin A, folic acid, vitamin B_{12}, niacin and zinc may also lead to hydrocephalus. Cerebeller hypoplasia has been observed due to bovine virus diarrhoea, hog cholera and feline panleukopenia virus. Some other congenital malformations are as under.

Anencephaly means absence of brain.

Microencephaly means small size of brain. *Cranioschisis* is failure of cranium to fuse which results in hernia of meninges and known as *meningocele*. Hernia of meninges and brain is known as *meningoencephalocele*.

ENCEPHALITIS

Encephalitis is the inflammation of brain characterized by purulent/ lymphocytic or proliferative changes. Encephalomyelitis is the inflammation of brain as well as spinal cord.

Etiology
- Bacteria
- *Listeria monocytogenes (L. ivanovii)* **main** cause
- *Haemophius* spp.
- *Pasturella* spp.
- Virus
- Mycoplasma
- Strychnine poisoning

Macroscopic and microscopic features
- Congestion
- Hemorrhage
- Small, tiny abscess
- Necrosis also known as encephalomalacia.
- Involvement of spinal cord leads to encephalomyelitis and of meninges is termed as meningoencephalitis.
- Tiny or micro abscess in cerebrum
- Infiltration by neutrophils and lymphocytes.
- Perivascular cuffing in Virchow Robin space by lymphocytes
- Necrosis of neurons.
- Satellitosis, neuronophagia
- Pleocytosis- Increase in number of white blood cells in cerebrospinal fluid.

ENCEPHALOMALACIA

Encephalomalacia is the necrosis of nervous tissue in brain characterized by loss of normal architecture and soft friable liquified mass.

Etiology
- Deficiency of copper, thiamine, vitamin-E.
- Poisons: Bracken fern, lead, mercury, salt poisoning, enterotoxaemia, mycotoxins.

Macroscopic and microscopic features
- Encephalomalacia- necrosis in brain.
- Myelomalacia necrosis in spinal cord.
- Poliomalacia is necrosis in brain gray matter.
- Leukomalacia is necrosis in brain white matter.
- Soft, friable liquified mass in brain.
- Congestion.
- Liquefactive necrosis
- Surrounded by neurological cells/ scavenger cells.
- Proliferation of small new capillaries

SPONGIFORM ENCEPHALOPATHY

Spongiform encephalopathy is characterized by the presence of vacuoles in grey and/or white matter.

Etiology
- Prion proteins
- Scrapie in sheep
- BSE in cattle

Macroscopic and microscopic features
- No characteristic gross lesion.
- Edema of brain or hydrocephalus
- Congestion
- Vacuolation in white and grey matter
- Vacuoles are usually in neurons, glial cells and in myelin

- Vacuoles are more extensive in medulla, pons and mid brain and gives brain "spongy form".

MENINGITIS

Meningitis is the inflammation of meninges, usually occurs alongwith encephalitis or encephalomyelitis and characterized by congestion and infiltration of neutrophils and mononuclear cells. Pachymeningitis is inflammation of durameter while leptomenigitis involves the piameter.

Etiology
- Virus *e.g.* swine fever
- Trauma
- Bacteria *e.g.* Pasturella, Listeria
- Toxoplasma
- Leptospira

Macroscopic and microscopic features
- Congestion
- Thickening of meninges.
- Petechial haemorrhage
- Infiltration of neutrophils and lymphocytes.
- Fibrosis

NEURITIS

Neuritis is the inflammation of nerves alongwith degenerative changes characterized by edema, infiltration of inflammatory cells.

Etiology
- Toxins
- Trauma
- Virus *e.g.* Marek's disease MD
- Lead and Mercury
- Bacteria *e.g.* Strangles
- Deficiency of vitamin E.

Macroscopic and microscopic features
- Wallerian degeneration
- Infiltration of neutrophils and lymphocytes.
- More destruction at distal end of the neuron.

Chapter 21
Pathology of Endocrine System, Eyes and Ear

PATHOLOGY OF HYPOTHALAMUS

The lesions in hypothalamus may cause diabetes insipedus characterized by polydypsia and polyuria with low specific gravity of urine. It occurs due to deficiency of antidiuretic hormone vasopressin.

Etiology/ Occurrence
- Lesions in hypothalamus and/or pituitary
- Adenoma and adenocarcinoma of pituitary
- Necrosis of hypothalamic nuclei due to larval migration

PATHOLOGY OF PITUITARY GLAND

HYPERPITUITARISM

Hyperpituitarism is increased secretion of hormone(s) from pituitary gland such as excessive secretion of somatotropic hormone may cause gigantism characterized by increased length of long bones, heavy and thick bones leading to large hands, feet, skull bones (*acromegaly*). Hyperpituitarism also increases adrenal cortical stimulating hormone leading to hyperplasia of adrenal cortex. Pituitary adenoma or adenocarcinoma is responsible for hyperpituitarism.

HYPOPITUITARISM

Hypopituitarism is decrease in pituitary hormone secretions due to atrophy, aplasia or hypoplasia of pituitary. Systemic diseases such as meningitis of bacterial or viral origin may also cause lesions in pituitary *e.g.* infectious canine hepatitis, hog cholera. It is characterized by dwarfism, genital hypoplasia and prolonged gestation period.

PATHOLOGY OF THYROID

HYPERTHYROIDISM

Hyperthyroidism is increased activity of thyroid gland leading to increased production of thyroxin characterized by tachycardia, increased basal metabolic rate, bulging of eyeballs and early maturity. It occurs due to presence of tumor in thyroid. Other signs included polydypsia, polyuria, and loss of weight, weakness, fatigue and hyperthermia.

HYPOTHYROIDISM

Hypothyroidism is reduced activity of thyroid gland characterized by decreased basal metabolic rate, obesity, retardation of growth and sexual development leading to cretinism. In adult, it is characterized by myxomatous mucoid degeneration in subcutaneous region giving floppy and edematous appearance. Hypothyroidism is caused by aplasia or hypoplasia of thyroid gland.

Goiter

Goiter is enlargement of thyroid gland, which may be accompanied by hypo- or hyperthyroidism. The enlargement of thyroid is due to hyperplasia, inflammation, or proliferation of connective tissue. The hyperplasia of gland is characterized by increased height and number to epithelial cells in acini of gland. It may be caused by deficiency of iodine, thiouracil toxicity and by use of goiterogenic substances such as soybean and cabbage. The goiter has been classified into 6 forms described as under:

Hyperplastic goiter

Due to iodine deficiency, there is hyperplasia of thyroid gland with reduction in thyroxin production. It occurs due to increased level of thyrotropic hormone from pituitary gland.

Familial goiter

There is hyperplasia of thyroid gland with reduced thyroxin secretion caused by defective or absence of enzymes responsible for thyroxin synthesis. It is not related with iodine deficiency but have congenital basis of occurrence

Colloid goiter

Colloid goiter is enlargement and distention of acini filled with colloid and flat epithelium caused by deficiency of iodine.

Adenomatous goiter

This is characterized by nodular enlargement of thyroid gland, with one or many hard nodules of variable in size and are characteristic adenoma of gland.

Toxic goiter

Toxic goiter is characterized by exophthalmus due to hyperthyroidism, enlargement of thyroid due to hyperplasia, and occurs as a hypersecretion of thyrotropic hormone from pituitary.

Equine goiter

Equine goiter is caused by excessive iodine levels in feed and occurs in new born foals with weakness from a goiterous mare. These foals are having enlarged thyroid gland.

LYMPHOCYTIC THYRODITIS

Lymphocytic thyroditis is characterized by infiltration of lymphocytes in gland causing destruction and is caused by autoimmune mechanism. The infiltration of lymphocytes is so severe that gives lymphofollicular appearance.

PATHOLOGY OF PARATHYROID GLAND

HYPOPARATHYROIDISM

Hypoparathyroidism is decreased activity of parathyroid gland characterized by decreased concentration of blood calcium and tonic spasms of muscles. It occurs due to infection, neoplasms, low calcium diets and hypersecretion of thyrocalcitonin.

HYPERPARATHYROIDISM

Hyperparathyroidism is the increased activity of parathyroid gland characterized by weakness, polydypsia, polyurea, hypercalcemia nephrocalcinosis, demineralization of bones, metastatic calcification in soft tissues and fibrous osteodystrophy. It may occur in adenoma or adenocarcinoma of parathyroid and hyperplasia of gland. Hyperparathyroidism is also associated with renal disease and chronic hypocalcemia to produce more parathormone hormone.

PATHOLOGY OF ADENAL GLANDS

HYPOADRENOCORTICISM

Hypoadrenocorticism is decreased activity of adrenal cortex characterized by atrophy, necrosis and decreased hormones leading to low blood pressure, decreased blood volume, hypoglycemia, gastrointestinal malfunction and hyperpigmentation in skin. It may occur in tuberculosis, histoplasmosis, amyloidosis, neoplasms and drug toxicity.

HYPERADRENOCORTICISM

Hyperadrenocorticism is increased activity of adrenal cortex characterized by hyperplasia and neoplasia of the gland leading to alopecia, muscle weakness, pendulous abdomen, obesity, polyuria, polydipsia, lymphopenia, eosinophilia, neutrophila and excessive secretion of 17- ketogenic steroids.

PATHOLOGY OF PANCREAS

Pancreatic islets or islets of Langerhans' are responsible for production of insulin, deficiency of which may cause hyperglycemia or diabetes mellitus. It is characterized by polyuria, glycosuria, hyperglycemia, polydypsia, loss of secretary granules in b-cells of pancreatic islets. It is caused by inflammation of pancreas causing excocrine pancreatitis. This condition may lead to arteriosclerosis in blood vessels of animals.

PATHOLOGY OF PINEAL GLAND

The pineal gland is responsible for secretion of melatonin hormone which inhibits gonadotropic hormone synthesis and release by pituitary and thus plays an important role in seasonal estrus/ reproductive capacity of animals. Degeneration and necrosis of gland may cause its decreased function but are not well reported. Adenoma of gland may be associated with increased sexual libido and activity.

PATHOLOGY OF EYE

Blepheritis is the inflammation of eyelids while *conjunctivitis* is used to describe the inflammatory condition of conjunctiva and *keratitis* for cornea. Inward turning of eyelid is known as *entropion* which may result in keratitis or conjunctivitis. Conjunctivitis is also caused by double row of eye lashes (*disctichiasis*).

DEVELOPMENTAL ANOMALIES

Aphakia is the absence of lens.

Microphakia is the small size of lens.

Hypoplasia of optic nerve is underdeveloped optic nerve with absence of optic nerve layer and ganglion cell layer of retina.

Agenesis of optic nerve is absence of optic nerve.

Coloboma is the congenital defect in the continuity of one of the tunics of the eye *i.e.* iris.

Congenital anophthalmos is the absence of the eye which may occur due to vitamin A deficiency in dam.

Congenital microphathalmos is the decreased size of eyes and may occur due to maternal vitamin A deficiency

Congenital opacity of cornea occurs in cattle and dogs due to effect of inherited recessive gene trait

Hemeralopia is day blindness which may occur in dogs due to single autosomal recessive gene.

KERATOCONJUNCTIVITIS

Keratoconjunctivitis is the inflammation of cornea and conjunctiva characterized by congestion of eyes, blindness, opacity and corneal edema.

Etiology
- Penetrating foreign objects *e.g.* Awns of wheat
- *Moraxella bovis*
- *Mycoplasma* spp.
- BHV-1, poxvirus
- *Rickettsia conjunctivae*
- *Chlamydia* spp.
- *Thelazia* spp.
- Allergy

Macroscopic features
- Congestion of conjunctiva leading to redness "pink eye".
- Edema, pain
- Increased lacrimation (Decreased lacrimation also causes conjunctivitis)
- Corneal opacity

CATARACT

Cataract is opacity of lens and is classified as under:

Subcapsular cataract is the opacity of lens due to abnormal proliferation of lens epithelium in anterior end as a result of injury.

Posterior polar cataract is opacity of lens due to abnormal growth of lens epithelium at posterior face of lens

Cortical cataract is opacity of lens due to disorganization of the lens fibers.

Nuclear cataract is the increased density of fibers of lens at the centre and occurs in old animals.

Morgagnian cataract is the liquefaction of cortical substance and has not been observed in animals.

Congenital cataract is seen in neonatal animals and occurs due to failure of closure of primary lens vesicle at the periphery of lens vesicle and is associated with Chediak - Higashi syndrome.

RETINITIS

Retinitis is the inflammation of retina caused by trauma, iritis, iridocyclitis and choroiditis. When it is associated with inflammation of choroids, it is known as chorioretinitis. It may lead to detachment of retina. *Iritis* is inflammation of iris. *Iridocyclitis* is the inflammation of iris and uvea. *Choroiditis* is inflammation of choroid.

The *chorioretinitis* is characterized by glaucoma occurs in canine distemper, feline panleukopenia, toxoplasmosis, tuberculosis, coccidioidomycosis, deficiency of vitamin A and bracken fern poisoning.

GLAUCOMA

Glaucoma is the intraoccular hypertension due to occlusion of the filtration angle and is caused by trauma, iridocyclitis, intraoccular hemorrhage and neoplasm. It may be unilateral or bilateral. It is characterized by enlargement of eye ball, opaque cornea and increase aqueous humor.

PATHOLOGY OF EAR

OTITIS EXTERNA

Otitis externa is inflammation of external ear caused by *Actinomyces bovis*, parasites and fungus and characterized by granulomatous inflammation.

Etiology
- *Actinomyces bovis*
- *Psoroptes communis* - mite
- *Otobius megnini* - tick
- Fungi- (otomycosis)

- Grass of wheat awns

Macroscopic and microscopic features
- Swelling and congestion leading to obstruction of ear canal.
- Excessive production of thick, tenacious and brownish wax.
- Granulomatous lesions filling the external auditory meatus
- Granulomatous lesions of actinomycosis in subcutaneous region around the cartilage.

OTITIS MEDIA

Otitis media is inflammation of middle ear including tympanic cavity and eustachian tube.

Etiology
- Infections from otitis externa or nasopharynx
- Mites
- Awns of wheat
- *Pasteurella* spp.

Macroscopic and microscopic features
- Occlusion of eustachian tube
- Purulent inflammation
- Suppurative inflammation

OTITIS INTERNA

Otitis interna is the inflammation of inner ear including membranous and osseous labyrinth. This is also known as *labyrinthitis.*

Etiology
- Infection from otitis media
- *Mycoplasma* spp.
- Mumps
- Measles

Macroscopic and microscopic features
- Disturbance in equilibrium
- Deafness
- Suppurative inflammation.

Chapter 22

Neoplasm

GENERAL CONSIDERATIONS

The word neoplasm has been derived from Greek language means "New formations or new growth" (Neo=new, plasm=growth). Thus, the neoplasm can be defined as *"A mass of tissue formed as a result of abnormal, excessive, uncoordinated, autonomous and purpose less proliferation of cells"*. The oncology is branch of science which deals with the study of tumours (Oncos=tumour, logos=study). The neoplasm is a new growth of cells that proliferate continuously without control, have resemblance to their embryonic stages and without any orderly arrangement and that serves no useful function of body. The growth of tumour persists in the same excess even after cessation of the stimuli/ etiology. A neoplasm is thus, characterized by the following key points.

1. Continuous growth
2. Resemblance to embryonic cells
3. No structural arrangement
4. No useful function
5. No clear etiology

The historical moments in the oncology are given in Table 1.1.

The tumours are reported even thousand years B.C. in the records of India and Egypt but Johannes Muller in the year 1838 was first to demonstrate that the tumour is composed of cells. In 1858, R. Virchow described cellular characteristics and in 1889 Hardley transplanted a neoplasm from one rat to another. Tyzzer established the genetic relatedness of tumours

Table 1.1. Historical milestones in neoplasms

Sl. No.	Year	Name of Scientist & Country	Development in area of neoplasms
1.	500BC	Jeevak (India)	Surgical removal of intestinal tumour
2.	1838	Muller (Germany)	Cellular nature of neoplasms
3.	1858	Leblanc (France)	Animal tumours have similar cellular composition
4.	1858	R. Virchow	Cellular characteristics of tumours
5.	1876	Novinsky (Russia)	Transplantability of canine venereal tumour
6.	1889	Hardley	Transplantation of neoplasm from one rat to another
7.	1903	Jenson (Denmark)	Reproduction of mouse mammary gland tumour through serial passage.
8.	1905	Bombay Veterinary College Scientists	Horn Cancer in bullocks
9.	1907	Tyzzer	Genetic relatedness of tumours in inbred mice
10.	1908	Ellerman and Bang (Denmark)	Transmissibility of avian lymphoid tumours
11.	1910	Rous	Transmission of Rous sarcoma of chicken by cell-free suspensions
12.	1910	Clunev (France)	Tumours experimentally produced by X-radiation
13.	1912	Murphy	Growth of rat tumours on chicken chorioallantoic membrane
14.	1914	Yamagiwa (Japan)	Carcinogenicity of coal tar by long-term application to skin of rabbits
15.	1924	Little and Strong	Development of inbred strains of mice for genetic analysis of tumours
16.	1932	Shope	Viral etiology of rabbit papilloma
17.	1933	Warburg	High rate of anaerobic glycolysis in tumour cells
18.	1936	Lucke	Virus induced renal carcinoma of frog
19.	1936	Bittner	Viral agent in milk causing mammary gland carcinoma of mice
20.	1943	Gross	Tumour specific antigens
21.	1947	Berenblum	Two stages in chemical carcinogenesis: initiation and promotion
22.	1951	Gross	Virus etiology of mouse lymphoma
23.	1962	Epstein and Barr	Herpes virus from Burkitt's lymphoma
24.	1964	Jarrett	Retrovirus as etiology of feline lymphosarcoma
25.	1969	Friedrich-Freksa	Chemical carcinogenesis induced altered enzyme patterns in liver
26.	1973	CM Singh (India)	Bovine lymphosarcoma/leukemia in buffaloes

in inbred mice in 1907 while in 1914 Yamagiwa found tar as one of the important cause of cancer in rabbits. Rous in the year 1910 described Rouse Sarcoma in fowls with a viral etiology. In 1932 Shope described papilloma due to transmissible viral agents while in 1936 Bittner's milk factor was associated with transplanted cancer in baby mice.

To understand the neoplasms, their characteristics and pathology, it is advisable to have a general idea about the growth disturbances. The neoplasm is also one of the growth disturbances or development related diseases. In brief, the important growth disturbances are defined as follows:

Agenesis

Complete absence of growth of an organ/ tissue.

Aplasia

Congenital disturbance with complete failure of development of an organ or tissue. Only primitive structure or rudimentary structure is present.

Hypoplasia

Failure of an organ to develop to its normal size.

Atrophy

Reduction in size of an organ/ tissue less than its former normal size. The reduction of size is either due to decrease in number or size of cells of an organ.

Hypertrophy

Increase in size of an organ or tissue due to increase in the size of cells of that organ.

Hyperplasia

Increase in size of an organ or tissue due to increase in the number of cells of that organ.

Metaplasia

Substitution of one cell type by another type of cells. *e.g.* Squamous metaplasia of oesophageal glands of poultry in Vitamin A deficiency (nutritional roup).

Dysplasia

Abnormal development of cells in a tissue/ organ.

Anaplasia

Reversion of cells to a more primitive or embryonic and less differentiated type.

In comparison to tissue growth as in case of hyperplasia or hypertrophy, a neoplastic growth does not obey the laws of the healing or normal tissue growth. The cells of a neoplasm continue to multiply indefinitely irrespective of any structural or functional requirements and form an ever increasing mass of tissue.

The macroscopic appearance of tumours is characterized by different size, shape, colour and consistency which depends on many factors such as location, type of tumour, blood supply, rate of growth and length of time tumour present in body. The size of a tumour varies from one mm to several centimeter diameter. The common warts/ papilloma over skin have smaller size while certain tumours have many centimeter diameter such as uterine tumours etc. The weight of tumour also varies from few milligram to several kg. A tumour of 48 kg was removed from uterus of a cow. The different shape of tumours are round, spherical, elliptical or multi lobulated. Some tumours have crab like structures which are formed as a result of its invasion to the surrounding tissue. The colour of tumours may be grayish white, yellow, red, brown or black. If tumour has fatty tissue it looks like yellow in colour while hemorrhage or congestion may give the pink or red colour to tumour; melanoma or melanosarcoma are characterized by black colour. The disintegration of hemoglobin gives brown colour to tumour due to presence of hemosiderin. The consistency of a tumour depends on the type of tissue involved. The tumour of bone is hard while connective tissue tumours are firm and dense or sclerotic. Brain tumours are mostly soft. If there is necrosis in mass of tumour it becomes soft and liquefied. In certain tumours, there are oedematous fluid which gives it watery consistency. Some tumours have mucin leading to its slimy consistency.

Microscopically, the tumour is composed of cells which resembles the type of tissue/ organ involved. The appearance of cells vary on degree of malignancy. *In benign tumours, the cells are of adult type while in malignant tumours these cells are having characteristics of embryonic stages.* This reversion towards embryonic type is also known as *anaplasia*. The more anaplastic cells we see in a tumour more malignancy will be there. However, it will depend on the degree of anaplasia which have following characteristics:

1. **Enlargement of nucleus:** The nucleus of tumour cell is enlarged which is indicative of a rapid cell growth and towards embryonic stage of the cell.

2. **Multiple nuclei in a cell:** The tumour cells having multiple nucleus are indicative of rapid cell division and such cells are known as *tumour giant cells*. Such cells are formed because of the fact that nucleus is dividing more rapidly than cytoplasm.

3. **Enlargement of nucleolus:** The increased size of nucleolus is also an indication of rapid cell growth; sometimes it becomes 2-3 times larger in size than normal.

4. **Increase number of mitotic figures:** If one finds more number of mitotic figures in a field under microscope, it is an indication of malignancy. More number of mitotic figures, the more severe malignancy will be there.

5. **Hyperchromasia of the cell:** The neoplastic cell takes intense colour and if it is more embryonic, it takes more intense colour and nucleus stains dark with hematoxylin.

6. **Embryonic type cells:** The neoplastic cell loses its resemblance to adult cells. The cell growth is not under control.

Classification, difference between benign and malignant neoplasms

The classification of neoplasms is summarized in Table 1.2.

Table 1.2. Classification of benign and malignant neoplasms

	Tissue of origin	Benign	Malignant
I	*Neoplasms of one parencymal cell type*		
(i)	*Epithelial neoplasms*		
1.	Squamous epithelium	Papilloma	Squamous cell carcinoma
2.	Transitional epithelium	Papilloma	Transitional cell carcinoma
3.	Glandular epithelium	Adenoma	Adenocarcinoma
4.	Basal cell layer	-	Basal cell carcinoma
5.	Melanoblasts	Melanoma	Melanocarcinoma
6.	Hepatocytes	Liver cell adenoma	Hypatocellularcarcinoma
7.	Placenta	-	Choriocarcinoma
(ii)	*Non-epithelial neoplasms (mesenchymal)*		
1.	Adipose tissue	Lipoma	Liposarcoma
2.	Fibrous tissue (adult)	Fibroma	Fibrosarcoma
3.	Fibrous tissue (embryonic)	Myxoma	Myxosarcoma
4.	Bone	Osteoma	Osteosarcoma
5.	Cartilage	Chondroma	Chondrosarcoma
6.	Smooth muscle	Leiomyoma	Leiomyosarcoma
7.	Skeletal muscle	Rhabdomyoma	Rhabdomyosarcoma
8.	Blood vessels	Hemangioma	Hemangiosarcoma
9.	Lymph vessels	Lymphangioma	Lymphangiosarcoma
10.	Meninges	Meningioma	Invasive meningioma
11.	Lymphoid tissue	Lymphoma	Malignant lymphoma
12.	Brain nerve sheath	Neurofibroma	Neurogenic sarcoma
13.	Brain nerve cell	Ganglioneuroma	Neuroblastoma
14.	Blood cells (lymphocytes)	-	Leukemia
15.	Mesothelium	-	Mesothelioma
II.	*Mixed neoplasms*		
	Salivary gland	Mixed salivary neoplasm	Malignant mixed salivary neoplasm
III.	*Neoplasms of more than one germ layer*		
	Gonads	Mature teratoma	Immature teratoma

1. Benign
2. Malignant (cancer)
3. Preneoplastic conditions
4. Neoplastic like malformations

1. Benign neoplasms

Neoplasms that are well differentiated, grow slowly by expansion and do not invade below basement membrane are called as benign neoplasms. They remain localized, encapsulated and can be removed by surgery. They are classified with addition of a *suffix-oma* to the cell type. *e.g.* Fibroma, Chondroma, Adenoma, Papilloma.

2. Malignant neoplasms

Neoplasms whose cells are anaplastic, metastasize and invade the adjacent tissues and destroy normal tissue. They are also called as *cancer* "like crab". They can adhere to any part of body. They are classified with suffix as carcinoma or sarcoma. Ectodermal origin- Carcinoma, Mesodermal origin- Sarcoma. *e.g.* Lymphosarcoma, Adenocarcinoma, Squamous cell carcinoma.

Some tumours are highly undifferentiated they are referred as "undifferentiated malignant tumours".

Table 1.3. Difference between benign and malignant tumours

Sl.No.	Characteristics	Benign	Malignant
1.	Growth rate	Slow	Rapid
2.	Growth limits	Circumscribed/covered	Unrestricted
3.	Mode of growth	Expansion	Invasion
4.	Differentiation	Good	Anaplasia
5.	Metastasis	Absent	Frequent
6.	Recurrence on surgery	Rare	Frequent
7.	Microscopic features	Resembles with tissue of origin	Poor resemblance with tissue of origin
8.	Basal polarity	Retained	Often lost
9.	Pleomorphism	Absent	Present
10.	Tumour giant cells	Absent	Present
11.	Anaplastic	Often absent	Present

3. Preneoplastic conditions

There are some preneoplastic lesions which predisposes the subsequent development of cancer. These are as follows:

a. *Chronic inflammatory conditions of liver* of old dogs have multiple nodules which are considered preneoplastic nodules and neoplastic cells do arise from such nodules. Such dogs have higher incidence of hepatocellular carcinoma.

b. *Intraepithelial neoplasia* are restricted to the epithelium only without infiltration in adjacent tissue. On cytology there are malignant features of the cells but with no invasion and they remain confined to epithelium. *e.g.* Uterine cervix, Solar keratosis, Bowen's disease of skin, Oral leucoplakia

c. *Role of pre neoplastic lesions* in squamous cell carcinoma, transitional cell carcinoma of bladder and malignant melanomas of skin and oral cavity is well established.

d. *Some benign tumours* like multiple adenoma of large intestine becomes malignant (adenocarcinoma) after sometime.

4. Neoplasia like malformations

A *hamartia* is a tissue defect of cells normally found in a particular area. *Hamartoma* is a tumour characterized by excessive focal overgrowth of mature cells in an organ. *Chorista* is a tissue defect of structures not found normally in that area. *Choriostoma* is tumour of such structures. *Teratoma* are made up of a number of parenchymal cell types arising from more than one germ layer.

ETIOLOGY

1. Instrisic or predisposing factors

(i) Heredity

Some chicken are susceptible for leucosis whole others are resistant for leucosis.

(ii) Age

Neoplasms are more common in old age.

(iii) Pigmentation

In white horses Melenosarcoma is common. Squamous cell carcinoma is common in hereford cattle.

(iv) Sex

No difference, tumours of genital tract are common in females.

2. Extrinsic factors

(i) Physical factors

Radium or UV-rays, X-rays, ionizing radiation

(ii) Chemical factors

A. Initiators
1. Coal-tar
2. Naturally occurring products e.g. Aflatoxins, Actinomycin D, Mitomycine, Safrole
3. Alkalating agents e.g. cyclophosphamide, chlorambucil, nitrosourea.
4. Polycyclic aromatic hydrocarbons- Tobacco, smoke, pollutants, methylcholanthrene, banzapyrene, benzanthracene
5. Aromatic amines- b-naphthylamine bezidine
6. Azodyes
7. Acylating agents- acetyl imidazole
8. Vinyl chloride monomer
9. Arsenic
10. Metals- Nickel, lead, cobalt, chromium
11. Insecticides- Aldrin, Dieldrin, Chlordane

B. Promoters
1. Phenols
2. Hormones- Estrogen
3. Drugs- Phenobarbital
4. Artificial sweetners- Saccharine
5. Colouring/ flavouring agents, preservatives

(iii) Virus
1. Papilloma virus
2. Polyoma virus
3. Adeno virus - Hamsters- Sarcoma
4. Poxvirus- Rabbit- Myxomatosis
5. Hepdna virus- Hepatitis B virus
6. Retrovirus
7. Herpes virus

NEOPLASTIC CELL GENESIS (CARCINOGENESIS)

Cell differentiation

Specialized cells derived from less specialized cells (embryonic cells) is controlled by specific gene. Cells become differentiated so that the genes that control embryonic characters are switched off and genes for more differentiated characters are activated. In neoplastic cells, the presence of abnormal genes (genetic mechanisms) or normal genes expressed at abnormal level (epigenetic mechanism) favour proliferation over differentiation.

Genetic mechanisms

Mutation in a somatic cell nucleic acid occurs to provide a stable and monoclonal population of cells.

Epigenetic mechanism

Genome is normal in cancer cell but transcription and translation is abnormal which is responsible for abnormal growth of cells.

In most tumours genetic mutation or genetic rearrangement occurs like DNA transcribe to mRNA and mRNA translated to protein (enzymes) which direct cells for proliferation. Changes occur in DNA as a result of direct chemical or radiation damage or there is insertion of viral genes to host DNA that induces cell proliferation through neutralizing normal growth controlling gene.

Tumours do not arise from completely differentiated cells such as neurons or keratinized epithelial cells, but stem cells (pluripotential) must be present for the growth of tumour. Neoplastic cells do not "dedifferentiate" but fail to respond to normal signals for differentiation.

VIRAL ONCOGENESIS

Oncogenes are the transforming genes present in host tumour cells of animal and man. It is also present in certain viruses. Experimentally, when they are incorporated in cells in culture it transforms the cells to multiply. When such genes are present in normal cells that are known as *cellular oncogenes (c-oncs)* or *proto-oncogenes,* which are present in a wide range of cells and has a physiological role of proliferation of cells through protein product.

Proto-oncogenes are converted into active oncogenes through following mechanisms:

1. **Point mutation:** Change in a single base pair of the nucleic acid.
2. **Translocation:** Transfer of one segment of chromosome to another chromosome.
3. **Gene amplification:** Extra copies of *c-oncs* are inserted leading to increased number of oncogenes.
4. **Inappropriate expression of proto-oncogenes:** When the expression of oncogenes is not in proper way and it gives rise to the products responsible for formation of tumours.
5. **Integration of viral DNA into host cell DNA:** Integration of viral DNA into host cell DNA causes adjacent gene activated for growth of the cell without control.

Cellular oncogenes of host cell can transcribe its copies in viral genome (retroviruses) and then it is known as *v- oncogenes (v-oncs)*. So *c-oncs* or *v-oncs* are closely related genes and have high degree of homology.

Antioncogenes

Antioncogenes are genes that suppresses the cellular proliferation. By inactivating antioncogene we can produce cancers. So neoplastic growth occurs either as a result of activation of oncogene or due to inactivation of antioncogene.

How the viruses cause cancers
1. A direct effect of gene (*v-oncs*).
2. A viral factor that affects a host gene (*c-oncs*).
3. A factor that inactivates the antioncogene.
4. Genes that do not affect the cell growth but influence the expansion/ metastasis.

There are many RNA and DNA viruses which can cause cancers.

1. Retrovirus

It produces cancers through 3 mechanisms.
i. RNA of Rous Sarcoma Virus utilizing reverse transcriptase converts into DNA (proviral DNA) which incorporated in host cell DNA. The *src* gene of the virus is thus responsible for transformation of the cells.
ii. Proviral DNA of avian leucosis virus has no oncogenes. However, it carries a viral RNA segment known as "Long Terminal Repeat (LTR)" present at the end of viral genome. This LTR has segments of promoters and enhancers, which activate transcription of viral genome to mRNA and activates the adjacent normal cell gene for growth and production of slow tumours. Gene (myc) of ALC virus is amplified and plays a role is transforming the cells.
iii. Some virus has a protein that transactivate the gene of proliferation and thus it increases the proliferation of gene to divide the cells.

2. Papova virus

These are the DNA viruses having two main genera Papilloma and Polyoma. Papilloma virus has *src, raf, myc* oncogene which produces warts/ benign tumours. These warts regress through cell mediated immune response. Polyoma produces multiple nodules in body.

3. Hepadna virus

Hepadna virus has *hap* oncogene causing hepatocellular carcinoma. It includes hepatitis-B virus and duck hepatitis virus.

4. Herpesvirus

DNA virus *e.g.* Marek's disease virus which causes polyneuritis and malignant lymphoma in poultry. This is the only virus for which a vaccine is available to control cancer.

Possible viral induced tumours

1. Pulmonary adenomatosis of sheep

It is progressive respiratory distress characterized by emaciation and proliferation of glandular cells. In this the squamous epithelium becomes metaplastic to cuboidal or columnar. Metastasis occurs in lymph nodes, skeletal muscles, kidneys and peritoneum.

2. Nasal adenocarcinoma of sheep.

3. Equine cutaneous histiocytoma

The *src* gene product of rouse sarcoma virus synthesizes protein kinase (60 kD) enzyme which stimulates DNA synthesis leading to mitosis. All vertebrate possess a cell gene related to *src* gene; which also produce similar protein kinase.

Over 20 retroviral oncogenes (*v-oncs*) have been identified. All have relatives in normal cells (proto oncogenes).

Some of the oncogenes are:
1. Rous Sarcoma Virus – *src*
2. Avian Leucosis Virus – *myc, myb, erb-B, erb-A*
3. Feline Leukemia Virus – *pim-1, myc*
4. Papilloma virus- *src,raf,myc*
5. Hepadna virus- *hap*
6. Reticuloendotheliosis- *rel*
7. Avian sarcoma virus- *yes, ros*
8. Feline sarcoma virus- *fes, fms*

NEOPLASTIC CELL METABOLISM

Normal regulation of programmed protein synthesis is lost in neoplastic cells. Gene expression and mRNA translation is being directed towards:

1. Purine synthesis to meet the requirement of mitosis
2. Defective sodium pump (ATPase) due to abnormal receptor molecules and surface glycoproteins on neoplastic cells.
3. Increased glycolysis
   a. Increased glycolysis may occur due to damage in self replicating DNA of mitochondira. *e.g.* Carcinogenic metabolite of benzopyrene have affinity to mitochondrial DNA.
   b. Enhanced glycolysis is also related to over production of inorganic phosphorus due to high rate of ATP hydrolysis. Inorganic phosphorus is required to phosphorylate glucose to glucose-6-phosphate.

ATP ADP + Pi   Stimulate glycolysis

   Hydrolysis

   c. Abnormal enzymes on cell surface may promote glycolysis. ATPase (Sodium pump, Na-K-dependent ATPase) is inefficient in cancer cells. Additional ATPs are required to pump out Na^+ which produces ADP and inorganic phosphorus that further stimulates glycolysis.

NEOPLASTIC CELL STRUCTURE

1. Anaplasia

Neoplastic cells are having anaplastic characters. More anaplasia represents more undifferentiated neoplasm.

2. Loss of contact

Neoplastic cells loss contact with neighbouring cells due to decreased adhesiveness. It helps in invasion and metastasis. Such cells bear more negative charge on surface, decrease in calcium content and presence of abnormal glycoprotein and glycolipids. Fibronectin is present on normal cell surface but it is absent or decreased in neoplastic cells. Fibronectin forms matrix for stabilization of cells and absence of matrix destabilizes tumour cells. Fibronectin suppresses invasiveness, absence of which increases invasiveness.

3. Neoplastic cell lack contact inhibition

Normally cell growth is inhibited after the fulfillment of function i.e. healing of wound due to contact and exchange of information which establishes check on cell growth. But in cancer cell such contact does not work because of absence of gap junctions. Vitamin A promotes proliferation of gap junctions and thus this vitamin helps in checking the growth/ spread of tumours.

4. Abnormal cytoskeleton of cells

Abnormal microfilament leads to defective actin polymerization while abnormal microtubules causes abnormal polymerization of tubulins leading to abnormal shape. Besides, unstable chromosome movements cause abnormality in cytoskeleton.

5. Chromosomal defects

Malignant cells are usually aneuploid i.e. cells having more or less than diploid number of chromosomes. This gives a pathologic karyotype in the form of chromosomal breaks or translocations. *e.g.* Plasmacytoma (tumour of B-lymphocytes) in which translocation of segments of chromosome 15 occurs to chromosome 12. This translocate carries the gene for production of monoclonal antibody in mice.

Thus gene for antibody production can be transported to chromosomes with gene of growth. The process of *monoclonal antibody* production is based on this principle.

SPREAD OF NEOPLASMS

I. Expansion

Benign tumours are encapsulated and surrounded by fibrous tissue and hence they do not infiltrate in neighbouring tissue. However, they expand as their growth increases.

II. Distant spread/ metastasis

Metastasis is the spread of tumours by invasion in such a way that detached tumour mass may form secondary tumour at the site of lodgment. Most of the malignant tumours metastasize except malignant tumour of central nervous system and basal cell carcinoma of skin. There are several methods of metastasis, which are as under:

1. Infiltration

Neoplastic cells infiltrate or invade the surrounding tissue. Various factors responsible for invasion are:

a. Growth of new cells so as to increase the size.
b. Lack of contact inhibition in malignant tumour cells.
c. Motility of malignant cells.
d. Secretion of lytic enzymes by some malignant cells.
e. Role of chemotactic factors and activation of complement.

2. Lymphatic spread

In general, epithelial tumours like carcinomas spread through lymphatic route. Cancer cells invade the wall of lymphatics which is known as lymphatic permeation and form tumour emboli. These cells are lodged in sub capsular sinus of lymph node and may grow. Nearest lymph node initially act as barrier filter and kill the tumour cells but later it provides fertile environment for growth of tumour cells. Sometimes lymphatic metastasis do not develop due to obliteration of lymphatics by inflammation; this is known as *skip metastasis*. Obstruction of lymphatics by tumour cells also disturbs the lymphatic flow and is responsible for metastasis at unusual sites. This is termed as *retrograde metastasis*. *e.g.* 1. Carcinoma of prostate to supra clavicular lymph node, 2. Metastasis in adrenals from lung cancer.

3. Hematogenous spread

Metastasis through blood is common route for most of the sarcomas (connective tissue tumours). However, some carcinomas (lung, mammary gland, thyroid, kidney) may spread through blood. Common sites of lodgment of tumour cells are liver, lungs, kidneys, brain and bones. Cancer cell invade the wall of capillaries to form tumour emboli. Blood borne metastasis appear as multiple and rounded nodules scattered in the organ.

4. Transcoelomic spread

The tumour cells invade serosal wall and enters in coelomic cavity and then tumour cells implant at another place. *e.g.* Peritoneal cavity- carcinoma of stomach/ ovary.

5. Spread along epithelial lined surfaces

Intact epithelium and mucous coat are quite resistant to penetration by tumour cells. The neoplasms of epithelium spread along the line of basement membrane without damaging it. *e.g.* 1. Spread of tumour through fallowpian tube from ovaries to endometrium, 2. Spread of tumour through bronchus to aveoli.

6. Spread via Cerebrospinal Fluid (CSF)

Tumour of meninges may spread through cerebrospinal fluid as the detached tumour cells metastasize at other sites in central nervous system through CSF.

7. Implantation

It is very rare method of spread of tumours. In this the tumour cells are implanted at another site inadvertently. *e.g.* 1. Surgeon's scalpel, needle, sutures may transfer tumour cells from one to another place in body. 2. Cancer of lower lip may metastasize to upper lip.

Process of metastasis

The process of metastasis includes 5 steps.

1. Penetration (Invasion):

The tumour cells penetrate or infiltrate in the adjoining tissue particularly in vascular space/ cavity.

2. Separation:

A group of tumour cells separate from primary tumour due to their lack of adhesiveness.

3. Dissemination:

The separated cells reach at distant places through stream of blood/ lymph or in cavity through amoeboid movement with a speed of 6.2 μm/ min.

4. Establishment:

At new site the tumour cells adapt in new environment for lodgment.

5. Subsequent Proliferation:

As the tumour cells lodge and adapt in new environment, it starts unrestricted growth at new site and forms secondary tumours.

TUMOUR IMMUNOLOGY

In some animals growth of neoplasm is very fast that leads to early death. In others, tumour growth is slow and the animal may survive several years. When malignant tumour is clinically manifested it takes 6 month to 1 year to cause death.

There are many systems/ functions in the body which works together to fight with neoplastic cells. These are described as under:

1. Nonspecific lysis and phagocytosis

Most tumour cells are phagocytosed by polymorphonuclear cells and macrophages. On contact, macrophages insert cytoplasmic processes into the tumour cells and transfer lysosomal enzymes into the cytoplasm of cancer cell leading to death of cell. Because in cancer cell decreased catalase and glutathione contents makes them susceptible to oxidative injury by macrophages. On the contrary reactive oxygen metabolites of neutrophils "respiratory burst"are mutagenic and may act as tumour promoter.

Natural killer cell

A population of immature lymphocytes which bears Fc receptor that causes lysis of neoplastic cells or virus infected cells.

Antibodies

Antibodies against tumour antigens also restrain the growth of tumour.

Escape of neoplastic cells from immunological destruction

1. Delayed immunostimulation

The tumour antigens appear late on the anaplastic/ neoplastic cell surface causing delayed immune response.

2. Antigenic modulation

Frequent change in antigenic determinants over neoplastic cell surface may escape the cell from immune response.

3. Antigenic overload

There are too many antigenic determinants on the neoplastic cell surface that leads to immune tolerance.

4. General Immunodeficiency

Neoplasia, in general, causes immunosuppression in body.

5. Specific immunodeficiency

There is lack of recognition of tumour antigens on neoplastic cells by the immunocytes that leads to suppression of specific immune response.

6. Humoral antibodies

Antibodies binds with tumour antigens and blocks the effect of more potent anti neoplastic action by another source.

Tumour antigens

Tumour cells develop certain biochemical alterations on their surface (protein change) that makes the "tumour" antigens". Tumour antigens are useful in differentiating between neoplastic or pre neoplastic cell. These tumour antigens may evoke immune response in body by humoral or cell mediated mechanism which may inhibit the tumour cell growth.

Types of tumour antigens

1. Fetal antigens and alpha fetoproteins produced by embryonic cells.

2. It is produced by liver cells but after birth it's production is stopped normally.
3. Differentiation antigen as in normal cells.
4. Viral antigens on cell surface. *e.g.* Retrovirus

Tumour antigens induced selective CMI response which destroys the malignant cells. During cytological or histological examination of biopsy material, if one finds lymphocytes along with cancer cells, the prognosis is considered as good.

Propionibacterium acnes (*Corynebacterium parvum*), BCG and filterate of G⁻ bacterial cultures are used to stimulate the reticulo-endothelial system against tumours. Macrophages attract and attach on tumour growth and remove it through phagocytosis. *e.g.* In ocular squamous cell carcinoma, intra tumour injection of BCG reduces growth by 71%.

In early tumour growth, tumour cells excrete some products that inhibits the macrophages. *e.g.* Macrophages also release certain soluble factors that are having anti tumour activities, such as tumour necrosis factor (TNF) which causes necrosis of tumour cells. It needs to be activated by *P.acnes* or LPS of G⁻ bacteria. It affects subcutaneous transplantation of tumour.

BENEFICIAL EFFECTS OF NEOPLASTIC CELLS

1. Monoclonal antibody production

Antibody production is done by B-cells but they have short life span. If fusion/ hybrids are produced between B-cells and myeloma cells (neoplastic B-cells) then this hybrid cells are capable of multiplying indefinitely and produce antibody indefinitely. After fusion they are kept in HAT medium (Hypoxanthine, aminopterin, thymidine)- either B or myeloma cell cannot survive, only clones will survive. Myeloma cells are from BALB/C mice. The clone will grow as tumour in peritoneal cavity; i/p fluid or ascites fluid have a good concentration of antibodies which are monoclonal in nature.

Advantages
1. High titre of monoclonal antibody.
2. Mono specificity.
3. Immortal clones may produce more quantity of antibody.
4. On mass scale in culture media one can produce even up to 1000 liters of antibody.
5. Monoclnal antibody is used for confirmatory diagnosis of diseases.

2. Cell culture

Cancerous cells are used for virus culture as cell lines specific for different organ/ cell. Such cell lines are serving very useful purpose as they are used in isolation, identification and characterization of viruses. Vaccines can be prepared from viruses using cell culture.

EPIDEMIOLOGY OF NEOPLASMS

Horn caner is commonest neoplasm of cattle in India; however, it may also occur is buffaloes and sheep. This neoplasm was first reported in 1905 from Bombay Veterinary College and since then it has been recorded from every part of the country. Adult cattle of 5-10 years of age are mostly suffer from horn cancer. It has been recorded in long horned animals with white coat. The prevalence of horn cancer was found highest in Kankrej 8.24% followed by in Gir (7.33%), Malvi (6.99%), Khillari (2.96) and others (1.11%). Working bullocks are comparatively more susceptible to horn cancer. In a study of 968430 cattle and buffaloes during 1966-70, neoplasm of horn has been recorded in 2652 animals including 2268 cattle and 384 buffaloes. More than 90% of affected animals were in the age group of 5-10 years.

A survey was carried out from 1995 to 1982 (17 years) on neoplasms in cattle and buffaloes and the prevalence of different neoplasms was recorded as squamous cell carcinoma (48.4%), fibroma (19.61%), melanoma (6.5%), lymphosarcoma (4.5%) and papilloma (4.2%). The occurrence of neoplasms in different animals were as 62.3% in bullocks, 19.4% in cows, 16% in buffaloes and 2.3% in bulls.

In dogs, a survey was conducted from (1940-1951) at Madras and 325 (13.5%) dogs were found to suffer from venereal tumour. Among various neoplasms diagnosed in dogs in Hisar (Haryana) are veneral neoplasm, papilloma, round cell sarcoma, adenocarcinoma, adenoma and lymphosarcoma. Canine venereal tumour was found more during summer (57.9%) as compared to winter (42.1%). The age group mainly involved was 1-5 years. Sex wise prevalence was 68.5% in females and 31.5% in males. In another survey, the frequency of different neoplasms in dogs was recorded as 42.2% of skin, 20.6% of mammary gland, 23.5% of genitalia and 13.2% of other organs.

A screening was conducted on neoplasms of equines from 1952 to 1973 in southern India, in which 69 horses and one donkey was found to be affected with neoplasms of skin and glands. Another survey conducted at Hisar from 1980-1988 suggested sarcoid as main tumour of horses. In Gujrat, a study of tumours in horses revealed 30% fibroma, 25% squamaous cell carcinoma, 16% fibrosarcoma, 6% papilloma and 6% melanoma.

CLINICOPATHOLOGICAL EFFECTS OF NEOPLASMS

Malignant neoplastic cells kill animals through many effects which are categorized into local and systemic effects.

1. Local effects

The main local effect is pressure on surrounding tissue. The tumour causes pain, ischemia, oedema and lymphatic blockade in surrounding tissue. The lumen of ducts are obstructed due to pressure from outside tumours. *e.g.* Squamous cell carcinoma of respiratory tract causes dyspnoea and hypoxia due to obstruction in pharynx. Tumors which cause obstruction in urinary tract or obstruction in bile ducts may lead to death.

2. Systemic effects

a. Cachexia

Cachexia is main characteristic feature of malignant tumours. In later stages, anorexia occurs in animals leading to loss of weight and lethariginess. Anorexia occurs due to depression of appetite centre in brain. A humoral factor is released by tumour cells that causes suppression of appetite centre in brain. Cytokines secreted by tumour cells or by altered macrophages (affected by neoplastic cell) are known as *cachectin* which causes suppression of gene that produces lipogenic enzymes responsible for fat deposition. Neoplastic cells act as amino acid trap and thus, drain out the essential amino acids leading to regression of skeletal muscles, liver, pancreas and other organs. Hepatocytes become atrophied.

b. Hypoglycemia

Hypoglycemia is characteristic feature of tumours of pancreas and other epithelial tumours. It is characterized by restlessness, weakness, tremors, episodes of collapse and seizures.

c. Anemia

Anemia is a common feature in all metastatic tumours. It is caused by:

i. Hemorrhage through invasion by cancer cells.
ii. Decreased erythropoiesis due to invasion of tumour cells in bone marrow.
iii. Increased erythrocyte fragmentation as many blood vessels pass though tumours. In highly vascular tumour, there are more chances of anemia.
iv. In hypersplenism, there is spleenomegaly due to excessive removal of RBC from circulation.
v. Iron deficiency due to tumour may leads to anemia.
vi. Due to anticancer therapy there is non regeneration of stem cells. It causes death of stem cells or dividing cells of bone marrow leading to anemia.
vii. Autoimmune anemia occurs in lymphoid neoplasms.
viii. Suppression of erythropoitin by kidneys.

d. Thrombocytopenia

In tumour patients thrombocyte production is reduced. *e.g.* In viral leukemia, platelet survival rate is reduced from 40-80% in dogs.

e. Thrombosis

Tumour cells produce procoagulants which are responsible for intra vascular coagulation and thrombi formation.

f. Hypercalcemia

In most of the malignant neoplasms, hypercalcemia occurs through 2 mechanism:

i. In solid tumours due to osteolytic metastasis excessive bone resorption occurs leading to calcium release that results in hypercalcemia.

ii. Tumour cell secrete proteins that increases parathyroid hormone leading to increase in calcium level in blood. Pseudohyperpara-thyroidism is associated with mammary gland cancer, fibrosarcoma, lymphosarcoma and adenocarcinoma in dogs and gastric carcinoma in horses.

g. Diarrhoea

Prolonged diarrhoea occurs in malignant neoplasms which is unresponsive to therapy and non associated with microorganisms. Neoplastic cell secretes vasoactive intestinal peptides that cause diarrhoea leading to death of the animal.

h. Fever

Some tumour cells release pyrogens that increases body temperature which is anti neoplastic in nature. In late stage of metastatic tumours fever is a characteristic feature.

DIAGNOSIS OF NEOPLASMS

- Symptoms and lesions
- Clinicopathological effects
- Immunological methods by using tumour markers
- Gross and microscopic features (histopathological examination)

PROGNOSIS OF NEOPLASMS

Grading of neoplasms

Grading and staging are two systems used to determine the prognosis and choice of treatment. Grading is defined as the macroscopic and microscopic degree of differentiation of tumour. Broder's grading is as under:

Grade I: Well differentiated tumour (less than 25% anaplastic cells)

Grade II: Moderately differentiated tumour (25-50% anaplastic cells)

Grade III: Low differentiated tumour (50-75% anaplastic cells)

Grade IV: Poorly differentiated tumour (more than 75% anaplastic cells)

Sometimes it is very difficult to identify the origin of tumour due to its poor differentiation. In such cases the common practice is to classify such tumours as under:
- Well differentiated
- Undifferentiated
- Keratinizing
- Non-keratinizing

Staging of neoplasms

Staging means extent of spread of tumour. Solid tumours are classified for the purpose of surgery. Various methods of staging of neoplasms are as under:

(i) TNM System

T (primary tumour)

T_0 = No evidence of tumour

T_1 = Tumour confined to primary site

T_2 = Tumour invades adjacent tissue

Lymph node (penetration/ metastasis)

(N = local lymph node)

N_0 = No evidence of tumour
N_1 = Regional node involvement
N_2 = Distant node involvement

Metastasis

(M = distal lymph node)

M_0 = No evidence of metastasis
M_1 = In same cavity/ place as primary tumour
M_2 = Distant metastasis
Stage I = T_1, N_0, M_0
Stage II = $T_1, N_0/ N_1, M_1$
Stage III = $T_2, N_1/ N_2, M_2$

(ii) American Joint Committee (AJC) Staging

It divides all cancers into stage 0 to IV taking into account 3 components: 1) Primary tumour, 2) Nodal involvement and 3) Distant metastasis

(iii) ABC Staging System

This system is mostly used to intestinal tumours. *e.g.* colon cancers. It was proposed by Duke's and thus also known as Duke's system. This system is helpful for surgical removal of cancer.

Stage A: When tumour is confined to sub mucosa and muscle and has a cure rate 100%.

Stage B: When tumour has penetrated the entire thickness of the wall into peri colic tissue and cure rate is 70%.

Stage C: It is characterized by lymph node metastasis and reduces the cure rate to 30%.

Animal tumours are classified as epithelial and non epithelial (Connective tissue tumours).

EPITHELIAL TUMOURS

PAPILLOMA

Papilloma is a benign tumour from an epithelial surface and involves squamous, transitional or columnar epithelium depending on the tissue of origin.

Etiology
- Papilloma virus of papovaviridae family.
- Macroscopic features
- Size small from few mm to 10 cm diameter from skin
- Peduculated or broad based (urinary bladder).
- Surface may be smooth or horny.
- Some times finger like projections.

Macroscopic and microscopic features
- Thick layers of epithelium.
- Layer of connective tissue present.
- Epithelium irregularly arranged.

Diagnosis
- Symptoms and lesions
- Histopathological examination

SQUAMOUS CELL CARCINOMA

Squamous cell carcinoma is a malignant tumour of squamous stratified epithelium. It is a common tumour of cattle in India; horn cancer is mostly seen in bullocks.

Etiology
- Exactly not known
- Possibly a virus
- Chronic irritation, trauma, paints, solar radiation
- Hormonal imbalances- Horn cancer, mostly occur in castrated animals

Macroscopic and microscopic features
- Papillary projections or cauliflower like growth.
- Broad base
- Soft and grey or pink in colour
- Horn cancer invade the frontal sinuses
- Eye cancer arises from nictitating membrane of cornea
- Stratum germinativum proliferate
- Concentric layers of keratin forms pearls *'Epithelial pearls'*
- Mitotic figures seen
- Thickening of prickle cell layer

Diagnosis
- Symptoms and lesions
- Histopathological examination

BASAL CELL CARCINOMA

Basal cell carcinoma is a malignant tumour of basal cells of Malpigian layer of epidermis or hair matrix. They are also known as *hair cell carcinoma* and are locally invasive with no metastasis.

Etiology
- Not known
- Common in dogs, horses, cats.

Macroscopic and microscopic features
- May occur singly and has broad base
- It is subcutaneous, rounded and encapsulated
- Firm in consistency
- Such skin shows alopecia and ulceration.
- Pleomorphic cells- round or cigar shaped
- Hyperchromatic nuclei
- Cells arranged in columns descended to dermis
- Prickle cells are not observed

- No hair, mitotic figures seen.

Diagnosis
- Symptoms and lesions
- Histopathological examination

ADENOMA AND ADENOCARCINOMA

Adenoma is benign and adenocarcinoma is malignant tumour of glandular epithelium. They may arise from any gland of the body.

Etiology
- Not known

Macroscopic and microscopic features
- Adenomas are nodular and encapsulated
- Clearly demarcated from surrounded tissues
- Pink in colour
- Polypoid in shape, may occlude gland or lumen of hollow organ.
- Adenomas are having single layer of columnar or cuboidal epithelial cells
- Such cells show papillary projections in adenocarcinoma
- Pleomorphic cells, mitotic figures seen
- Small nucleus, with fine chromatin and fine nucleoli
- Such cells grouped into masses and invasive to basement membrane.

Diagnosis
- Symptoms and lesions
- Histopathological examination

SEBACEOUS GLAND ADENOMA

This is a benign tumour of sebaceous gland in skin and commonly observed in dogs at head, neck, eyelids, prepuce, tail and back.

Etiology
- Not known

Macroscopic and microscopic features
- Small tumours, lobulated
- Grayish yellow in colour
- Tumours are greasy in touch.
- Large polyhedral cells
- Fat droplets in cytoplasm
- Nucleus small and round with fine chromatin
- Cells are grouped in masses separated by connective tissue stroma.

Diagnosis
- Symptoms and lesions
- Histopathological examination

PERIANAL ADENOMA OF DOG

Perianal adenoma is modified benign tumour of sebaceous glands located at anal ring. These are commonly seen in dogs.

Etiology
- Not known

Macroscopic and microscopic features
- Single or multilobular/ nodular
- Firm, encapsulated
- Situated laterally or above the anus.
- Epithelial cells arranged in lobules
- Polyhedral with giant granular acidophilic cytoplasm
- Cells are large and rounded
- Malignant tumours characterized by mitotic figures and anaplasia of the cells.

Diagnosis
- Symptoms and lesions
- Histopathological examination

SWEAT GLAND ADENOMA

Sweat gland adenoma is benign tumour of sweat glands of skin of face and is common in dogs.

Etiology
- Not known

Macroscopic and microscopic features
- Solid nodules small in size
- Hard to touch
- Grey in colour.
- There may be columnar or cuboidal cells arranged in glandular fashion
- Acinis may have lumen or solid
- Cells have acidophilic and faintly granular cytoplasm
- Nucleus round or oval
- Secretion accumulated, then cyst adenocarcinoma/ cystadenoma.

Diagnosis
- Symptoms and lesions
- Histopathological examination

CHOLANGIOCELLULAR CARCINOMA

Cholangiocellular carcinoma is the tumour of bile duct commonly occurs in cattle and sheep.

Etiology
- Not known
- More common in liver fluke infected animals
- Aflatoxins

Macroscopic and microscopic features
- Small in size and multiple
- Round and encapsulated
- Yellowish white in colour

- Consist acini lined by columnar cells containing mucin
- Cyst like spaces filled with neoplastic cells
- Nucleus located at the base of cells
- Cells are surrounded by collagenous stroma.

Diagnosis
- Symptoms and lesions
- Histopathological examination

HEPATOCELLULAR CARCINOMA

Hepatocellular carcinoma is tumour of hepatic ells and observed in cattle and sheep.

Etiology
- Not known
- Aflatoxin
- Liver fluke infection.

Macroscopic and microscopic features
- Single, projected as brownish or greenish nodule
- Round or ovoid
- Hepatic cells arranged in columns
- Cells are large and polyhedral with acidophilic granular cytoplasm
- Nucleus is very large, central and pale staining
- Numerous mitotic figures
- Tumour giant cells are seen
- Divided by connective tissue stroma.

Diagnosis
- Symptoms and lesions
- Histopathological examination

Neoplasm

PAPILLOMA/ MALIGNANT DUCT PAPILLOMA OF MAMMARY GLAND

Papilloma or malignant duct papilloma is a tumour of duct epithelium of teat canal commonly seen in bitches.

Etiology
- Not known

Macroscopic and microscopic features
- Tumours are soft or hard, cystic
- Grayish white in colour
- Enlarged teats
- Hard swelling
- Tumour arises from lining epithelium of teat canal
- May be single
- Cells are cuboidal/ columnar forms papillary projections
- Cells contain eosinophilic material
- Anaplastic cells have hyperchromasia
- Cells arranged in acinar or multi acinar form in malignant papilloma.

Diagnosis
- Symptoms and lesions
- Histopathological examination

ADENOMA AND ADENOCARCINOMA OF THYROID

Adenoma of thyroid is common in horses. It is the benign tumour of thyroid. Adenocarcinoma is malignant tumour of thyroid commonly seen in old dogs.

Etiology
- Goiter
- Iodine deficiency may predispose.

Macroscopic and microscopic features
- Small, rounded and encapsulated tumour

- Adenoma may cause pressure atrophy on rest of the gland
- Adenocarcinoma is multiple, unilateral, solid or cystic and highly invasive.
- Formation of acini
- Columnar or cuboidal cells forms solid mass
- Nucleus oval, hyperchromatic
- Mitotic figures are common.

Diagnosis
- Symptoms and lesions
- Histopathological examination

GRANULOSA CELL TUMOUR OF OVARY

Granulosa cell tumour arises from ovary mesenchyma and common in cattle. These tumours are seen in younger animals.

Etiology
- Not known

Macroscopic and microscopic features
- Single, very large even up to 20 cm diameter
- Rounded, lobulated projected on the surface of ovary
- Yellow in colour.
- Tumour cells are arranged in columns, clusters or compact alveoli as irregular mass or pseudo glands
- In lumen, hyaline acidophilic material
- Several mitotic figures are seen.

Diagnosis
- Symptoms and lesions
- Histopathological examination

SEMINOMA

Seminoma is a malignant tumour of epithelium of seminiferous tubules of testes. It is common in dogs and bulls. It is more commonly seen in castrated and cryptorchid animals.

Neoplasm

Etiology
- Castration or cryptorchidism may predispose.

Macroscopic and microscopic features
- White or grey in colour
- Lobulated as bulging from testes
- Areas of necrosis may be seen.
- Epithelial cells are arranged as sheets or islands separated by thin strands of fibrous tissue
- Cells are round, large, uniform in size with acidophilic and granular cytoplasm
- Mitosis are numerous.

Diagnosis
- Symptoms and lesions
- Histopathological examination

MELANOMA AND MALIGNANT MELANOMA

Melanoma arises from melanoblasts situated in stratum germinativum of epidermis. Common in animals specially in old grey or white horses.

Etiology
- Not known
- Mostly seen in dark coloured cattle, buffalo, sheep and goats

Macroscopic and microscopic features
- Vary in size few mm diameter to several cm diameter
- Black or brown in colour
- Rounded, nodular, flat and pedunculated
- Firm and smooth
- On section, shiny black surface is seen
- Malignant melanomas are soft.
- Collection of pigment laden cells covered by fibrous tissue

- Cells are polyhedral or oval or elongated
- In malignant melanomas, cells are anaplastic and may not have melanin
- Nucleus is large and vesicular
- Several mitotic figures are seen

Diagnosis
- Symptoms and lesions
- Histopathological examination

VENEREAL SARCOMA

It is a transmissible venereal tumour in bitches or dogs seen at glans penis or vagina. Histogenic classification is not clear but may be a reticuloendothelial in origin.

Etiology
- Not known. But it is transmissible in abraded mucous membrane through coitus

Macroscopic and microscopic features
- Solitary/ multiple
- Spreads like a cauliflower
- Pink in colour
- Soft in consistency
- Ulcerated and blood stained discharge.
- Cellular mass, uniform in size and shape
- Round and polyhedral cells
- Finely granular acidophilic cytoplasm
- Numerous mitotic figures
- Nucleus large, round and central hyperchromatic.

Diagnosis
- Symptoms and lesions
- Histopathological examination

ADAMANTINOMA

Adamantinomas are tumours arising from enamel organ. It is more common in cattle.

Etiology
- Not known

Macroscopic and microscopic features
- Arises from alveolar border of maxilla or mandible
- Soft nodule
- Round or lobulated
- Dense fibrous stroma having epithelial neoplastic ameloblasts
- Arranged in cyst or solid masses.
- Columnar epithelial cells with a giant basophilic cytoplasm
- Cells arranged in the form of a cyst
- Cyst may contain acidophilic debris.

Diagnosis
- Symptoms and lesions
- Histopathological examination

CONNECTIVE TISSUE TUMOURS (NON-EPITHELIAL TUMOURS)

FIBROMA AND FIBROSARCOMA

Fibroma is a benign and fibrosarcoma is malignant tumour of fibrous connective tissue.

Etiology
- Not known
- 20% of skin tumours are fibropapilloma of gum, vagina, rectum or glans penis origin

Macroscopic and microscopic features
- Hard
- Common in horse, dogs

- Size from tiny nodules to large even upto several cm diameter
- Congestion
- Interlacing bundles of fibrous connective tissue
- Nuclei of such cells are spindle shape
- Blood vessels, lymphocytes and monocytes are seen
- Increased number of mitotic figures (Malignant giant cells) in fibrosarcoma.

Diagnosis
- Symptoms and lesions
- Histopathological examination

MYXOMA AND MYXOSARCOMA

Myxoma is tumour of fibrous tissue capable of producing mucin and anaplasia. These are observed mostly on subcutaneous, subserous and submucous surfaces.

Etiology
- Unknown
- Myxomatosis virus in rabbits

Macroscopic and microscopic features
- Rounded, bunch of grapes like structures
- Slimy in touch due to mucin content
- Present on subcutaneous, subserous or submucosal surfaces.
- Spindle shaped cells
- Cells lying in basophilic mucinous matrix
- Pleomorphism
- Several mitotic figures
- Infiltration of inflammatory cells.

Diagnosis
- Symptoms and lesions

Neoplasm

- Histopathological examination

LIPOMA AND LIPOSARCOMA

Lipoma is a tumour of fat cells and seen in subcutaneous, subserosa, mesentery or submucosa. Lipoma is common in old aged animals while liposarcoma, the malignant tumour of fat cells is very rare.

Etiology
- Unknown

Macroscopic and microscopic features
- Size vary from small nodule (1-2 mm dia) to large big mass (several cm diameter)
- Mostly spherical and lobulated
- On section, cut surface is oily
- Yellow in colour
- Polyhedral cells may have a large fat globule or several small ones with marginal nucleus.
- Connective tissue divides the mass into lobules
- In malignancy, anaplastic cells have little fat.

Diagnosis
- Symptoms and lesions
- Histopathological examination

CHONDROMA AND CHONDROSARCOMA

Chondroma is a benign and chondrosarcoma is malignant tumour of cartilage cells. These are rare in animals. In dogs, chondroma are reported in mammary gland.

Etiology
- Not known
- Common in sheep, arises from osteochondral junction of scapula, ribs, humerus and femur

Macroscopic and microscopic features
- Chondromas are multinodular

- Encapsulated and rounded
- Bluish white in colour
- Section shows translucent appearance
- Calcification may be observed
- Rounded or ovoid cells in bluish matrix
- Cells are arranged mostly as single.
- Strands of fibrous connective tissue forms lobules
- Chondrosarcoma cells are pleomorphic
- Several mitotic figures

Diagnosis
- Symptoms and lesions
- Histopathological examination

OSTEOMA AND OSTEOSARCOMA

Osteoma is benign and osteosarcoma is malignant and hard tumour of bone. This is rarely seen in animals. On skull, scapula or pelvic bones, they are known as *compact osteoma* while on long bones they are called as *spongy osteoma.*

Etiology
- Not known
- Rare in occurrence

Macroscopic and microscopic features
- Nodular, encapsulated
- Found on skull, scapula, pelvic bones or head of long bones.
- Round or ovoid in shape
- White, yellow or pink in colour.
- Osteoid tissue with lamellar arrangement
- Confused with exostosis
- Osteosarcoma have pleomorphic cells
- Tumour giant cells
- Several mitotic figures
- Several new blood vessels

Diagnosis
- Symptoms and lesions
- Histopathological examination

LEIOMYOMA AND LEIOMYOSARCOMA

Leiomyoma is a benign tumour of smooth muscle found in different organs like uterus, vagina, stomach, intestines, urinary bladder, esophagus etc. Such tumours are commonly seen in cow, dog and poultry. Leiomyosarcoma is malignant neoplasm of smooth muscles.

Etiology
- Not known

Macroscopic and microscopic features
- Small size tumours with broad base
- Firm, lobulated and pink in colour.
- Muscle bundles arranged in all directions and planes
- Muscle bundles separated by fibrous tissue with blood vessels
- Nucleus becomes cigar shaped and contain filamentus chromatin
- Leiomyosarcoma have anaplastic cells with shorter chromatin
- Mitotic figures are common.
- Such tumours are invasive to adjacent tissues.

Diagnosis
- Symptoms and lesions
- Histopathological examination

RHABDOMYOMA AND RHABDOMYSARCOMA

Rhabdomyoma is a benign and rhabdomyosarcoma is malignant tumour of skeletal and cardiac muscles and are rare in animals.

Etiology
- Not known

Macroscopic and microscopic features
- Found in tongue, chest, sternal muscles, neck region, cardiac muscles
- Broad based.
- Striated muscles grow on different directions
- Fibrous tissue divides the muscle bundles into lobules
- In Rhabdomyosarcoma, the anaplastic cells are pleomorphic, polyhedral and spindle shaped.
- Presence of tumour giant cells.

Diagnosis
- Symptoms and lesions
- Histopathological examination

HEMANGIOMA AND HEMANGIOSARCOMA

Haemangioma is benign while hemangiosarcoma is malignant tumour of blood vessels.

Etiology
- Not known

Macroscopic and microscopic features
- Usually single
- Vary in size few mm diameter to several cm diameter.
- Dark red in colour and confused with haematoma
- Bleeding is severe on rupture or injury.
- Many capillaries are seen
- Usually single cell lined capillaries
- Lumen filled with newly formed endothelial cells
- Pleomorphism in endothelial cells
- Such cells grouped into masses in malignant tumours
- Numerous mitotic figures are seen.

Diagnosis
- Symptoms and lesions
- Histopathological examination

Neoplasm

MESOTHELIOMA

Mesothelioma is a tumour of mesothelial lining cells of serous cavities specially of peritoneum and pleura. Such tumours are found in thorax and abdomen.

Etiology
- Not known
- Macroscopic features
- Pink in colour and hard
- Multiple, nodular and scattered in cavity
- Found in thorax and/or abdominal cavity.
- Collection of cells resembling epithelial cells
- Cells have acidophilic granular cytoplasm and large vesicular nucleus
- Numerous blood vessels in tumour
- A core of fibrous tissue present
- Mitotic figures may be seen.

Diagnosis
- Symptoms and lesions
- Histopathological examination

MASTOCYTOMA

Mastocytoma is a tumour of mast cells commonly seen in dogs in subcutaneous tissue of hind legs.

Etiology
- Not known

Macroscopic and microscopic features
- Usually single and have a size of about 8-12 cm diameter.
- Nodular, pedunculated
- Hard, pink or grey in colour
- Ulceration over tumour is common.
- Pleomorphic mast cells
- Inflammatory cells like neutrophils and lymphocytes are

also seen
- Darkly stained cells
- Cytoplasm is more than in lymphocytes
- No or little cytoplasmic granules
- Few mitotic figures

Diagnosis
- Symptoms and lesions
- Histopathological examination

LYMPHOMA AND LYMPHOSARCOMA

Lymphoma is a benign and lymphosarcoma is a malignant neoplasm of lymphoid cells primarily found in lymph nodes.

Etiology
- Not known
- Possibly a retrovirus

Macroscopic and microscopic features
- Tumours in several lymph nodes and spleen.
- Obliteration of lymph vessels/ blood vessels.
- Common in dogs (canine venereal tumour), cat and cattle.
- Enlargement of lymph nodes.
- Spleen is enlarged, soft and friable.
- Liver enlarged and pale.
- Immature pleomorphic lymphoid cells.
- Mitotic figures are seen.
- Tumour giant cells are seen.
- In blood, number of immature lymphoid cell increases and known as *Leukemia*.

Diagnosis
- Symptoms and lesions
- Histopathological examination

Chapter 23
Viral Diseases

FOOT AND MOUTH DISEASE

Foot and mouth disease is a contagious viral disease of cloven footed animals caused by a picorna virus and characterized by presence of vesicles in oral mucosa and foot.

Etiology
- RNA virus of picornaviridae family
- Picorna virus
- Serotypes A, O, C, SAT-1, SAT-2, SAT-3, Asia-1, serotype 'O' is most common in India.

Pathogenesis

Inhalation is the main route of infection in ruminants; however, ingestion of contaminated feed and water, inoculation of contaminated vaccines, insemination with contaminated semen and contact with fomites such as clothing, instruments etc. may also transmit the infection. When animal gets infected through respiratory tract, viral replication starts in pharynx followed by viremic spread to other tissues and organs like epithelium of mouth. Viral excretion commences about 24 hours prior to the onset of clinical form of disease and continues for several days. The aerosols of infected animals contain large amount of virus particularly of swine. Large amount of virus is excreted in milk. In cattle and sheep, virus may be detectable up to 2 years and 6 months of exposure, respectively.

Characteristic symptoms
- Fever (102-104°F)
- Drooling of saliva
- Vesicular mouth lesions

- Lameness due to formation of vesicles on coronets

Macroscopic and microscopic features
- Presence of vesicles on tongue, lips, cheeks and palate
- Damaged vesicle leaves a raw surface having red areas due to congestion
- Gastroenteritis
- **Myocarditis-** *Tigroid appearance*
- Enlargement of spleen.
- Hydropic degeneration in stratum spinosum cells of epidermis
- Presence of micro vesicles
- Infiltration of neutrophils
- Hyaline degeneration and necrosis of muscles of myocardium
- Infiltration of neutrophils and mononuclear cells in myocardium.

Diagnosis
- Symptoms and lesions
- Immunodiagnostic tests for demonstration of antigen/antibody- CFT, ELISA
- Isolation of virus and its typing
- Demonstration of virus in affected tissues using electronmicroscopy

VESICULAR STOMATITIS

Vesicular stomatitis is a contagious viral disease of animals caused by vesiculovirus and characterized by the presence of vesicles in oral cavity, necrosis and intercellular oedema. It is also known as *sore mouth* of cattle.

Etiology
- Vesiculovirus of rhabdoviridae family.
- RNA virus with 70-175 nm size, bullet shape

Viral Diseases

Pathogenesis

Transmitted through insects from infected to susceptible animals. There is viremia and virus settles in oral mucosa causing vesicular glossitis.

Clinical Symptoms
- Hypersalivation
- Rubbing of lips with manger

Macroscopic and microscopic features
- Vesicles on tongue
- Vesicles on snout of pigs
- Intercellular oedema in malpighian layer
- Necrosis of epithelial layer
- Infiltration of neutrophils and mononuclear cells

Diagnosis
- Symptoms and lesions
- Detection of antibody or antigen using ELISA

VESICULAR EXANTHEMA

Vesicular exanthema is a viral disease of swine characterized by fever and vesicle formation in snout, lips, nostrils, tongue, feet and mammary gland.

Etiology
- Calcivirus of 35-40 nm diameter

Pathogenesis

The source of infection is infected pig or pork and virus spreads among susceptible animals through direct contact. Viremia lasts for 3-4 days and virus localizes in buccal mucosa and skin.

Clinical Symptoms
- Fever
- Vesicles on mouth, snout, teats, claws
- Anorexia

- Rupture of vesicle leads to ulcer

Macroscopic and microscopic features
- Vesicles on snouts, lips, tongue
- Vesicles on coronary band and mammary gland
- Rupture of vesicles
- Ruptured vesicles covered by brown and dry dead tissue
- Ulcer on secondary bacterial infection.
- Vesicles, hydropic degeneration on stratum spinosum layer of epidermis
- Infiltration of mononuclear cells

Diagnosis
- Symptoms and lesions
- Detection of antibody or antigen using ELISA

RINDERPEST

Rinderpest is an acute contagious viral disease of cattle and buffaloes caused by morbillivirus and characterized by erosive mouth lesions and erosions and hemorrhagic enteritis. It has been eradicated from India.

Etiology
- Morbilli virus of paramyxoviridae family.
- RNA virus
- Very fragile virus, sensitive to glycerol.

Pathogenesis

Virus enters in body through inhalation, penetrates the epithelium of upper respiratory tract and multiplies in tonsils and mandibular and pharyngeal lymph nodes. From there it enters in blood mononuclear cells, which disseminate the virus to other lymphoid organs, lungs and epithelial cells of mucous membrane. The virus has high affinity for lymphoid tissue and alimentary tract mucosa. In tissues, there is pronounced destruction of lymphocytes. Viremia develops within 2 to 3 days after which virus can be demonstrated in lymph nodes, spleen, bone marrow and mucosa of respiratory and digestive tract. There is marked leucopenia due to viral replication and destruction of lymphoid tissue. Due to destruction of epithelial lining of mucous membranes, there is presence of erosions in the form of "Zebra" stripes in caecum, colon and rectum which is considered characteristic of rinderpest. Intra cytoplasmic and intra nuclear eosinophilic inclusion bodies are commonly seen in epithelial cells.

Characteristic symptoms
- Fever (105-107°F)
- Diarrhoea, melena
- **Erosive mouth lesions**
- Skin eruptions
- Conjunctivitis
- Mortality up to 80%

Macroscopic and microscopic features
- Erosions on oral mucosa
- Bran like deposits on erosions, on removal haemorrhagic raw surface is present
- Hemorrhage in intestines leading to *"Zebra markings"*
- Petechial hemorrhage in bladder, vagina and other mucous membrane
- Congestion of conjunctivae.
- Erosions in epithelium of oral and gastrointestinal mucosa
- Infiltration of mononuclear cells
- Congestion and hemorrhage in intestines
- Depletion of lymphoid cells in peyer's patches
- Lymphocytolysis in spleen and lymph nodes.

Diagnosis
- Symptoms and lesions
- Immunodiagnostic tests for demonstration of antigen/antibody- AGPT, CIEP, ELISA

- Isolation of virus

MALIGNANT CATARRHAL FEVER

Malignant catarrhal fever is an infectious disease of cattle caused by herpes virus and characterized by catarrhal and mucopurulent conjunctivitis, presence of erosions/ ulcers on nostrils, oral mucosa, intestines and enlargement of lymph nodes.

Etiology
- DNA virus of herpesviridae family
- Herpes virus

Pathogenesis

It is caused by herpes virus which is strongly associated with cells. The disease is transmitted through wild beast and sub clinically infected sheep to cattle. In circulating blood it is attached to leucocytes, especially mononuclear cells. After entry, the virus attacks and replicates in lymphoid tissues (e.g. lymph nodes, peyers patches and spleen). Many lymphocytes are destroyed in germinal centers leading to their depletion. The incubation period is very long and there is no clear information about pathogenesis of disease. There is generalized lymphadenopathy and lympho-pro liferative response involves T_h and T_c cells. There is most constant finding is marked perivascular coughing of mononuclear cells, mainly monocytes.

Characteristic symptoms
- Fever (105-107°F)
- Drooling of saliva
- Ulcerative mouth and nasal lesions
- Diarrhoea, dysentery with melena
- Conjunctivitis
- Enlargement of superficial lymph nodes

Macroscopic and microscopic features
- Conjunctivitis, rhinitis

- Mucopurulent exudate in eyes and nostrils
- Erosions and ulcers on oral and intestinal mucosa
- Liver and kidneys enlarged and mottled
- Necrosis of epithelium and intense lymphocytic infiltration in mucosa of upper respiratory tract, oral mucosa and abomasum
- Infiltration of eosinophils in mucosa and submucosa of gastrointestinal tract.

Diagnosis
- History of sheep rearing with cattle
- Symptoms and lesions
- Immunodiagnostic tests for demonstration of antigen/ antibody- AGPT, ELISA
- Isolation of virus through co-cultivation of peripheral blood lymphocytes

BOVINE VIRAL DIARRHOEA/ MUCOSAL DISEASE

Bovine viral diarrhoea is a contagious viral disease of cattle caused by pestivirus and characterized by hypoplasia of cerebellum, ulcers in oral and nasal mucosa, oesophagus, abomasum and intestines.

Etiology
- Pestivirus of Togaviridae family.

Pathogenesis

The virus spreads by direct or indirect contact with infected animals. Overcrowding and transportation play an important role in spread of virus through oral and nasal route. The virus also spreads through contaminated food and water, urine and nasal discharge. After entry virus multiplies in lymphocytes which leads to viremia. From circulation, virus reaches in the mucous membrane of alimentary tract. In buccal cavity, it causes inflammation and edema which is manifested by ulcerative stomatitis and enteritis. However, pathogenesis of the lesions remains obscure.

Characteristic symptoms
- Fever (105-107°F)
- Drooling of saliva
- Ulcerative mouth and nasal lesions
- Diarrhoea, dysentery with melena

Macroscopic and microscopic features
- Hypoplasia of cerebellum
- Ulcers in oral and nasal mucosa
- Ulcers and hemorrhage in mucosa of gastrointestinal tract
- Ulcers in esophagus
- Hemorrhage in vagina, epicardium and sub cutaneous tissue.
- Necrosis, ulcer, and infiltration of lymphocytes in oesophagus.
- Hemorrhage in intestines
- Ulcers in intestines
- Infiltration of mononuclear cells

Diagnosis
- Symptoms and lesions
- Immunodiagnostic tests for demonstration of antigen/antibody- AGPT, ELISA
- Isolation of virus

POX
Pox is an infectious viral disease of animals caused by members of poxviridae family and characterized by the presence of pock lesions on hair less parts of the skin.

Etiology
- Sheep- Ovi pox virus, Capri pox virus
- Goat- Capri pox virus
- Cow- Cow pox virus
- Buffalo- Buffalo pox virus

- Camel- Camel pox virus
- Swine- Swi pox virus

Pathogenesis

The disease is transmitted by direct contact with affected animals and through the hand of the milkers, insects and milking machine. Generally virus enters through small abrasions of skin. Following incubation period of 3-7 days, the pock lesions appear on skin which comprises of erythema, followed by papules, vesicles, pustule and scab; on detach and slough off it may leave scar.

Characteristic symptoms
- Fever (105-107°F)
- Pock lesions on hairless parts of skin like papule, vesicle, pustule, scab and scar

Macroscopic and microscopic features
- Presence of pock lesions on hair less parts of body including papule, vesicle, pustule, scab and scar.
- Cow- Pock lesions on teats
- Buffaloes- Face, teats
- Sheep and Camel- Whole body
- Necrosis of stratum spinosum epithelium of epidermis
- Infiltration of mononuclear cells in dermis and epidermis
- Presence of intracytoplasmic inclusions

Diagnosis
- Symptoms and lesions
- Immunodiagnostic tests for demonstration of antigen/antibody- AGPT, ELISA
- Isolation of virus

INFECTIOUS BOVINE RHINOTRACHEITIS

Infectious bovine rhinotracheitis is an infectious viral disease of cattle caused by herpes virus and characterized by respiratory disease, conjunctivitis, encephalitis in calves and abortions and mastitis in cows.

Etiology
- DNA virus of Herpesviridae family
- Bovine herpes virus –1 (BHV-1)

Pathogenesis

The main source of infection is nasal exudate and coughed up droplets, genital secretions, semen and foetal fluid/ tissues. Aerosol or droplet infection causes respiratory disease. In genital from, venereal transmission occurs. In respiratory disease, after entry virus multiplies in nasal cavity and upper respiratory tract resulting in rhinitis, laryngitis and tracheitis. There is extensive loss of cilia in trachea. This leaves the tracheal epithelium covered with microvilli, which has an adverse effect on the defense mechanism of respiratory tract. The virus spreads from nasal mucosa through trigeminal ganglion, resulting in a non-suppurative encephalitis. Through peripheral leucocytes, virus may reach to placenta and foetus in pregnant animals causing abortion. The foetus is highly susceptible to the herpes virus infection.

Characteristic symptoms
- Fever (106°F)
- Nasal discharge
- Abortions in late gestation
- Conjunctivitis
- Infectious pustular balanoposthitis in bulls
- Infectious pustular vulvovaginitis in cows

Macroscopic and microscopic features
- Rhinotracheitis, pneumonia, mucopurulent exudate in trachea.
- Pustules in vulva/ vagina, glans penis and prepuce
- Ulcers in vulva/ vagina

Viral Diseases

- Necrotic lesions in liver of aborted foetus
- Hyaline membrane pneumonia
- Erosions/ ulcers in mucosa of upper respiratory tract
- Ulcers on vulval mucous membrane
- Infiltration of lymphocytes
- Presence of intranuclear inclusions in mucosal epithelium
- Necrotic lesions in liver, spleen and kidneys of aborted foetus

Diagnosis
- Symptoms and lesions
- Immunodiagnostic tests for demonstration of antigen/ antibody- AGPT, ELISA
- Isolation of virus

ROTAVIRUS INFECTION

Rotavirus causes acute gastroenteritis in neonates of animals characterized by yellowish watery diarrhoea, shortening of villi, dehydration, malabsorption and maldigestion.

Etiology
- Rotavirus belonging to family Reoviridae
- Double stranded RNA
- 11 segments in genome

Pathogenesis

The disease spreads either through direct contact or through contaminated water, milk and fomites. The virus infects mature epithelial cells of the small intestine due to presence of receptors in the form of beta-galactosidase on the brush border of the epithelium or the receptors of immunoglobulins (IgG) are utilized by the virus. Only differentiated columnar epithelial cell lining of apical half of villi are susceptible. The virus does not enter and replicate in immature/ proliferating cells in crypts because these cells lack receptors for the virus. Epithelial cells develop cisternae (wide spaces) in endoplasmic reticulum with swollen mitochondria. The viral particles appear in distended cisternae and lysosomes. The epithelial cells are vacuolated and desquamated in the lumen of the intestine. Villi thus become atrophic and shortened resulting in malabsorption and maldigestion. The death of affected calves occurs due to dehydration.

Characteristic symptoms
- Fever (104-106°F)
- Watery yellowish diarrhoea, dysentery with melena
- Dehydration

Macroscopic and microscopic features
- Congestion of intestines
- Presence of desquamated cells mixed catarrhal exudate in the small intestines
- Enlargement of mesenteric lymph nodes
- Increased number of goblet cells in villi
- Shortening of the length of villi
- Fusion of two adjacent villi
- Infiltration of mononuclear cells in mucosa and submucosa
- Congestion and hemorrhage

Diagnosis
- Symptoms and lesions
- Immunodiagnostic tests for demonstration of antigen/antibody- AGPT, CIEP, ELISA
- Isolation of virus
- Demonstration of virus antigen in intestinal tissue sections using immunoperoxidase technique.

CORONAVIRUS INFECTION

Coronavirus infection causes acute gastroenteritis in neonates of animal characterized by damage in villi as well as crypts leading to mal digestion, mal absorption, shortening of villi, haemorrhage in small and large intestines.

Etiology
- Coronavirus

Pathogenesis

The disease spreads either through direct contact or through contaminated water, milk and fomites. The virus infects both mature and immature epithelial cells of the small intestine. Epithelial cells of crypts and villi develop cisternae (wide spaces) in endoplasmic reticulum with swollen mitochondria. The viral particles appear in distended cisternae and lysosomes. The epithelial cells are vacuolated and desquamated in the lumen of the intestine. Villi thus become atrophic and shortened resulting in malabsorption and maldigestion. The death of affected calves occurs due to dehydration and loss of blood.

Characteristic symptoms
- Fever (104-106°F)
- Diarrhoea, dysentery with melena
- Dehydration

Macroscopic and microscopic features
- Congestion of small and large intestines
- Presence of mucohaemorrhagic exudate along with desquamated cells in intestine
- Enlargement of mesenteric lymph nodes
- Increase number of goblet cells on villous surface
- Shortening of villi and crypts
- Hemorrhage from exposed villi
- Fusion of two adjacent villi
- Congestion and hemorrhage in mucosa and submucosa
- Infiltration of mononuclear cells in mucosa and submucosa

Diagnosis
- Symptoms and lesions
- Immunodiagnostic tests for demonstration of antigen/antibody- CFT, ELISA

- Isolation of virus
- Demonstration of virus antigen in intestinal tissue sections using immunoperoxidase technique

PARAINFLUENZA-3 INFECTION

Parainfluenza-3 virus causes respiratory disease in cattle, sheep and goat characterized by rhinitis and bronchopneumonia

Etiology
- Parainfluenza-3 virus
- Secondary invaders
- Corynebacterium
- Streptococci
- *Pasturella multocida*

Pathogenesis

It is one of the important pathogenesis of both animal and man. Infection occurs through the respiratory route and virus multiplies in respiratory epithelium resulting in viremia with short courses of fever, rhinitis and nasal discharge, lacrimation, coughing and dyspnoea.

Characteristic symptoms
- Fever (105-107°F)
- Nasal discharge
- Sneezing, coughing

Macroscopic and microscopic features
- Congestion of nasal mucosa
- Mucopurulent exudate in upper respiratory tract
- Congestion and consolidation of lungs
- Congestion of mediastinal lymph nodes
- Lobular distribution of lesions in lungs
- Infiltration of mononuclear cells in alveoli around the bronchi
- Proliferation of septal cells present in inter alveolar spaces

- Presence of giant cells in alveoli
- Presence of intra cytoplasmic and intra nuclear eosinophilic inclusions

Diagnosis
- Symptoms and lesions
- Immunodiagnostic tests for demonstration of antigen/antibody- AGPT, ELISA
- Isolation of virus
- Demonstration of viral antigen in respiratory tract epithelium using immunoperoxidase technique.

BOVINE IMMUNODEFICIENCY

Bovine immunodeficiency is an infectious viral diseases of cattle caused by lentivirus and characterized by lethargyness, abscess formation, abomasitis, lymphosarcoma and immunosuppression.

Etiology
- Lentivirus of retroviridae family
- RNA virus having reverse transcriptase enzyme

Pathogenesis

The virus mainly spreads through insect bites; though the possibility of vertical transmission cannot be ruled out. The virus replicates in macrophages and lymphocytes and remains cell associated as infection is life long leading to lymphocytolysis and immunosuppression.

Characteristic symptoms
- Letharginess
- Abscess formation
- Mastitis, dermatitis, pneumonia or digestive disorders as a result of immunosuppression.

Macroscopic and microscopic features
- Subcutaneous nodules of lymphoid follicles

- Abscess on skin
- Pododermatitis
- Lymphadenopathy
- Lymphosarcoma
- Lymphocytosis or lymphopenia
- Lymphocytic encephalitis and meningitis

Diagnosis
- Symptoms and lesions
- Detection of virus antigen/ antibody using ELISA
- Demonstration of viral antigen in lymphocytes using immunoperoxidase technique
- Demonstration of virus using electronmicroscopy.

BOVINE LEUKEMIA

Bovine leukemia is an infectious viral disease of cattle caused by oncornavirus characterized by malignant lymphoma in lymph nodes, lymphocytosis with immature lymphocytes in blood. It is also known as bovine lymphoma or malignant lymphoma.

Etiology
- Oncorna virus of retroviridae family
- Type C oncorna virus having reverse transcriptase, RNA virus

Pathogenesis

The virus is transmitted horizontally and infects lymphocytes leading to their proliferation. The proviral DNA of virus incorporated in host cell DNA inducing neoplastic growth of the cells.

Characteristic symptoms
- Lymphocytosis
- Enlargement of superficial lymph nodes
- Weakness, emaciation, cachexia

Macroscopic and microscopic features
- Enlargement of lymph nodes (mesenteric, pelvic and sublumbar)
- Dehydrated, emaciated and cachectic carcass
- Immature lymphocytes in blood
- Mitotic figures, anaplastic cells in lymph nodes
- Heavy lymphocytic infiltration in myocardium

Diagnosis
- Symptoms and lesions
- Detection of antigen/ antibody using ELISA
- Demonstration of viral antigen in affected tissue using IFT or immunoperoxidase technique
- Demonstration of virus using electronmicroscopy

EPHEMERAL FEVER

Ephemeral fever is a viral disease of animals characterized by three days sickness, oedematous lymph nodes, hydropericardium, hydrothorax, pulmonary emphysema, tendovaginitis, and congestion of abomasal folds and focal necrosis of muscle.

Etiology
- Vesiculovirus of Rhabdoviridae family
- Bullet shaped RNA virus

Pathogenesis

The virus is transmissible through insects and after an incubation period of 2-10 days, viremia sets in. Thereafter, virus localizes in the joints, lymphocytes and muscles.

Clinical Symptoms
- Three day sickness
- Shifting lameness
- High fever which subsides after 3 days
- Stiffness of joints

Macroscopic and microscopic features
- Hydrothorax, hydropericardium
- Edematous lymph nodes
- Rhinitis, tracheitis, pulmonary emphysema
- Congestion of abomasum
- Vascular enlargement/ congestion
- Emphysema in lungs
- Focal necrosis of muscle
- Petechiae in peripheral nerves

Diagnosis
- Symptoms and lesions
- Detection of antigen and antibody using ELISA
- Demonstration of viral antigen in affected tissues using immunoperoxidase technique.

BLUE TONGUE

Blue tongue is an infectious viral disease of sheep caused by orbivirus and characterized by oedema and congestion of face, congestion and cyanosis of tongue, endothelial hyperplasia and arteritis.

Etiology
- Orbivirus of Reoviridae family
- dsRNA virus
- Serotype 1, 2, 9, 15, 18, 23 in India

Pathogenesis

Blue tongue is transmitted by biting of insects including culicoids and other mosquitoes and ectoparasites like *Malophagus ovinus*. The infection has also been transmitted by insemination from an infected male, since virus is present in the semen. After infection, viral replication starts in hemopoietic cells which results in viremia and subsequent replication in endothelial cells of blood vessels throughout the body. The damage of endothelial cells leads to development of hyperemia, hemorrhage, edema and thrombosis.

Characteristic symptoms
- Fever (105-107°F)
- Edema of face
- Cyanosis of tongue
- Signs of mosquito bite on skin

Macroscopic and microscopic features
- Edema and congestion of face, head, neck
- Edema and cyanosis of tongue
- Petechial haemorrhage on oral and nasal mucosa
- Hemorrhage on coronets leading to pododermatitis
- Hemorrhage in abomasum and intestines.
- Hemorrhage and infiltration of mononuclear cells in tongue
- Hyperemia of vascular corium of skin in coronets
- Hemorrhage in muscles of coronets
- Hemorrhage and infiltration of neutrophils in abomasum and intestines.

Diagnosis
- Symptoms and lesions
- Immunodiagnostic tests for demonstration of antigen/antibody- AGPT, CIEP, ELISA
- Isolation of virus

CONTAGIOUS ECTHYMA

Contagious ecthyma is a highly infectious viral disease of sheep and goats characterized by the presence of pustular and scabby lesions on muzzle and lips.

Etiology
- Contagious ecthyma virus belongs to poxviridae family
- Similar to pseudo-cow pox virus
- Very resistant virus

Pathogenesis

Virus transmitted through direct and indirect contact with contaminated materials like feed, fences, manure, bedding. Infected lambs may transmit the virus through suckling on teats and udder of dam. Lesions develop on mouth as papule and then pustules. These are covered with thick tenacious scabs covering a raised area of ulceration.

Characteristic symptoms
- Pustular and scabby lesions on muzzle, nostrils and lips
- Pustular lesions on coronets, ears, anus, vulva, prepura
- Morbidity is high, mortality low

Macroscopic and microscopic features
- Pustular lesions on muzzle, lips and nostrils
- Gastroenteritis
- Bronchopneumonia
- Ulcers in nasal mucosa, oesophagus, abomasum and small intestines.

Diagnosis
- Symptoms and lesions
- Immunodiagnossis- ELISA
- Demonstration of antigen in tissue sections using immunoperoxidase techniques

OVINE PULMONARY CARCINOMA (PREVIOUSLY PULMONARY ADENOMATOSIS)

(Pulmonary adenomatosis) or Jaagsiekte is an infectious viral disease of sheep caused by a lentivirus and characterized by metaplasia of alveolar epithelium to cuboidal or columnar giving it an appearance of gland.

Etiology
- Lentivirus of Retroviridae family
- RNA virus, having reverse transcriptase enzyme

Viral Diseases

Pathogenesis

It has a very long incubation period (1-3 years). It is transmitted through direct contact or droplet infection for a long period of time. The disease may also be vertically transmitted from mother to lambs. After entry virus multiplies and localizes in lungs. There is development of oedematous growth in the alveolar epithelium due to metaplasia. As a result there is interference of oxygen exchange resulting to hypoxia and anoxia.

Characteristic symptoms
- Chronic nasal discharge
- Weakness, wasting

Macroscopic and microscopic features
- Nodular foci in lungs
- Congestion and consolidation of lungs
- Later stages characterized by fibrosis.
- Lymphoid follicles in lungs
- Proliferation and hypertrophy of alveolar epithelial cells leading to cuboidal or columnar epithelium giving it a shape of gland
- Thickening of alveolar wall
- Adenomatosis in bronchial and mediastinal lymph nodes.

Diagnosis
- Symptoms and lesions
- Immunodiagnostic tests for demonstration of antigen/ antibody- ELISA
- Demonstration of viral antigen in lung tissues using IFT or immunoperoxidase technique.

MAEDI/ VISNA

Maedi is an infectious chronic viral disease of sheep caused by lentivirus and characterized by encephalomyelitis and pneumonia.

Etiology
- Lentivirus of Retroviridae family
- RNA virus having reverse transcriptase enzyme

Pathogenesis

The disease is mainly transmitted through respiratory route. Mononuclear cells of infected sheep contain virus including mononuclear cells of colostrums and milk through which lambs get infected. The virus replicates in the macrophages which leads to cell associated viraemia and dissemination of the virus to the brain and other organs. The virus can not be trapped by antibodies. Antibodies are produced very slowly as a result; these antibodies are insufficient in selecting antigenically different virions. So the virus can spread between cells much faster than it can be neutralized by antibodies.

Characteristic symptoms
- Chronic nasal discharge
- Wasting
- Aimless movements

Macroscopic and microscopic features
- Lungs have dense and rubbery consistency
- Lungs enlarged 2-5 times
- Cut surface is dry with no exudate
- Congestion of meninges and brain
- Enlargement of mediastinal lymph nodes, adhesive pleuritis.
- Zones of demyelination with destruction of para ventricular white matter in cerebellum and cerebrum
- Gliosis and lymphocytic infiltration in brain and meninges
- Thickening of the alveolar wall due to proliferation of mononuclear cells and fibroblasts
- Alveolar lining cells become swollen and becomes cuboidal in shape.
- Intra cytoplasmic inclusions in macrophages.

Diagnosis
- Symptoms and lesions
- Immunodiagnostic tests for demonstration of antigen/antibody- ELISA
- Demonstration of viral antigen in macrophages and/or lung tissue using immunoperoxidase technique.

PESTE DE PETITS IN RUMINANTS (PPR)
Peste de Petits ruminants (PPR) is an infectious viral disease of small ruminants caused by morbilli virus and characterized by giant cell pneumonia, erosive stomatitis and enteritis.

Etiology
- Morbilli virus of Paramyxoviridae family
- RNA virus, very frazile virus

Pathogenesis
Infection is mainly trasnmitted by inhalation through close contact with infected animals. After entry virus penetrate retropharyngeal lymph nodes and mucosa and multiplies there that leads to viremia. The virus reaches mucous membrane of alimentary and respiratory tract where it proliferates and causes damage to them. There is inflammation of mucosa leading to enteritis, diarrhoea, dehydration and death in young animals. Due to inflammation of lungs, giant cell pneumonia and respiratory distress develops. In PPR, lymphoid necrosis is not high as in rinderpest. Most of sheep and some adult goats recover and they carry antibodies that provide life long immunity.

Characteristic symptoms
- Fever (105-107°C)
- Diarrhoea, melena
- Erosive mouth lesions
- Skin eruptions
- Conjunctivitis
- Mortality up to 80%

Macroscopic and microscopic features
- Congestion and consolidation of lungs
- Hemorrhagic/ erosive enteritis
- Erosive mouth lesions
- Erosine lesions in large intestine in strips along payers patches giving rise to *"Zebra markings"* in large intestine
- Giant cell pneumonia
- Erosions in oral mucous membrane
- Erosions in intestinal mucous membrane
- Hemorrhage and congestion in intestines
- Infiltration of mononuclear cells
- Depletion of lymphoid cells in lymph nodes.

Diagnosis
- Symptoms and lesions
- Immunodiagnostic tests for demonstration of antigen/ antibody- AGPT, CIEP, ELISA
- Isolation of virus
- Demonstration of viral antigen in lung and intestinal tissue using immunoperoxidase technique.

SWINE FEVER (HOG CHOLERA)

Swine fever is an acute contagious viral disease of pigs caused by pestivirus of Togaviridae family and characterized by gluing of eyes, congestion and widespread haemorrhage in visceral organs.

Etiology
- Pestivirus of Togaviridae family
- RNA virus

Pathogenesis

Pig is the only domestic animal which is naturally infected by the virus. Infection is usually acquired by ingestion but inhalation is also a possible route. The source of virus is always infected pig and its products. In infected pig, virus is found in all excretions and secretions of body. After ingestion, virus reaches in the tonsils, where primary multiplication of virus occurs within few hours of infection. Then virus is transported through lymphatics and enter in blood capillaries resulting in an initial viraemia by about 24 hours of infection. As time goes on, virus spreads to different tissues like spleen, peripheral and visceral lymph nodes, bone marrow, peyer's patches. The virus causes destruction of endothelial cells, lymphoreticular cells, macrophages and epithelial cells. Virus causes hydropic degeneration and proliferation of vascular endothelium which results in occlusion of blood vessels leading to congestion, hemorrhage and infarction in arterioles, venules and capillaries. In small and medium sized arteries, thrombosis is also seen. At early stages, there is leucopenia followed by leucocytosis.

Characteristic symptoms
- Fever (105-106°F)
- Gluing of eyes
- Hurdling
- Congestion of skin with eruptions
- Mortality up to 100%

Macroscopic and microscopic features
- Gluing of eyes
- Congestion and hemorrhage in kidneys, lymph nodes, urinary bladder, skin, spleen, lungs and large intestines
- Button ulcers in large intestines
- Erythema and cyanosis on ventral abdomen and thorax skin.
- Perivascular cuffing in brain by lymphocytes, monocytes and plasma cells
- Intranuclear, round, homogenous acidophilic inclusion in neurons
- Hemorrhage in spleen, lymph nodes and kidneys
- Necrosis of mucosa and submucosa in intestines leading to formation of ulcers and infiltration of mononuclear cells.

Diagnosis
- Symptoms and lesions
- Immunodiagnostic tests for demonstration of antigen/antibody- AGPT, CIEP, ELISA
- Demonstration of viral antigen in affected tissues using immunoperoxidase technique.
- Isolation of virus

TRANSMISSIBLE GASTROENTERITIS

Transmissible gastroenteritis is contagious viral disease of pigs caused by corona virus and characterized by vomiting, diarrhoea, dehydration with high mortality.

Etiology
- Corona virus
- RNA virus

Pathogenesis

Transmission of virus occurs through inhalation and ingestion. Virus infects mature enterocytes of intestinal villi causing their necrosis and desquamation leading to atrophy of villi.

Characteristic symptoms
- Diarrhoea
- Vomiting
- Dehydration
- Morbidity and mortality 100%

Macroscopic and microscopic features
- Dehydrated carcass
- Curdled milk in stomach
- Congestion of small intestine
- Petechiae in intestines
- Shortening and fusion of villi, villous atrophy
- Cuboidal epithelium on villous surface

Viral Diseases

- Absence of microvilli, vacuolation in epithelial cells
- Infiltration of mononuclear cells in mucosa and submucosa

Diagnosis
- Symptoms and lesions
- Detection of viral antigen in faeces or antibody in serum using ELISA
- Demonstration of viral antigen in enterocytes using immunoperoxidase technique
- Demonstration of virus using by electronmicroscopy

PSEUDORABIES

Pseudorabies is a viral disease of animals, mainly of swine and characterized by itching, in coordination, tremors, convulsions, paralysis and encephalitis.

Etiology
- Herpes virus- *Herpes suis*
- DNA virus

Pathogenesis

After intranasal or entry through skin, the virus takes 7-8 days to localize in peripheral nerves. Where it causes necrosis of muscles and fascia and travels to spinal cord and brain to cause encephalomyelitis.

Clinical Symptoms
- Fever, itching
- In coordination of hind limbs
- Tremors, paralysis, convulsions
- Scratching due to itching
- Respiratory failure leads to death

Macroscopic and microscopic features
- Encephalitis

- Scratch wounds due to itching
- Enlargement of lymph nodes
- Necrosis of nerve fibers and ganglion
- Lymphocytic infiltration
- Intranuclear inclusion in nerve cells, ganglion and schwann cells
- Focal necrosis of pharyngeal mucosa, tonsils, lymph nodes, lungs and liver

Diagnosis
- Symptoms and lesions
- Detection of antigen and/or antibody using ELISA
- Demonstration of viral antigen in affected tissues using immunoperoxidase technique.

EQUINE INFLUENZA

Equine influenza is contagious viral diseases of horses caused by orthomyxovirus and characterized by fever, coughing and pandemic occurrence of the disease.

Etiology
- Influenza A virus of orthomyxoviridae family
- Very unstable virus, frequent antigenic drift and shift

Pathogenesis

Virus spreads through inhalation and multiplies in respiratory epithelium causing erythema, edema and focal erosions. There is very mild and short viremia.

Characteristic symptoms
- Fever (101 – 106°F)
- Coughing
- Nasal discharge
- Oedema and pain in superficial lymph nodes

Viral Diseases

Macroscopic and microscopic features
- Erosions in upper respiratory mucosa
- Peribronchitis, bronchitis
- Bronchopneumonia
- Hyaline membrane formation on bronchiolar and alveolar epithelium
- Peribronchitis, bronchitis and bronchopneumonia

Diagnosis
- Symptoms and lesions
- Detection of antigen/ antibody using hemagglutination, hemagglutination inhibition test, ELISA
- Demonstration of viral antigen in affected tissue using immunoperoxidase technique
- Demonstration of virus in tissue/ secretions using electronmicroscopy

EQUINE INFECTIOUS ANEMIA

Equine infectious anemia is a viral disease of horses caused by lentivirus and characterized by icterus, anemia, hyperemia and oedema of sub cutis of the ventral wall of abdomen, pleura, heart, spleen and lymph nodes.

Etiology
- Lentivirus of Retroviridae family
- RNA virus having reverse transcriptase enzyme

Pathogenesis

The disease is transmitted mechanically by the bite of mosquito (Culex) or biting flies (Stomoxys, Tebanus). It can also be transmitted by unsterilized needles, comb, saddle, etc. through minute transfer of blood from infected animal. After entry virus multiples in various organs like spleen, kidneys, lymph nodes and liver. After 30 days of viremia virus attacks erythrocytes and cause their destruction. It also causes destruction of endothelial cells of blood vessels, peripheral nerves, meninges, and brain tissue leading to the development of nervous signs. The hemolytic anemia develops due to hemolysis and phagocytosis of erythrocytes by reticuloendothelial system. Virus antibody complex may be deposited on the renal glomerulus causing glomerulonephritis.

Characteristic symptoms
- Anemia
- Icterus
- Chronic wasting/ weakness
- Edema of dependent parts of body

Macroscopic and microscopic features
- Edema in ventral abdomen
- Petechial or ecchymotic haemorrhage on pleura, peritoneum and serosa of visceral organs
- Enlargement of spleen, liver and lymph nodes
- Increased red marrow in bones specially in long bones.
- Congestion, hemorrhage and oedema in visceral organs
- Infiltration of immature lymphoid cells in liver, kidneys, heart etc.
- Erythro-phagocytosis in spleen
- Dilatation of sinusoids due to congestion and filled with lymphoid cells.

Diagnosis
- Symptoms and lesions
- Immunodiagnostic tests for demonstration of antigen/ antibody- ELISA
- Demonstration of viral antigen in affect tissues using immunoperoxidase technique.

EQUINE ENCEPHALOMYELITIS

Equine encephalomyelitis is an arboviral disease characterized by circling movements, high fever, paralysis, neuronophagia and perivascular cuffing. This is also known as **staggers, borna** *disease* or *forage poisoning*.

Etiology
- Group A arbovirus of alphavirus
- Western, eastern and Venezuelan strains

Pathogenesis
The virus spreads through mosquitoes and birds, reptiles and rodents are the resinous of the virus. With an incubation period of 10-15 days, clinical signs of fever and aimless walking appear in horse.

Clinical Symptoms
- Aimless walking, circling movements
- Fever
- Paralysis

Macroscopic and microscopic features
- No characteristics gross lesions
- Congestion of meninges and brain
- Encephalomalacia
- Neuronophagia, chromatolysis
- Perivascular cuffing by lymphocytes
- Intra nuclear acidophilic inclusion bodies in neurons

Diagnosis
- Symptoms, lesions
- Detection of antigen or antibody using ELISA
- Demonstration of viral antigen in nerve cells using immunoperoxidase technique.

EQUINE VIRAL ARTERITIS

Equine viral arteritis is an infectious disease of horse, mules and donkeys characterized by palpebral oedema, abortion, enteritis and pneumonia.

Etiology
- Pestivirus of Togaviridae family
- RNA virus 40-70 nm diameter

Pathogenesis
Virus reaches in body through inhalation and viraemia occurs causing severe damage to small arteries in intestines, lymph nodes and adrenals that leads to diarrhoea and abdominal pain. It causes severe myometritis, conjunctivitis and pulmonary oedema.

Clinical Symptoms
- Edema in limbs
- Conjunctivitis
- Abortion
- Diarrhoea
- Panleucopenia

Macroscopic and microscopic features
- Enteritis
- Palpebral oedema
- Pneumonia, enlargement of mediastinal lymph nodes
- Placentitis
- Hydrothorax
- Widespread edema in lungs placenta with congestion and hemorrhage.
- Arteritis in cecum and colon-characterized by deposition of eosinophilic material in media with cellular infiltration

Diagnosis
- Symptoms and lesions
- Detection of antigen and antibody using ELISA
- Demonstration of viral antigen in affected tissues using immunoperoxidase technique.

AFRICAN HORSE SICKNESS

African horse sickness is an acute viral disease of horses caused by orbivirus and characterized by fever, conjunctivitis, and oedema of lungs, heart and neck. This is also known as *equine plague*.

Etiology
- Orbivirus of reoviridae family
- dsRNA with 10 segments

Pathogenesis
Virus enters in body through inhalation and after an incubation period of 7-10 days, it causes edema in lungs with laboured breathing. There is several liters of water accumulates in thorax.

Clinical Symptoms
- Fever
- Dyspnoea
- Coughing
- Foamy discharges from nostrils

Macroscopic and microscopic features
- Hydrothorax
- Pulmonary edema
- Sub endocardial hemorrhage
- Conjunctivitis
- Pulmonary edema characterized by separation of interlobular tissue from alveoli
- Infiltration of mononuclear cells in inter alveolar spaces
- Sub endocardial hemorrhage
- Necrosis in liver

Diagnosis
- Symptoms and lesions
- Demonstration of antibody or antigen using ELISA

- Demonstration of viral antigen in affected tissues using immunoperoxidase technique.

EQUINE VIRAL ABORTION (EHV INFECTION)

Equine viral abortion is caused by herpes virus and characterized by death of foetus, abortion, retained placenta and post parturient metritis.

Etiology
- Equine herpes virus-1 of herpesviridae family
- DNA virus

Pathogenesis

The virus spreads through inhalation or ingestion of contaminated material. On entry, virus affects the macrophages and remains in latency till suitable conditions. It affects the placenta, foetus causing placentitis and death of foetus near completion of gestation that results in abortion.

Characteristic symptoms
- Abortion in late gestation
- Retained placenta
- Vaginal discharges

Macroscopic and microscopic features
- Necrotic lesions on lung, liver and lymph nodes of aborted foetus
- Metritis
- Placentitis
- Necrosis in liver of aborted foetus
- Intranuclear eosinophilic inclusion bodies in hepatocytes, spleen, lymph nodes and bronchioles
- Interlobular oedema in lungs
- Bronchopneumonia

Diagnosis
- Symptoms and lesions
- Detection of viral antigen/ antibody using ELISA
- Demonstration of viral antigen in affected tissue by immunoperoxidase technique
- Demonstration of virus using electronmicroscopy

RABIES

Rabies is a viral disease of animals mainly affecting carnivores like dogs, wolves, foxes caused by a lyssa virus and characterized by encephalitis, and presence of intra cytoplasmic inclusions in nerve cells.

Etiology
- Lyssa virus of Rhabdoviridae family
- Bullet shaped, RNA virus

Pathogenesis

The source of infection is always an infected animal and method of spread is almost always by bite of a rabid animal. The virus may appear in the milk of affected animals but spread through this means remains doubtful. After entry of the virus, there is incubation period of 1 week to 1 year with a mean of 1-2 months. Several factors play role in establishing rabies include virulence of the strain, quantity of infectious virus in saliva and susceptibility of the species. Length of incubation period depends on anatomical distance between bite site and the central nervous system, severity of the bite and amount of infectious virus in the saliva.

After entry virus first replicates in the muscle cells and sheds into extra-cellular spaces. Then virus enters into nervous system at motor end plates and binds to receptors for acetylcholine (Ach). After reaching peripheral/ central nerves, the virus spreads within axon of nerve cells to the ventral horn cells of spinal cord @ 3-4 mm/ hour. Virus multiplication occurs first in the spinal cord and then spreads to the brain and from where it is disseminated throughout the central nervous system. During dissemination to central nervous system, there is no viremia. Direct trans neural transfer of virus from cell bodies of neurons and dendrites to adjacent axon terminals is a mechanism of dissemination of rabies in the central nervous system. Brain stem, cerebral cortex and hippocampus are mainly affected by rabies virus and destruction of these regions gives rise to clinical symptoms of rabies. There is centrifugal spread via nerves throughout the body including salivary gland, cornea and tonsils. The virus replicates rapidly in salivary gland and such saliva is the major source of infection for susceptible animals. When there is irritation phenomenon (induced by virus in the nerve cells) occurs, which causes external i.e. furious form and when destruction of neurons occurs resulting in paralysis *i.e.* paralytic/ dumb form.

Characteristic symptoms
- Drooling of saliva
- Moving aimlessly
- **Eating of non food materials**

Macroscopic and microscopic features
- No characteristic gross lesions except some wooden or non food items present in the stomach of dog.
- In other animals, lesions of bite on skin must be present
- Necrosis of neurons, neuronophagic nodules, perivascular cuffing with lymphocytes in brain particularly hippocampus
- Proliferation of lymphocytes, plasma cells, glial cells replacing neurons form *Babes nodules*
- Intra cytoplasmic eosinophilic inclusions '*Negri bodies*'

Diagnosis
- History of bite
- Symptoms and lesions
- Immunodiagnostic tests for demonstration of antigen/ antibody- IFT, ELISA

- Isolation of virus
- Mouse inoculation test

INFECTIOUS CANINE HEPATITIS

Infectious canine hepatitis is an infectious viral disease of dogs caused by adenovirus characterized by necrotic lesions in liver and intra nuclear inclusions in hepatocytes.

Etiology
- Mastadenovirus of adenoviridae family
- DNA virus

Pathogenesis

The excretion of virus occurs in urine and infection spreads mainly through naso-oral and conjunctiva routes. Initial infection occurs in tonsils and peyer's patches. There is viremia and infection of endothelial and parenchymal cells in many tissues leading to hemorrhage and necrosis, especially in the liver, kidneys, spleen and lungs. Chronic kidney lesions and corneal clouding *"blue eye"* results from immune- complex reactions.

Characteristic symptoms
- Fever (104-106°F)
- Vomiting, diarrhoea
- Icterus
- Conjunctivitis

Macroscopic and microscopic features
- Enlargement and congestion of liver
- Presence of focal necrotic patches
- Thickening of the wall of gall bladder
- Enlargement of spleen
- Hyperemia of conjunctiva
- Necrosis of hepatocytes leading to formation of focal necrotic foci
- Infiltration of mononuclear cells

- Intra nuclear inclusions in hepatocytes and Kupffer cells of liver, kidneys and brain
- Congestion, vascular dilatation of sinusoids

Diagnosis
- Symptoms and lesions
- Demonstration of intra nuclear inclusions in hepatocytes
- Immunodiagnostic tests for demonstration of antigen/ antibody- AGPT, CIEP, ELISA
- Demonstration of viral antigen in hepatocytes using immunoperoxidase technique.

Canine Distemper

Canine distemper is an infectious viral disease of dogs caused by a morbilli virus and characterized by catarrhal and purulent exudate in nasal mucosa, purulent bronchopneumonia, and vesicular/ pustular dermatitis.

Etiology
- Morbillivirus of Paramyxoviridae family
- RNA virus, very frazil virus

Pathogenesis

The route of infection is through inhalation of aerosol droplets from infected animal. After entry of virus through respiratory tract, it starts multiplication in respiratory epithelium and alveolar macrophages. Thereafter virus spreads to the tonsils and bronchial lymph nodes. Before appearance of clinical manifestations, the virus circulates in blood associated with lymphocytes and spreads to various tissue like bone marrow, spleen, brain and other lymphoid tissues. Viral replication causes direct damage to neurons and astrocytes. Indirect damage to oligodendroglial cells results in demyelination which leads to encephalitis.

In distemper encephalitis and extensive demyelination of neurons occur in chronic cases as a result of local antiviral response. The brain macrophages ingest these immune complexes and infected cells as a result they release free radicals and other toxic products. These products damage neighbouring cells especially oligodendroglia and cause demyelination. This demyelination develops as a result of autoimmune attack. In this syndrome antibodies are induced against myelin proteins which causes tissue destruction.

Characteristic symptoms
- Fever (105-107°F)
- Mucopurulent nasal discharge
- Vesicles and pustules on abdominal skin
- Foot pad becomes hard due to hyperkeratinization

Macroscopic and microscopic features
- Catarrhal and purulent exudate in upper respiratory tract
- Lobular pneumonia
- Congestion and consolidation of lungs
- Hyperkeratinization of foot pad skin
- Presence of pustules on lower abdomen
- Bronchopneumonia characterized by infiltration of neutrophils in alveoli around bronchioles
- Presence of intracytoplasmic and intra nuclear eosinophilic inclusions in epithelial cells of upper respiratory passage, bronchioles, urinary bladder, stomach, skin and in circulating neutrophils

Diagnosis
- Symptoms and lesions
- Demonstration of intra nuclear and intra cytoplasmic inclusions in hepatocytes, epithelium of bronchioles, skin and in circulating neutrophils.
- Immunodiagnostic tests for demonstration of antigen/antibody- AGPT, CIEP, ELISA
- Demonstration of viral antigen in hepatocytes and respiratory tract epithelium using immunoperoxidase technique.

CANINE PARVOVIRAL INFECTION

Parvovirus causes acute gastroenteritis in dogs characterized by necrotising enteritis and myocardial necrosis

Etiology
- Canine Parvovirus of Parvoviridae family
- DNA virus

Pathogenesis

Young dogs are mostly affected. Infection enters in body through oropharyngeal route and virus starts replication in pharyngeal lymphoid tissues. From here virus is distributed to other organs and tissues via blood stream. Cells that are in 'S' phase of cell cycle have receptors for virus and are infected and killed or prevented from entering mitosis. There is development of characteristic leucopenia involving all white blood cells- lymphocytes, neutrophils, monocytes and platelets due to their destruction.

Rapidly dividing intestinal epithelial cells in crypts are very susceptible to infection. The loss of cells from villous tips continues in normal fusion but the failure in replacing these cells with cells from crypts leads to greatly shortened, non absorptive villi and hence resulting in diarrhoea.

Characteristic symptoms
- Fever (104-106°F)
- Diarrhoea, dysentery with melena
- Dehydration

Macroscopic and microscopic features
- Congestion of intestines
- Presence of mucohemorrhagic exudate mixed with desquamated cells in lumen of intestines
- Necrosis in myocardium
- Enlargement of mesenteric lymph nodes
- Necrosis of villous and crypt epithelial cells

Viral Diseases

- Dilatation of crypts
- Intranuclear inclusions in intestinal epithelium
- Infiltration of mononuclear cells in mucosa and sub mucosa of intestines
- Myocardial necrosis surrounded by infiltration of mononuclear cells.

Diagnosis
- Symptoms and lesions
- Demonstration of intranuclear inclusions in intestinal epithelial cells
- Immunodiagnostic tests for demonstration of antigen/ antibody- AGPT, CIEP, ELISA
- Demonstration of viral antigen in intestinal epithelium using immunoperoxidase technique

FELINE LEUKEMIA

Feline leukemia is an infectious viral disease of cats caused by oncorna virus and characterized by malignant lymphoma, lymphocytosis and immunosuppression. It is also known as feline lymphoma or feline lymphosarcoma.

Etiology
- Oncorna virus of retroviridae family
- Type C oncorna virus, RNA virus has reverse transcriptase

Pathogenesis

The virus is transmitted horizontally through salivary and nasal secretions of sick cats. It affects lymphocytes causing their proliferation leading to production of neoplastic growth.

Characteristic symptoms
- Enlargement of superficial lymph nodes
- Lymphocytosis
- Chronic diarrhoea
- Abortion

Macroscopic and microscopic features
- Enlargement of lymph nodes (mesenteric, lumbar)
- Enteritis
- Anemia
- Placentitis
- Lymphocytosis
- Anaplastic lymphoid cells in lymph nodes

Diagnosis
- Symptoms and lesions
- Detection of viral antigen/ antibody using ELISA
- Demonstration of viral antigen using immunoperoxidase technique
- Demonstration of virus using electronmicroscopy

Chapter 24
Bacterial Diseases

TUBERCULOSIS

Tuberculosis is a chronic bacterial disease of cattle, buffaloes, sheep, goat and pigs caused by *Mycobacterium* sp. and characterized by presence of tubercle nodules in lungs, spleen and lymph nodes.

Etiology
- *Mycobacterium tuberculosis*
- *M. bovis*

Pathogenesis

Disease spreads through contact with infected animals or their discharges or morbid tissues. The infected animals release the organisms through sputum at coughing and contact animals get infection through droplet inhalation. Besides sputum, faeces, urine, vaginal discharges, semen, milk, lymph and wound discharges may act source of infection. It is also transmitted through contaminated instruments, utensils and beddings. After entry through inhalation or ingestion, bacilli localizes at the point of entry and produce typical tubercle in associated lymph nodes. Mostly pharyngeal and mesenteric lymph nodes are affected. From lymph nodes, infection may extend across body cavities, blood vessels and lymph vessels. The inhaled organism enter in the bronchial tree after lodging in bronchi a tissue reaction takes place. Neutrophilic infiltration is there and when neutrophils are necrosed, macrophages come to destroy the organism but they fail then many macrophages becomes elongated to form epithelioid cells, the hall mark of granulomatous inflammation. Some macrophages are joint together to form giant cells to destroy the acid fast bacilli. As a consequence of this some bacilli are phagocytosed and are destroyed. A zone of lymphocytes, macrophages, epithelioid cells, giant cells and fibrous connective tissues are formed around the central necrosed area.

Characteristic symptoms
- Low grade fever
- Progressive wasting/ weakness, loss of production
- Coughing

Macroscopic and microscopic features
- Consolidation of lungs
- Nodules of tubercle present in lungs containing cheesy mass
- Granulomatous lesions in spleen, lymph nodes, liver and intestines.
- Tubercle on pleura and mesentery (*pearly disease*).
- Granulomatous lesions characterized by the presence of tubercles in different organs
- Tubercle consists of central caseative necrosed area surrounded by macrophages, lymphocytes, epithelioid cells and giant cells
- In older cases central necrosed area is calcified and surrounded by fibrous tissue capsule.

Diagnosis
- Symptoms and lesions
- Tuberculin testing of animals
- Immunodiagnostic tests for demonstration of antigen/ antibody- ELISA
- Demonstration of acid fast bacilli in impression smears of tubercle or in tissue sections of lungs and lymph nodes.

PARATUBERCULOSIS (JOHNE'S DISEASE)

Paratuberculosis is a chronic bacterial disease of bovines, ovines and caprines caused by *Mycobacterium paratuberculosis* and characterized by dehydration, emaciation, chronic diarrhoea and thickening of the intestine (*corrugations*).

Etiology
- *Mycobacterium paratuberculosis*

Pathogenesis

Faeces containing the organism is primary source of infection which is acquired by ingestion of contaminated feed and water. It has very long incubation period (15-18 months). The organism has also been isolated from genitalia and semen of infected bulls. Following infection, organism localizes in intestinal mucosa and its associated lymph nodes. The organism penetrate the intestinal mucosa and set up residence within macrophages. The organism multiplies intracellularly without killing host cells and are resistant to intracellular digestion. They grow inside macrophages and distributed through out body. The primary site for bacterial multiplication is terminal ileum and the large intestine leading to decreased absorptive surface, chronic diarrhoea and malabsorption.

Characteristic symptoms
- Chronic diarrhoea
- Progressive wasting/ weakness, loss of production
- Hide bound condition

Macroscopic and microscopic features
- Emaciation, cachexia
- Thickening of the intestinal wall
- Presence of '*rugae*' or transverse folds thickened due to chronic inflammatory changes
- Corrugations cannot be removed even after stretching of intestinal wall
- Lymph nodes (Mesenteric) are also enlarged.
- Infiltration of macrophages, epithelioid cells and lymphocytes in mucosa and sub mucosa
- Presence of acid fast bacilli in epithelioid cells

- Absence of caseative necrosis and calcification in cattle. However, it is present in sheep and goat.
- Nests of epithelioid cells in mesenteric lymph nodes.

Diagnosis
- Symptoms and lesions
- Demonstration of acid fast bacteria in rectal pinch
- Johnin testing of animals
- Immunodiagnostic tests for demonstration of antigen/ antibody- ELISA
- Demonstration of organisms in tissue sections using special stains and immunoperoxidase technique.

BRUCELLOSIS

Brucellosis is an infectious bacterial disease of animals caused by *Brucella* sp. and characterized by abortion in late gestation and formation of granulomatous lesions in genital organs, joints and fetal liver.

Etiology
- *Brucella abortus*
- *Br. ovis*
- *Br. meletensis*
- *Br. canis*

Pathogenesis

The brucella organism spreads through ingestion of contaminated feed and water with aborted foetal contents or foetal membrane. It is also transmitted through inhalation and may pierce the intact or abraded skin or conjunctivae. Congenital infection may also occur. After entry, bacteria multiply in reticuloendothelial cells in regional lymph nodes. The organism enter and travel through intestinal epithelial cells overlaying peyer's patches by endocytosis and then enters into lymphatics. The brucella organism has specific affinity with female and male reproductive organs, placenta, foetus and mammary glands.

The organism can also localize in other organs like lymph nodes, spleen, liver, joints and bones. The bacteria proliferates intracellularly and it has high affinity with erythritol sugar which is present in abundance in placenta and foetus. This organism causes abortions in animals in late gestation.

Characteristic symptoms
- Orchitis
- Accumulation of fluid in scrotum
- Abortion in late gestation (7-9 month)
- Retention of placenta

Macroscopic and microscopic features
- Edema of chorion, thickened and leathery chorion/ placenta
- Edema of foetus, serosanguinous fluid in body cavity
- Pneumonia, necrotic foci in liver
- Enlargement of scrotum in males
- Induration of mammary gland in cows.
- Infiltration of phagocytic cells, epithelioid cells and lymphocytes surrounded by fibrous tissue proliferation
- Fetal broncho pneumonia
- Organism in chorionic epithelial cells
- In males, proliferation of fibrous tissue which compresses or replaces the epididymis.

Diagnosis
- Symptoms and lesions
- Immunodiagnostic tests for demonstration of antigen/ antibody- CFT, SAT, ELISA, DIA
- Isolation of bacteria
- Demonstration of organisms in tissue sections using special stains.

HEMORRHAGIC SEPTICEMIA

Hemorrhagic septicemia is a highly contagious and infectious disease of animals caused by *Pasteurella multocida* and *Mannheimia hemolytica* and characterized by oedematous swelling in neck region, dyspnoea, pneumonia and wide spread haemorrhage in visceral organs.

Etiology
- *Pasteurella multocida*
- *Mannheimia hemolytica*

Pathogenesis

The disease spreads by ingestion of contaminated feed and water. The saliva of affected animals contains large number of organisms during the early stages of the disease. The organism is normal inhabitant in the terminal bronchioles and alveoli and it can't invade the lungs because of pulmonary defense but due to stress like malnutrition, long transportation, climatic changes, the organism become virulent and destroys the mononuclear leucocytes of bloods and macrophages of lungs. Due to death of macrophages vasoactive substances are released to cause inflammation and fibrin deposition. The other secondary invaders like PI-3 virus, bovine herpes virus and bacteria cause significant change. Death occurs due to hypoxia and toxaemia. It has been reported that primarily there is infection of PI-3 virus which is precipitated by bacteria resulting in septicemia.

Characteristic symptoms
- High fever (105-107°F)
- Edema in throat and brisket region
- Dyspnoea
- Ghar-ghar sound on respiration

Macroscopic and microscopic features
- Edema consisting of gelatinous material in neck and brisket region
- Serosanguinous fluid in peritoneal and pleural cavity

- Swollen and enlarged lymph nodes
- Pericardial hemorrhage
- Haemorrhagic gastroenteritis
- **Lungs are congested and consolidated** *"Marbling"*.
- Fibrinous bronchopneumonia
- Congestion and hemorrhage in lymph nodes, spleen, liver, kidneys and myocardium
- Congestion and haemorrhage in intestinal mucosa and sub mucosa
- Infiltration of neutrophils, macrophages and lymphocytes.

Diagnosis
- Symptoms and lesions
- Demonstration of bipolar bacteria in blood smears on methylene blue staining
- Isolation of bacteria
- Immunodiagnostic tests for demonstration of antigen/antibody- ELISA

BLACK QUARTER

Black Quarter is an acute disease of cattle and sheep caused by *Clostrium chauvei* and characterized by lameness, hot painful swelling in thigh muscles producing crepitating sound on pressure and accumulation of serosanguinous fluid in affected area.

Etiology
- *Clostridium chauvei*
- Gram positive, anaerobe

Pathogenesis

The organism is transmitted through contaminated soil. Route of entry is through alimentary tract mucosa after ingestion of spores in contaminated feed. In case of sheep, the disease is generally occurs by wound infection. After ingestion and germination of the spores, the bacteria multiplies in the intestines and crosses the intestinal mucosa and enters in general circulation to get deposited in various tissues/ organs including skeletal muscles. In skeletal muscles the organism remains in dormant stage until damage to the muscle sets up an appropriate anaerobic environment for their germination and proliferation and release of certain toxins locally which causes necrosis and gas gangrene of muscles.

Characteristic symptoms
- High fever (104-107°F)
- Swelling in thigh muscles
- Crepitating sound on pressure

Macroscopic and microscopic features
- Accumulation of serosanguinous fluid in thigh muscles producing crepitating sound on pressure
- The affected area looks like greenish or bluish
- Edema of subcutaneous tissue
- Affected muscles have porous appearance due to presence of gas
- Black colour of muscles is due to iron sulfide (FeS)
- Fibrino hemorrhagic pericarditis, pleurisy and ulcerative endocarditis.
- Degeneration and coagulative necrosis of muscles
- Streaks of hemorrhage between fibers
- Presence of 'Rod' shaped bacteria, edema and infiltration of leucocytes.

Diagnosis
- Symptoms and lesions
- Demonstration of Gram positive bacteria in exudate
- Isolation of bacteria
- Immunodiagnostic tests for demonstration of antigen/ antibody- ELISA
- Demonstration of organism in muscle tissue section using special stains.

ENTEROTOXAEMIA

Enterotoxaemia is an acute disease of sheep, goat and camel caused by *Clostridium perfringens* and characterized by endocardial haemorrhage, gastroenteritis and pulpy kidneys.

Etiology
- *Clostridium perfringens* type D-sheep
- *Clostridium perfringens* type A-camel.

Pathogenesis

The organism is normal inhabitant of gut in animals. When there is anaerobic condition develops in gut due to over feeding, this organism starts proliferation and production of toxins. The toxins are readily absorbed through stomach and intestines to cause disease in animals.

Characteristic symptoms
- Over filled stomach
- Sudden mortality
- Hyperglycemia

Macroscopic and microscopic features
- Enlarged pulpy kidneys
- Congestion of abomasum and intestines
- Hemorrhage on endocardium and pericardium
- Congestion and edema of lungs.
- Cloudy swelling and necrosis of tubular epithelium in kidneys
- Congestion in liver, spleen and intestines
- Endocardial haemorrhage
- Oedema in lungs.

Diagnosis
- History of over feeding
- Symptoms and lesions
- Demonstration of toxin in intestinal/ stomach contents on mouse inoculation test

- Isolation and identification of causative organism.

BRAXY

Braxy is an acute fatal disease of sheep caused by *Clostridium septicum* and characterized by oedema, necrosis and hemorrhage in abomasum.

Etiology
- *Clostridium septicum*

Pathogenesis

It is a soil borne infection and mostly occurs in sheep vaccinated with enterotoxaemia vaccine. The organism gets entry through ingestion of spores. The ingested spores are localized in stomach and germinate under anaerobic conditions due to over feeding of lush green feed or high amount of grains leading to abomasitis.

Characteristic symptoms
- Over filled stomach
- Sudden mortality
- History of enterotoxaemia vaccination

Macroscopic and microscopic features
- Edema of abomasal folds
- Congestion and hemorrhage in abomasum
- Necrosis of abomasal mucosa
- Congestion and necrosis in intestines.
- Microscopic features
- Congestion and hemorrhage of abomasal mucosa
- Presence of 'Rod' shaped organism in mucosal epithelium of abomasum
- Necrosis and presence of ulcers in abomasal mucosa.

Diagnosis
- History of over feeding and enterotoxaemia vaccination
- Symptoms and lesions

- Demonstration of toxin in intestinal/ stomach contents on mouse inoculation test
- Isolation and identification of bacteria

TETANUS

Tetanus is a bacterial disease of animals caused by the toxins of clostridia and characterized by prolonged spasmodic contractions of muscles, stiffness and immobilization. It is also known as *"lock jaw"*.

Etiology
- *Clostridium tetani*
- Gram positive, anaerobe, rod shaped, produces toxins

Pathogenesis

It occurs as a sequel to a wound that allows the growth of anaerobic *Clostridium tetani*, which releases neurotoxins. This neurotoxin fixes the gray matter of the brain and spinal cord and causes stiffness of muscles leading to asphyxia and death.

Clinical Symptoms
- Convulsions
- Immobilization
- Stiffness of muscles
- Lock jaw

Macroscopic and microscopic features
- Presence of wound or history of wound.
- Stiffness of muscles
- Gram positive organism in wound.
- Necrosis in muscles and gray matter of brain.

Diagnosis
- Symptoms and lesions
- Presence of wound and bacteria

SWINE ERYSEPALAS

It is an important disease of pigs caused by a Gram-positive bacteria and characterized by arthritis, vegetative endocarditis and rhomboid shaped erythematous skin lesions. It is also known as *"diamond skin disease"*.

Etiology
- *Erysepalothrix rhusiopathie*
- Gram-positive, rod shaped, pleomorphic

Pathogenesis
Infection enters through skin or ingestion and causes bacteremia or septicemia. The organism then localizes in joints, skin and heart valves to produce lesions.

Clinical Symptoms
- Arthritis
- Erythema on skin, later sloughing of skin and patches on abdomen.

Macroscopic and microscopic features
- Arthritis
- Erythema or sloughing of skin
- Vegetative endocarditis- nodular mass of over growth on valves
- Hypertrophy of left ventricle
- Infiltration of lymphocytes in joint capsules
- Fibrinous exudate with necrosis, leucocytic infiltration and colonies of bacteria in heart lesions.
- Necrosis in skin sections.

Diagnosis
- Symptoms and lesions
- Isolation of bacteria
- Demonstration of bacteria in tissue sections using special stains.

LISTERIOSIS

Listeriosis is an acute infectious disease of animals caused by *Listeria* sp. and characterized by congestion of meninges and brain, presence of micro abscess in brain and lymphocytic leptomeningitis.

Etiology
- *Listeria monocytogenes (L. ivanovi)*

Pathogenesis

Listeria is transmitted by ingestion of contaminated materials. Silage is considered as one of the important organism. Besides, it is normal inhabitant of bowl of many animals. There are certain predisposing factors including nutritional deficiencies, silage feeding, weather change and long duration flood etc. The organism penetrates the epithelial cells of intestines, conjunctiva, urinary bladder etc. The organism has a lucein rich protein on their surface known as internalins, which is required for penetration into epithelial cells. Internalins bind with E-cadherin on host epithelial cells. They multiply in epithelial cells, destroy the cells and are released then they are phagocytosed by macrophages and multiply there. The activated macrophages can phagocyte and kill bacteria. The centripetal movement of bacteria in trigeminal nerve eventually make them to reach medulla oblongata. The listeria organism is excreted in faeces in animals even in absence of disease.

Characteristic symptoms
- High fever (105-107°F)
- Circling movements
- Abortion
- Torticollis

Macroscopic and microscopic features
- Congestion and/or haemorrhage in meninges
- Foci of softening/ micro abscess in medulla
- Small necrotic foci/ abscess in visceral organs.

- Microabscess in brain
- Infiltration of mononuclear cells and neutrophils
- Perivascular cuffing by lymphocytes, eosinophils, histiocytes and neutrophils
- Softening of brain/ liquifactive necrosis.

Diagnosis
- Symptoms and lesions
- Isolation and identification of bacteria
- Immunodiagnostic tests for demonstration of antigen/ antibody- ELISA
- Demonstration of bacteria in tissue sections using special stains.

SALMONELLOSIS

Salmonellosis is an infectious disease of calves, lambs and piglets caused by *Salmonella* sp. and characterized by septicemia, wide spread hemorrhage on visceral organs, typhoid nodules in liver and hemorrhagic enteritis.

Etiology
- *Salmonella enteritidis* var. Typhimurium (*S.* Typhimurium)
- *Salmonella enteritidis* var. Dublin (*S.* Dublin)
- *Salmonella enteritidis* var. Cholaraesuis (*S.* Cholaraesuis)

Pathogenesis

It is transmitted horizontally by direct or indirect contact. Infection is acquired by ingestion of materials contaminated with faeces of clinically ill animals. After entry, bacteria adhere to intestinal cells through fimbriae/ pilli and colonize in small intestine then they penetrate enterocytes (intestinal cells) for further multiplication. They cross lamina propria and continue to proliferate both free and within macrophages and are transported to mesenteric lymph nodes. Further multiplication leads to septicaemia and spread of the bacteria to various organs/ tissues like spleen, liver, meninges, brain and joints. It may cause mild enteritis to fatal enteritis with septicemia.

Characteristic symptoms
- Fever (102-105°F)
- Weakness, icterus, anemia
- Diarrhoea, melena
- Dehydration

Macroscopic and microscopic features
- Haemorrhage in intestines
- Petechiae on kidneys *"Turkey egg appearance"*
- Edema of spleen and lymph nodes
- Button ulcers in intestines of piglets
- **Focal necrosis and reactive granuloma in liver** *"Typhoid nodules"*.
- Necrosis and desquamation of intestinal mucosal epithelium
- Necrosis in liver and infiltration by neutrophils, macrophages and lymphocytes
- Congestion and edema in spleen and lymph nodes.

Diagnosis
- Symptoms and lesions
- Isolation of bacteria
- Immunodiagnostic tests for demonstration of antigen/antibody- SAT, ELISA
- Demonstration of bacteria in tissue sections using special stains.

COLIBACILLOSIS

Colibacillosis is an infectious disease of new born animals caused by *E. coli* and characterized by enteritis, swelling of lymph nodes and peyer's patches, pneumonia and hemorrhage on endocardium.

Etiology
- *Escherichia coli*

Pathogenesis

The disease is transmitted through contaminated feed and water. Discharges of aborted foetus, vaginal discharges, umbilical infection and intrauterine infection may act as source of infection for newly born animals. The colonization of organism in gut depends on the immune status animals. The cell wall of *E.coli* consists of lipopolysaccharide which causes fever mediated through the production of host cytokines including TNF and IL-1. *E.coli* also secretes substances that suppresses phagocytosis by neutrophils. The endotoxins secreted by *E.coli* is an ADP- ribosyltransferase which generate excess c-AMP to cause diarrhoea and dehydration.

Characteristic symptoms
- Fever (103-106°F)
- Diarrhoea, dehydration
- Nasal discharges
- Naval ill

Macroscopic and microscopic features
- Swollen umblicus
- Swelling of joints
- Suppurative nephritis
- Congestion and hemorrhage in intestines
- Congestion of lungs and mesenteric lymph nodes
- Hemorrhage in endocardium.
- Necrosis and desquamation of mucosal epithelium in intestine
- Infiltration of neutrophils and mononuclear cells
- Infiltration of neutrophils in kidneys forming micro abscess
- Catarrhal bronchopneumonia
- Congestion and reactive hyperplasia in lymph nodes.

Diagnosis
- Symptoms and lesions
- Isolation of bacteria
- Immunodiagnostic tests for demonstration of antigen/antibody- ELISA
- Demonstration of organisms in tissue sections using special stains.

STRANGLES

Strangles is an acute infectious disease of horses caused by streptococci and characterized by abscess in pharyngeal and maxillary lymph nodes, pericarditis, pleurisy, suppurative pneumonia, presence of abscess on liver, kidneys and spleen.

Etiology
- *Streptococcus equi*

Pathogenesis

The disease spreads through inhalation; the most important source of infection is nasal discharge. The bacteria reaches on pharyngeal and nasal mucosa and causes acute pharyngitis and rhinitis. Drainage to lymph nodes leads to formation of abscess. Guttural pouches are filled with pus. Then infection spreads in other organs and causes suppuration in kidneys, brain, liver, spleen, tendon sheath and joints. After an attack, strangles has subsided and purpura hemorrhagica may develop due to the development of sensitivity to streptococcal proteins.

Characteristic symptoms
- Fever (104-107°F)
- Abscess in throat region
- Dyspnoea

Macroscopic and microscopic features
- Abscess in pharyngeal and sub maxillary lymph nodes
- Abscess in liver, kidneys and spleen
- Suppurative pericarditis

- Suppurative pneumonia
- Empyema.
- Infiltration of neutrophils in liver, kidneys, spleen, pericardium and lungs
- Degeneration and necrosis in liver along with accumulation of neutrophils
- Lymphoid depletion in spleen.

Diagnosis
- Symptoms and lesions
- Isolation of bacteria
- Immunodiagnostic tests for demonstration of antigen/antibody- ELISA
- Demonstration of organisms in tissue sections using special stains.

GLANDERS

Glanders is an infectious disease of equines caused by *Burkholderia* sp. characterized by ulcers in nasal passage, miliary nodules in lungs, edema of lymph nodes, lymphangitis and lymphadenitis.

Etiology
- *Burkholderia mallei*

Pathogenesis

The disease is transmitted through ingestion of contaminated feed and water and also through utensils particularly watering troughs, contaminated by nasal discharge/ sputum. Rarely spread through direct contact or grooming tools. Spread through inhalation can also occur. The organism invades the intestinal wall and causes septicemia (acute form) or bacteraemia (chronic form). The organism may invade the regional lymph nodes by pharyngeal lymph nodes and proliferate there. The respiratory mucosa and lungs are most commonly affected but disseminated lesions may occur. Nasal involvement is indicated by a copious and persistent nasal discharge. In cutaneous form there is development of lesions along the lymphatics resulting in lymphangitis and lymphadenitis.

Characteristic symptoms
- Fever (103-105°F)
- Dyspnoea
- Discharge of pus from lymph vessels and lymph nodes
- Ulcer in nasal passage

Macroscopic and microscopic features
- Abscess in superficial lymph nodes and discharge of oily pus from lymph vessels in hind legs
- Abscess in lungs and liver
- Pleurisy with purulent exudate
- Ulcers and deposition of purulent exudate in nasal passage
- Enlargement of lymph nodes
- Punched out ulcers in lungs.
- Centrally aggregates of neutrophils surrounded by histiocytes in lungs
- Infiltration of neutrophils in and around necrotic foci in liver, kidneys and intestines.
- Edema in lymph nodes

Diagnosis
- Symptoms and lesions
- Mallein testing of equines
- Isolation of bacteria
- Immunodiagnostic tests for demonstration of antigen/antibody- ELISA, CFT
- Demonstration of organism in tissue sections using special stains.

ANTHRAX

Anthrax is an acute septicemic disease of animals caused by *Bacillus* sp. and characterized by sudden death, absence of rigor mortis, tary colour blood from natural openings and widespread hemorrhage.

Etiology
- *Bacillus anthracis*

Pathogenesis

The infection occurs through ingestion or inhalation of spores/ vegetative forms of the organism or entry of bacteria through broken skin. After entry the spores germinate and localize for multiplication and spread by means of lymphatics to lymph nodes and then in blood stream, causing severe septicaemia. The bacteria possesses both capsule and exotoxin. Due to presence of capsule phagocytic cells become unable to destroy them. The exotoxin is lethal in nature, it causes edema and tissue damage. The exotoxin has 3 components-
1. Edema factor (EF) or factor I is adenyl cyclase which causes increase in cellular c-AMP level that causes electrolyte and fluid loss.
2. Protective antigen (PA) or factor II is a fragment of exotoxin and has anti-phagocytic activity.
3. Lethal factor (LF) or factor III stimulates macrophages for production of oxidizing radicals and cytokines. Mainly IL-1 and TNF-α, which induce shock and death.

Characteristic symptoms
- High fever (105-107°F)
- Hemorrhage from natural orifices
- Dyspnoea
- Tary colour blood
- Sudden mortality up to 90%

Macroscopic and microscopic features
- Post mortem examination of animals suspected for anthrax

Bacterial Diseases

should not be conducted.
- Blood smear examined for anthrax bacilli
- Discharge of blood from vagina, anus and mouth
- Tary colour of blood
- Enlargement of spleen
- Widespread hemorrhage on serous surfaces of visceral organs
- Subcutaneous oedema
- Anthrax bacilli and spores in blood smear
- Spleen shows haemorrhage and accumulation of blood in red pulp
- Hemorrhage in lymph nodes, liver, lungs and kidneys
- Degenerative and necrotic changes in kidneys and liver.

Diagnosis
- Symptoms and lesions
- Demonstration of bacteria in blood smear
- Immunodiagnostic tests for demonstration of antigen/antibody- ELISA, AGPT (Ascoli test)
- Animal inoculation test causes death of mouse within 24 hrs.

CAMPYLOBACTERIOSIS

Campylobacteriosis is an infectious disease of cattle and sheep caused by *Campylobacter* sp. and characterized by early abortion, suppurative metritis, cervicitis and vaginitis.

Etiology
- *Campylobacter foetus*

Pathogenesis

The bacteria is natural inhabitant of reproductive tract of bovines. In case of males, it is confined to prepucial cavity and mucosa of glans penis and distal portion of urethra. In females, lumen of vagina, cervix, uterus and oviduct harbor the bacteria.

Infection spreads through coitus or AI due to use of infected semen. From bull to bull transmission occurs through artificial vagina at breeding centers. After entry in females, the bacteria multiplies in the cervix and reaches to uterine horn and oviduct within 7-14 days. In the cervix, the organism metabolizes amino acids and other organic acids. The organism is protected from phagocytes because it is covered with mucous. This organism causes abortion at 5 month of gestation because the organism impairs the supply of oxygen and some nutrients (amino acids) required for implantation of embryo leading to abortion.

Characteristic symptoms
- Abortion in mid gestation (5 month)
- Mucopurulent vaginal discharge
- Retention of placenta

Macroscopic and microscopic features
- Abortions at 4-5 month of gestation
- Purulent exudate in uterine discharges- yellowish
- Congestion of vagina
- Oedema in foetus
- Necrotic foci in liver
- Oedematous placenta.
- Infiltration of neutrophils, macrophages and lymphocytes in uterine mucosa
- Enlargement of uterine glands
- Necrosis in placenta
- Suppurative endometritis, cervicitis and vaginitis.

Diagnosis
- Symptoms and lesions
- Isolation of bacteria
- Immunodiagnostic tests for demonstration of antigen/ antibody- ELISA
- Demonstration of organisms in tissue sections using special stains.

ACTINOBACILLOSIS

Actinobacillosis is a disease of cattle caused by *Actinobacillus* sp. and characterized by granulomatous lesions in tongue, lymph nodes and presence of colony of organism (palisade of Indian club like structures) in between the inflammatory exudate. This is also known as *wooden tongue*.

Etiology
- *Actinobacillus lignieresii*

Pathogenesis

The organism is normally present in the oral cavity of cattle and sheep. Infection occurs when there is traumatic injury of oral mucosa. When condition become favourable to the causative organism due to injury, it reaches to regional lymph nodes and nasal mucosa. The organism has affinity with soft tissues and thus affects soft tissue of head and neck. There is acute inflammatory changes and subsequent granulomatous reaction including necrosis and suppuration.

Characteristic symptoms
- Anorexia, pain in tongue due to hardening
- Sporadic occurrence
- Drooling of saliva

Macroscopic and microscopic features
- Enlargement of tongue due to granuloma formation.
- Nodular lesions may also appear in rumen, skin, lungs and liver
- Flooding of pus from lesions present in tongue.
- Presence of colony of organism palisade of Indian club like structures surrounded by neutrophils, mononuclear cells and lymphocytes
- Such lesions are surrounded by fibrous tissue
- Muscle tissue of tongue is replaced by fibrous tissue.

Diagnosis
- Symptoms and lesions
- Isolation of bacteria
- Demonstration of organisms/ colony in tissue sections.

ACTINOMYCOSIS

Actinomycosis is a disease of cattle, buffaloes and camels caused by *Actinomyces* sp. and characterized by suppurative osteomyelitis of mandible and Miliary nodules in lungs. This is also known as *lumpy jaw*.

Etiology
- *Actinomyces bovis*

Pathogenesis

The causative organism is a normal inhabitant of the bovine buccal cavity and infection occurs through wounds in buccal mucosa due to sharp edged objects. After entry from buccal cavity, it causes rarefaction of bone followed by osteomyelitis characterized by chronic suppurative and granulomatous reaction.

Characteristic symptoms
- Anorexia due to pain in jaw
- Abscess in mandible and swelling of jaw
- Discharging of pus from lesion

Macroscopic and microscopic features
- Lumpy jaw
- Swelling of jaw at mandible
- Miliary nodules in lungs and mammary gland
- Discharging of pus from jaw.
- Suppurative osteomyelitis of mandible
- Central liquefactive necrosed area which is having colonies of the organism surrounded by mononuclear and lymphocytic cells

- Colonies are known as *sulphur granules*, bigger in size than actinobacillosis and may take Gram positive stain.

Diagnosis
- Symptoms and lesions
- Isolation of bacteria
- Demonstration of organisms/ colony in tissue sections using special stains.

BOTRIOMYCOSIS (STAPHYLOCOCCOSIS)

Botriomycosis is an infectious disease of animals caused by staphylococci and characterized by suppurative granulomatous lesions in udder, jaw, shoulder or sternal region.

Etiology
- *Staphylococcus aureus*

Pathogenesis

The causative agent is transmitted through contamination of infected animals. The organism possesses number of virulent factors which include surface proteins for adherence, enzyme for protein degradation and toxins for host cell damage. *S. aureus* has receptors for fibrinogen, fibronectin and vintronectin on their surface through which it binds with host endothelial cells. The toxin produced by bacteria contains coagulase, fibrinolysins, hyaluronidase, hemolysins and endotoxins. The lipases destroy the skin surface and thus help the bacteria in abscessation.

Characteristic symptoms
- Hardening of udder
- Papillary projections from jaw
- Yellow pus discharge from lesion

Macroscopic and microscopic features
- Hard and nodular enlargement of udder
- Hard over growth in lower jaw or at shoulder or sternal region

- Yellow pus discharges from lesions
- Enlargement of lymph nodes.
- Infiltration of neutrophils, macrophages and lymphocytes surround the necrotic lesion which contain colony of organism
- On Gram's stain, Gram positive cocci are seen.

Diagnosis
- Symptoms and lesions
- Isolation of bacteria
- Demonstration of organisms in tissue sections using special stains.

NECROBACILLOSIS

Necrobacillosis is an infectious disease of animals caused by *Spherophorus necrophorus* and characterized by necrosis of liver, foot rot, diphtheria and enteritis.

Etiology
- *Spherophorus necrophorus*

Pathogenesis

The causative organism is a common inhabitant of the oral cavity. It produces a variety of toxins including exo- and endtoxins which are the cause of necrosis, edema, laryngitis and dyspnoea. There is formation of diphtheritic membrane over oral mucosa. In sheep it causes abscess formation in foot.

Characteristic symptoms
- Nasal discharge
- Coughing
- Sneezing
- Diarrhoea
- Lameness

Macroscopic and microscopic features
- Presence of diphtheritic membrane of tongue and phar-

ynx in calves
- On removal of diphtheritic membrane, ulcer is left
- Necrotic areas in trachea
- Suppurative pneumonia
- Necrotic lesions in esophagus, rumen, abomasum, liver, spleen and heart
- Necrotic lesions and gangrenous foot.
- Necrosis and infiltration of neutrophils in liver
- Necrosis and bronchopneumonia in lungs
- Necrosis of epithelium, ulcer and infiltration of neutrophils in tongue
- Congestion in lungs and liver.

Diagnosis
- Symptoms and lesions
- Isolation of bacteria
- Immunodiagnostic tests for demonstration of antigen/antibody- ELISA
- Demonstration of organisms in tissue sections using special stains.

NOCARDIOSIS

Nocardiosis is a bacterial disease of animals caused by gram-positive bacteria and characterized by pneumonia, mastitis, lymphangitis and lymphadenitis. This is also known as *"Bovine Farcy"*.

Etiology
- *Nocardia asteroids*
- Gram-positive, acid fast, aerobic, filamentus

Pathogenesis

Organism enter via soil contamination of wounds and causes local subcutaneous oedema which also spreads to lymph nodes. Lesions may break skin to form abscess and sinuses connecting two abscesses. This is pyogranuloma formation.

Clinical Symptoms
- Purulent nasal discharge
- Discharge from lymphatics and lymph nodes *"Farcy"*
- Mastitis and abortion

Macroscopic and microscopic features
- Granulomatous lesions in lungs
- Mastitis- hardness of udder
- Lymphatics discharging pus
- Enlargement of lymph nodes, spleen and liver with abscess.
- Granulomatous lesion in lungs- in central area acid-fast organism surrounded by neutrophils, macrophages, lymphocytes and giant cells.
- Tangled colonies of organism in necrotic debris.
- Purulent exudate

Diagnosis
- Symptoms and lesions
- Isolation and identification of bacteria
- Demonstration of organisms in tissue sections using special stains.

PSEUDOTUBERCULOSIS

Pseudotuberculosis is a chronic disease of sheep, goat and camel caused by *Corynebacterium pseudotuberculosis* and characterized by pyogranulomatous lesions in lymph nodes. This is also known as **caseous lymphadenitis.**

Etiology
- *Corynebacterium pseudotuberculosis* or *C. ovis*
- Gram-positive, diphtheroid bacillus

Pathogenesis

Infection enters through abraded skin or oral mucous membrane and involves the local lymph nodes. The organism is intracellular and survive within macrophages due to presence of a toxic lipid. It terms absecess and caseation in lymph nodes, lungs, liver, kidney, brain, skin and spinal cord.

Clinical Symptoms
- Enlargement of lymph nodes
- Discharge of thick green pus from lymph nodes
- Nodular lesions on skin (camels)
- Paraplegia/ paralysis of hind legs

Macroscopic and microscopic features
- Enlargement of lymph nodes
- Nodules on skin
- Caseous mass on cut of lesion, onion like concentric laminated mass
- Discharge of pus
- Caseous necrosis surrounded by epithelioid cells, lymphocytes and covered by fibrous connective tissue
- Concentrically laminated mass with no giant cells
- Calcification

Diagnosis
- Symptoms and lesions
- Isolation and identification of causative organisms
- Demonstration of bacteria in tissue sections using special stains.

YERSINIOSIS

Yersiniosis is an infectious disease of animals caused by *Yersimia* sp. and characterized by abortion in cattle, necrotic hepatitis and arteritis. This is often confused with brucella induced abortions in cattle as yersimia serologically cross reacts with brucella.

Etiology
- *Yersinia enterocolitica*
- *Yersinia pseudotuberculosis*

Pathogenesis
Yersinia have a protein 'invasin' on their cell wall which binds with host cell integrins that helps in attachment and multiplication of organism inside the host cells. It causes necrosis, pus formation and formation of nodules in liver. This organism also causes placentitis leading to abortion.

Clinical Symptoms
- Abortion in cattle, sheep and goat
- Diarrhoea in pigs

Macroscopic and microscopic features
- White/ gray nodules on placenta and liver of aborted foetus
- Enteritis, ulcers in ileum
- Enlargement of mesenteric lymph nodes
- Necrotic foci in liver, spleen, lymph nodes and lungs
- Necrotic lesions in liver surrounded by macrophages, lymphocytes, epithelioid cells and covered by fibrous capsule
- Necrosis in intestines, spleen, lymph nodes

Diagnosis
- Symptoms and lesions
- Isolation and identification of bacteria
- Immunodiagnostic tests for detection of antigen/ antibody using SAT/ ELISA
- Demonstration of organisms in tissue sections using special stains.

BLACK DISEASE

Black disease is an infectious disease of sheep, cattle and buffaloes caused by *Clostridium nouyi* and characterized by necrotic hepatitis, hydropericardium and black discolouration of skin.

Etiology
- Clostridium nouyi
- Gram positive, rod, anaevobes
- Predisposed by *Fasciola hepatica* and *Fasciola gigantica* infection

Pathogenesis
The damage caused by metacerearial liver fluke in liver provides anaerobic environment favourable for growth of clostridial organism. The causative agent is normally present in intestine and it reaches in liver through metacercariae. The organism produces alpha and beta toxin which causes hepatic necrosis.

Clinical Symptoms
- Fever (105-107°F)
- Sudden death

Macroscopic and microscopic features
- Focal or diffused streaks of necrosis in liver along the track of liver fluke migration
- Petechial on endocardium, epicardium with hydropericardium
- Black discolouration of subcutaneous/ skin
- Necrosis in liver, infiltration of neutrophils
- Congestion, hemorrhage
- Presence of gram positive rods in necrotic lesions

Diagnosis
- Symptoms and lesions
- Isolation and identification of organism and its toxin
- Demonstration of organisms in tissue sections/ smear using special stains.

BOTULISM

Botulism is a fatal disease of animals caused by toxins of *Clostridium botulinum* and characterized by paralysis and sudden death.

Etiology
- *Clostridium botulinum*
- Neurotoxin C_1 and C_2
- Predisposing factor- phosphorus deficiency leading to pica.

Pathogenesis

Disease occurs on ingestion of contaminated materials such as bone chewing, bone meal, food of animal origin. The preformed toxins of botulinum in these materials act on peripheral nerve endings to cause their blockage leading to paralysis.

Clinical Symptoms
- Paralysis
- Sudden death

Macroscopic and microscopic features
- No characteristics gross lesion
- No characteristic gross lesion

Diagnosis
- History
- Symptoms
- Very difficult to establish diagnosis.

Chapter 25
Chlamydial Diseases

CHLAMYDIOSIS

Chlamydiosis is an infectious disease of animals caused by Chlamydia sp. and characterized by encephalitis, polyarthritis and pneumonia in calves and abortions in cows and sheep.

Etiology
- *Chlamydia psittacii*

Pathogenesis

Chlamydial infection spreads through inhalation of contaminated dust from infected birds. Organism multiplies in lungs and through blood it spreads to liver, spleen, kidneys, brain, joints and placenta to cause pathology.

Characteristic symptoms

Calves
- Fever, dyspnoea
- Nasal discharge, hypersalivation
- Swelling of joints

Cows and Sheep
- Abortion at 7-9th month of gestation
- Subcutaneous edema in foetus

Macroscopic and microscopic features

Calves
- Serofibrinous peritonitis
- Enlargement of spleen

- Congestion of brain and spinal cord
- Edema of synovial tissues
- Congestion and consolidation of lungs

Cows and Sheep
- Abortion
- Subcutaneous oedema in foetus
- Enlargement of lymph nodes, spleen
- Fibrino purulent exudate in placenta
- Lobular pneumonia
- Congestion of brain and spinal cord
- Fibrinous exudate in synovial fluid
- Fibrino-purulent placentitis
- Bronchopneumonia
- Epithelization of alveolar cells

Diagnosis
- Symptoms and lesions
- Detection of antigen/ antibody using ELISA
- Demonstration of chlamydial organism in synovial fluid, foetal stomach contents and lung tissue using special stains and immunoperoxidase techniques.
- Demonstration of chlamydial inclusions in tissue sections/ impression smears.

Chapter 26
Rickettsial Diseases

ANAPLASMOSIS

Anaplasmosis is an infectious disease of animals caused by a rickettsia and characterized by icterus, enlargement of spleen, pale tissues, thin watery blood and petechiae over serous membranes.

Etiology
- *Anaplasma centrale*
- *A. marginale*
- *A. ovis*

Pathogenesis

The disease is transmitted through bite of tick (Boophilus), biting flies (Tabanus) and also in some cases due to mosquitoes. It is intra cellular organism and multiplies inside the erythrocytes by binary fission. The infected erythrocytes are engulfed by the cells of reticuloendothelial system (spleen, bone marrow). The process of erythrophagocytosis cause extra vascular haemolysis leading to anemia. It also causes autoimmune reaction leading to lysis of erythrocytes.

Characteristic symptoms
- High fever (105-107°F)
- Anemia
- Icterus
- Macroscopic features
- Anemia, icterus
- Enlarged and yellow liver

- Petechiae on epicardium
- Enlargement of spleen
- Catarrhal exudate in intestines
- Gall bladder distended with granular bile.

Macroscopic and microscopic features
- Presence of organism in erythrocytes
- Hemorrhage in liver, kidneys and myocardium
- Necrosis in kidneys
- Haemosiderosis in spleen.

Diagnosis
- Demonstration of organism in blood smear
- Symptoms and lesions
- Immunodiagnostic tests for demonstration of antigen/antibody- ELISA

Chapter 27
Mycoplasmal Diseases

CONTAGIOUS BOVINE PLEUROPNEUMONIA (CBPP)

Contagious bovine pleuropneumonia (CBPP) is an infectious disease of cattle caused by *Mycoplasma* sp. and characterized by cuprous pneumonia, pleurisy and dilation of lymph vessels.

Etiology
- *Mycoplasma mycoides*

Pathogenesis

The infection spreads through inhalation of droplets from infected animals. The recovered animals act as source of infection at least for a period of 3 years. After entering through respiratory tract the organism reaches to bronchioles. It may remain in retropharyngeal gland from where it may spread in whole body. The organism from bronchioles enter into interlobular septa and causes inflammation followed by edema which causes dilation and subsequent thrombosis of lymph and blood vessels prior to development of pneumonic lesions. Death occurs due to anoxia and toxaemia.

Characteristic symptoms
- Fever (104-106°F)
- Dyspnoea
- Nasal discharge

Macroscopic and microscopic features
- Congestion and consolidation of lungs with fibrinous adhesions in pleura
- Serofibrinous exudate in thoracic cavity

- Dilation of lymph vessels in lungs
- Marbled appearance on cut surfaces of lungs.
- Thrombosis, ischemia and necrosis surrounded by fibrosis
- Thickening of alveolar septa due to serofibrinous exudate
- Congestion and consolidation of lung due to thickening of outer alveolar septa
- Serofibrinous pericarditis.

Diagnosis
- Symptoms and lesions
- Isolation of mycoplasma, nipple shaped colony on media
- Immunodiagnostic tests for demonstration of antigen/antibody using ELISA
- Demonstration of organisms in tissue sections using immunoperoxidase technique

CONTAGIOUS CAPRINE PLEUROPENUMONIA (CCPP)

Contagious caprine pleuropenumonia (CCPP) is an infectious disease of goats caused by *Mycoplasma* sp. and characterized by catarrh of upper respiratory tract, unilateral or bilateral pleuropneumonia, pleurisy and pericarditis.

Etiology
- *Mycoplasma mycoides*

Pathogenesis

The disease is readily spread by inhalation but organism does not survive for long period out side the animal body and its pathogenesis is just like CBPP.

Characteristic symptoms
- Fever (103-106°F)
- Dyspnoea
- Nasal discharge

Macroscopic and microscopic features
- Rhinitis and catarrh of upper respiratory tract
- Congestion and consolidation of lungs
- Pleurisy with gelatinous exudate
- Fibrinous pericarditis
- Edema and congestion of bronchial and mediastinal lymph nodes.
- Adhesions of lungs with pleura
- Congestion, infiltration of mononuclear cells in inter alveolar spaces; formation of lymphoid aggregates
- Deposition of fibrin in alveoli
- Fibrinous pericarditis
- Oedema and congestion in lymph nodes.

Diagnosis
- Symptoms and lesions
- Isolation of mycoplasma, nipple shaped colony on media
- Immunodiagnostic tests for demonstration of antigen/antibody- ELISA
- Demonstration of organisms in tissue sections using immunoperoxidase technique

MYCOPLASMAL ABORTION

Mycoplasmosis specially abortions in cattle due to mycoplasma is a disease of adult cattle caused by several species of *Mycoplasma* sp. and characterized by abortions in pregnant animals, mastitis and pneumonia and polyarthritis in foetus.

Etiology
- *Mycoplasma mycoides*
- *M. bovigenitalium*

Pathogenesis

Pathogenesis is not exactly known. However, this organism is considered to be non-pathogenic for animals. But in a state of immunosuppression, it may cause illness as opportunistic pathogen.

Characteristic Symptoms
- Abortion in cattle
- Mucous discharge from vagina
- Hard swelling of udder in mastitis

Macroscopic and microscopic features
- Abortion in cattle
- Bronchopneumonia in foetus
- Edema of placenta
- Lymphoid infiltration and aggregation of lymphocytes in placenta, uterus and in mammary gland.
- Lymphofollicular reaction in lungs and liver in foetus.

Diagnosis
- Serological examination-detection of antibody or antigen
- Isolation of mycoplasma using ELISA
- Demonstration of organism in tissue sections using immunoperoxidase technique

Chapter 28
Spirochaetal Diseases

LEPTOSPIROSIS

Leptospirosis is an infectious disease of animals caused by spirocheate *Leptospria* sp. and characterized by widespread haemorrhage in visceral organs, nephritis, icterus, hepatitis and anemia.

Etiology
- *Leptospira icterohaemorrhagiae*
- *L. pomona*

Pathogenesis

The organism is transmitted through direct contact with urine of infected animals or ingestion of urine contaminated feed or water. It can also be transmitted through aborted fetuses and infected uterine discharges. The organism enters through abraded skin and mucous membrane and reaches in blood and multiplies rapidly in blood producing septicemia and high rise in body temperature. Thereafter the organism localizes in the kidneys leading to acute or chronic nephritis. In kidneys, it multiplies in proximal convoluted tubules (PCT) and is excreted in urine which acts as source of infection.

Characteristic symptoms
- High fever (105-107°F)
- Anemia
- Icterus
- Abortion, mastitis
- Hemoglobinuria

Macroscopic and microscopic features
- Anemia, icterus
- Hemoglobinuria
- Blood mixed milk
- Hemorrhage in liver, kidneys, lungs and lymph nodes
- Enlargement of spleen and kidneys
- Abortion
- Grayish white foci on visceral organs.
- Necrosis and hyperplasia of kupffer's cells in liver
- Necrosis of tubular epithelium and formation hyaline in tubules of kidneys along with lymphocytic infiltration
- Haemosiderosis in spleen
- Encephalitis.

Diagnosis
- Symptoms and lesions
- Demonstrations of leptospira in urine samples under dark field microscopy
- Isolation of leptospira
- Immunodiagnostic tests for demonstration of antigen/ antibody- ELISA
- Demonstration of organism in tissue sections using special stains

Chapter 29
Prion Diseases

SPONGIFORM ENCEPHALOPATHY

Spongiform encephalopathy is an infectious disease of animals caused by prion proteins and characterized by presence of vacuoles in brain.

Etiology
- Prion proteins
- Sheep- Scrapie or Ovine spongiform encephalopathy
- Cattle- Bovine spongiform encephalopathy (Mad cow disease)

Pathogenesis

Scrapie is also known as ovine spongiform encephalopathy. The principle means of transmission of disease is from infected mother to their lambs early in life; placental transmission has also been reported. The incubation period of disease is very long (2-5 year). The clinical form is restricted in adults. The prion proteins (PrP) occur normally in the central nervous system of all domestic animals and man bounded with neuronal surface. Animal susceptible to prion disease have a gene (PrP gene) which encodes for normal "Prion protein (PrP)" or "cellular prion protein (PrPc). In scrapie prion protein (PrPsc)/ scrapie associated fibril protein (SAI) is generated which are resistant for protease digestion. Accumulation of PrPsc in neural tissues appears to be the cause of the pathology in prion disease. When prion protein contaminated meat and bone meal are fed to the cattle as part of their concentration, the agent (prion) got introduced into cattle. Prion protein (PrP) on reaching brain slowly and progressively converted into and abnormal form

(PrP sc) and this abnormal protein causes development of lesions including vacuolation in nerve cells.

Characteristic symptoms
- No characteristic symptom
- Circling movements of animal
- Itching in skin in sheep suffering from scrapie

Macroscopic and microscopic features
- No gross lesion
- Presence of large vacuoles in the cytoplasm of neurons in medulla oblongata, midbrain and spinal cord
- Brain looks like sponge
- Inflammatory changes like infiltration of cells, congestion, haemorrhages are absent
- Occasionally accumulation of lymphocytes in Vircho-Robin spaces.

Diagnosis
- History of case
- Symptoms and lesions
- Vacuoles in neurons
- Histopathological examination of brain tissue

Chapter 30
Fungal Diseases

RINGWORM

Ringworm is a fungal disease of skin affecting animals characterized by popular skin lesions in circular form discharging serus exudate.

Etiology
- *Microsporum canis*- dogs
- *M. gypseum*- dogs, horse, pig
- *Trichophyton verrucosum*- bovines
- *T. equinum*- horses

Pathogenesis

The fungi enter in skin through abrasion and the hyphae appear in stratum corneum after germination and invade the hair follicles. The hyphae growth and spore formation in stratum corneum leads to hyperkeratosis and the fungus spreads centrifugally from the point of primary invasion leading to ring shaped lesion.

Characteristics Symptoms
- Ring shaped lesions on skin
- Serum's discharge from lesions
- Hyperkeratosis, severe itching
- Loss of hairs

Macroscopic and microscopic features
- Ring shaped lesions on skin of face, around eyes, neck and shoulder

- Loss of hairs with raised, dry, crusty and grayish white masses
- Hyperkeratosis
- Presence of hyphae in hair follicles
- Hyperkeratosis of skin

Diagnosis
- Symptoms and lesions
- Demonstration of hyphae in hair follicles/ skin scrapings
- Demonstration of fungus in lesions using Wood's lamp
- Isolation of fungus in SDA media

CANDIDIASIS

Candidiasis is a fungal disease of animals caused by *Candida albicans* and characterized by a variety of manifestations including mastitis, chronic pneumonia, vaginal discharges, abortion and oesophagitis.

Etiology
- *Candida albicans*
- Yeast like cells, oval, 3.5-5.5m size

Pathogenesis

The fungus may enter through inhalation, ingestion or through abraded mucous membrane. It causes rumenitis and oesophagitis in calves with chronic lesions. It is thought to occur as a result of heavy antibacterial therapy and may cause mastitis, pneumonia and/or abortion.

Characteristic Symptoms
- Cutaneous granulomatous lesions in dogs and cats
- Difficulty in ingestion
- Hard udder
- Vaginal discharges/ abortion

Macroscopic and microscopic features
- Chronic pneumonic lesions- nodules in lungs
- Oesophagitis
- Cutaneous nodular lesions
- Rumenitis
- In tissue sections presence of candida as round or oval budding cells with pseudomycelia.
- Chronic granulomatous lesions

Diagnosis
- Symptoms and lesions
- Demonstration of candida in skin scrapings or lesions
- Isolation of fungus

RHINOSPORIDIOSIS

Rhinosporidiosis is a fungal disease of cattle and buffaloes caused by *Rhinosporidium* sp. and characterized by polypoid growth on nasal mucosa and dyspnoea.

Etiology
- *Rhinosporidum seeberi*

Pathogenesis

Fungus enters through abraded skin/ mucous membrane and causes hyperplasia of stratum spinosum.

Characteristic Symptoms
- Dyspnoea
- Sneezing
- Mucopurulent nasal discharge

Macroscopic and microscopic features
- Nasal polyps from small size to several centimeters in diameter filling whole nasal cavity.
- Papular lesions on conjunctival sac, ears and vagina.
- Fibromyxomatous lesion with numerous blood vessels

- Presence of white specks consists of sporangia filled with endospores.

Diagnosis
- Symptoms and lesions
- Microscopic examination of nasal polyps
- Demonstration of causative fungi in tissue sections using special stains

ASPERGILLOSIS

Aspergillosis is a fungal disease of animals characterized by granulomatous pulmonary lesions, abortion and lobar pneumonia in foetus.

Etiology
- *Aspergillus fumigatus*
- Dark green conidia

Pathogenesis

Aspergillus enters in body through mouldy grains or inhalation. In lungs fungi causes chronic granuloma formation leading to nodules with caseation and fibrosis.

Characteristic Symptoms
- Nasal discharge
- Sneezing/ coughing
- Abortion in ewes

Macroscopic and microscopic features
- Tubercle like granulomatous lesions in lungs
- Abortion in ewes and cattle
- Lobar pneumonia in aborted foetus
- Granulomatous lesions in lungs
- Fungus can be demonstrated in lesions

Diagnosis
- Symptoms and lesions
- Microscopic examination of tissue sections to demonstrate fungus using special stain

BLASTOMYCOSIS

Blastomycosis is a systemic fungal disease of animals caused by *Blastomyces dermatitidis* and characterized by chronic granulomatous lesions in skin and other internal organs including lymph nodes, liver, spleen, kidneys, lungs and intestines.

Etiology
- *Blastomyces dermatitidis*
- Yeast like bodies in tissues

Pathogenesis
Organism causes chronic granulomatous inflammation of skin and internal organs.

Characteristic Symptoms
- Nodules on skin
- Debilitating condition of animal
- Lameness
- Swelling and hardness of superficial lymph nodes

Macroscopic and microscopic features
- Presence of nodules on skin, lymph nodes, lungs, kidneys and liver
- Papule or pustule on skin
- Presence of yeast like bodies in chronic granulomatous lesions

Diagnosis
- Symptoms and lesions
- Identification of fungus in tissue sections using special stains

COCCIDIOIDOMYCOSIS

Coccidioidomycosis is a systemic fungal disease of animals characterized by granulomatous lesions in lymph nodes and lungs.

Etiology
- *Coccidioides immitis*
- Spherical bodies- sporangia

Pathogenesis

Desert rodents normally inhabit the fungus and excrete large number of spherules through faeces in soil, which germinate and multiply in soil after rain. When the ground dries, large number of arthroconidia are produced and released in air. Animals get infection through air during grazing that produces lesions in lungs and lymph nodes.

Characteristic Symptoms
- Nasal discharge
- Sneezing or coughing
- Nodular lesions on skin

Macroscopic and microscopic features
- Nodular lesions in lungs and lymph nodes
- Thick, yellow, gelatinous pus in lesion
- Abscess wall shows granulation tissue
- Granulomatous lesions in mediastinal, bronchial, submaxillary, retropharyngeal and mesenteric lymph nodes
- Granulomatous lesions in lungs

Diagnosis
- Symptoms and lesions
- Demonstration of fungus in tissue sections using special stains

CRYPTOCOCCOSIS

Cryptococcosis is a systemic fungal disease of animals characterized by nervous disorders including encephalitis, meningitis and presence of granuloma in eyes, sinuses and nasal septum.

Etiology
- *Cryptococcus neoformans*
- Spherical or ovoid shape, thick walled, single or budding, 3-8 mm diameter.

Pathogenesis
The organism is normally found in soil. Cryptococcosis occurs in animals through inhalation or implantation. In cows, it can enter through teat canal. It slowly reaches to the central nervous system due to its tropism to nervous tissue. Presence of capsule saves the organism from phagocytosis.

Characteristic Symptoms
- Nervous signs including in coordination of movements, staggering gait.
- Sneezing or coughing

Macroscopic and microscopic features
- Encephalitis
- Pneumonia
- Granuloma in nasal mucosa and meninges
- Granulomatous lesions in eyes, sinuses and nasal septum
- Mastitis
- Enlargement of lymph nodes
- Encephalitis and meningitis
- Pleocytosis
- Granulomatous lesions in lymph nodes
- Presence of cryptococcus in tissue sections

Diagnosis
- Symptoms and lesions
- Demonstration of fungus in tissue sections using special stains
- Isolation of fungus

HISTOPLASMOSIS

Histoplasmosis is a systemic fungal disease of animals characterized by chronic pneumonia, spleenomegaly, hepatomegaly, leucopenia and ulcers in intestines.

Etiology
- *Histoplasma capsulatum*
- Intracellular, chlamydocondia- round, thick walled structure 7-15 m diameter.

Pathogenesis

Air borne infection of histoplasma reaches to the lungs where it is phagocytosed by the reticuloendothelial cells that disseminate the infection in different organs/ tissues.

Characteristic Symptoms
- Leucopenia
- Diarrhoea
- Anemia
- Sneezing/ coughing
- Pyrexia
- Dyspnoea
- Emaciation
- Enlarged abdomen

Macroscopic and microscopic features
- Spleenomegaly
- Hepatomegaly
- Ulcers in intestines
- Lymphadenopathy

- Ascites
- Organism packed in macrophages
- Granulomatous lesions in lungs, liver, spleen and lymph nodes

Diagnosis
- Symptoms and lesions
- Demonstration of fungus in macrophages in tissue sections using special stains
- Isolation of fungus

MUCOUS MYCOSIS

Mucous mycosis is caused by *Absidia* sp. and characterized by chronic inflammation of lymph nodes, lung, uterus and placenta.

Etiology
- *Absidia corymbifera*

Pathogenesis
Not clear

Characteristic Symptoms
- Abortion
- Chronic wasting- progressive weakness

Macroscopic and microscopic features
- Granulomatous lesions in lungs, lymph nodes placenta, uterus
- Thick, hard, tubercle like nodules
- Cheesy exudate with calcification
- Reddish gray exudate with pus flukes in interplacentome space.
- Granulomatous lesions in lungs, lymph nodes
- Infiltration of neutrophils, macrophages, lymphocytes, eosinophils, giant cells.
- Calcification of centrally caseative necrosed area.

Diagnosis
- Symptoms and lesions
- Demonstration of fungus in tissues
- Isolation of fungus.

DEGNALA DISEASE

Degnala disease is a non-infectious disease of animals caused by mycotoxins and characterized by dry gangrene on extremities such as tip of ear, tail and hooves with sloughing of hooves.

Etiology
- *Fusarium tricinctum*
- Mycotoxins of fungus
- Paddy straw infested with fungus is source of mycotoxin.

Pathogenesis

Ingestion of mycotoxin in feed causes vasoconstriction leading to infarction, necrosis at extremities. Saprophytes invade and form dry gangrene.

Characteristic Symptoms
- Dry gangrene on tail, ear, scrotum and hooves
- Sloughing of skin
- Lameness

Macroscopic and microscopic features
- Sloughing of skin from hooves leaving raw wound surface
- Gangrene at tail, ears and scrotum
- Loss of architectural details
- Necrosis
- Edema with slight mononuclear infiltration

Diagnosis
- Symptoms and lesions
- Detection of toxin in feed

Chapter 31
Parasitic Diseases

TRYPANOSOMIASIS

Trypanosomiasis is an infectious disease of animals caused by protozoan parasite and characterized by emaciation, enlargement of spleen and lymph nodes, petechiae on serous membranes, ulceration on tongue and gastric mucosa and gelatinous exudate in subcutaneous region.

Etiology
- *Trypanosoma evansi*

Pathogenesis

The disease is mainly transmitted through bite of flies like Tabanus, Stomoxys, Haematopota etc. The carrier animals remain as potential source of infection. The pathogenesis of disease is not completely known. After entering in mammalian host, trypanosomes multiply in blood stream by binary fission leading to parasitemia. The parasites has variable surface glycoproteins which cause continuous exposure of immune system leading to hyperplasia of spleen and lymph nodes. In chronic cases, due to formation of antigen- antibody complexes glomerulonephritis and vasculitis is seen.

Characteristic symptoms
- High fever (105-107°F)
- Dyspnoea
- Paraplegia, emaciation
- Edema in dependent parts of body
- Conjunctivitis, keratitis

Macroscopic and microscopic features
- Emaciated carcass
- Enlargement of spleen and lymph nodes
- Gelatinous exudate in subcutaneous region
- Ulcerative keratitis
- Congestion of abomasum and intestines
- Petechiae on kidneys, liver and heart
- Ulcers in tongue and abomasum.
- Presence of flagellate parasite in blood smear
- Hyperplasia of lymphoid follicles in lymph nodes and spleen
- Congestion in intestines
- Erosion and ulcers in abomasum.

Diagnosis
- Demonstration of protozoan parasite in blood smear
- Symptoms and lesions
- Immunodiagnostic tests for demonstration of antigen/antibody- ELISA

THEILERIOSIS

Theileriosis is an infectious disease of animals caused by protozoan parasite and characterized by enlargement of lymph nodes, pulmonary edema, hemorrhage in kidneys and liver, ulcers in abomasum and catarrhal enteritis.

Etiology
- *Theileria annulata*

Pathogenesis

The parasite is transmitted through bite of ticks of genus Hyalomma. The disease can also be transmitted mechanically by inoculation of blood and tissue suspension made from spleen, lymph nodes and liver of infected animals. After entry the organism at sporozoit stage remains in blood circulation and enters in erythrocytes but they don't multiply. The multiplication occurs in lymphocytes where it forms schizonts. Infected lymphocytes are ruptured and schizonts are released and other lymphocytes are affected. Later some schizonts are differentiated unto merozoites. The rapidly multiplying schizonts are causing severe damage to lymphoid cells through their lysis.

Characteristic symptoms
- High fever (105-107°F)
- Anemia
- Enlargement of superficial lymph nodes

Macroscopic and microscopic features
- Anemia
- Pulmonary oedema
- Enlargement of lymph nodes and spleen
- Erosions and ulcers in abomasum
- Hemorrhage in epicardium
- Catarrhal enteritis
- Lymphoid depletion
- Presence of parasites in erythrocytes or its developmental stages in lymphocytes
- Perivascular lymphoid proliferation
- Congestion in intestines
- Proliferation of goblet cells.

Diagnosis
- Demonstration of protozoan parasite in blood smear/ lymph node biopsy
- Symptoms and lesions
- Immunodiagnostic tests for demonstration of antigen/ antibody- ELISA

BABESIOSIS

Babesiosis is an infectious disease of animals caused by

protozoan parasite and characterized by hemoglobinuria, anemia, petechiae and ecchymoses in serous membranes, icterus, pulmonary oedema and gastroenteritis.

Etiology
- *Babesia bigemina*
- *B. bovis*

Pathogenesis

The disease is transmitted from sick to healthy animal through ticks following trans ovarian route. The incubation period of disease is 5-10 days. After infection, the parasite multiplies in peripheral blood and there is intra-vascular haemolysis leading to hemoglobinuria. The infected erythrocytes liberate some enzymes which interact with the components of blood and leads to increased erythrocyte fragility, hypertensive shock and disseminated intra ocular coagulation.

Characteristic symptoms
- High fever (105-107°F)
- Anemia, icterus
- Hemoglobinuria

Macroscopic and microscopic features
- Anemia, icterus
- Hemoglobinuria
- Enlargement of spleen and liver
- Edema in lungs
- Petechiae and ecchymoses in kidneys, lungs, liver and spleen
- Congestion in gastrointestinal tract
- Presence of pear shaped Babesia organism in erythrocytes
- Hemorrhage in liver, kidneys, lungs and spleen
- Hemosiderosis in spleen
- Necrosis of tubular epithelium in kidneys and presence of hyaline casts.

Diagnosis
- Demonstration of protozoan parasite in blood smear
- Symptoms and lesions
- Immunodiagnostic tests for demonstration of antigen/antibody- ELISA

TRICHOMONIASIS

Trichomoniasis is a protozoan parasitic disease of animals caused by *Trichomonas* sp. characterized by abortion, vaginitis, metritis and balanitis in cattle and gastroenteritis in horses.

Etiology
- *Trichomonas foetus*- cattle
- *T. faecalis*- horses
- *T. suis*- swine
- *T. gallinae*- poultry

Pathogenesis

Following coitus, cow gets infection from bull that causes vaginitis, endometritis, placentitis, foetal infection and abortion in early gestation. Abortion followed by pyometra due to invasion of secondary bacterial infection.

Characteristic Symptoms
- Abortion
- Retention of placenta
- Sterility
- Pyometra

Macroscopic and microscopic features
- Vaginitis
- Gastroenteritis in horses
- Metritis- Pyometra
- Abortion during 3-5 month of gestation
- Balanitis in bulls

- Infiltration of neutrophils in uterus.
- Presence of trichomonads in tissue sections of uterus.

Diagnosis
- Symptoms and lesions
- Demonstration of trichomonads in prepuceal washing and vaginal discharges
- Demonstration of trichononades in uterine tissue sections

TOXOPLASMOSIS

Toxoplasmosis is a protozoan parasitic disease of animals characterized by encephalitis, foetalization of lungs, ulcers in intestines, necrosis in liver and abortion.

Etiology
- *Toxoplasma gondii*
- Immunosuppression predisposes animals and reactivation of parasites to cause disease.

Pathogenesis

Transmission of parasite occurs through ingestion of contaminated meat or feed. The sporozoites penetrate intestinal wall and multiply. Thereafter, they reach to the other organs through blood stream. In brain it causes encephalitis; infection may also occur in foetus as congenital that leads to pneumonia, enterocolitis and skin lesions.

Characteristic Symptoms
- Convulsions
- Nasal discharge
- Nervous signs- staggering gait, incoordination in moments.

Macroscopic and microscopic features
- Necrosis in brain and liver
- Nodules in lungs
- Ulcers in intestines

- Edema in placenta
- Lymphocytic infiltration in brain, pancreas, lungs and myocardium.
- Coagulative necrosis in liver
- Fetalization of lung alveolar lung epithelium becomes cuboidal or columnar.
- Granulomatous inflammation in intestines.

Diagnosis
- Symptoms and lesions
- Serological examination- ELISA
- Demonstration of parasites

COCCIDIOSIS

Coccidiosis is protozoan parasitic disease of animals characterized by gastroenteritis, hepatitis and typhlitis.

Etiology
- Cattle
- *Eimeria bovis*
- *E. zuernii*
- Sheep and goats
- *E. ovina*
- *E. parva*
- *E. intricata*
- Pigs
- *E. scrofae*
- *E. suis*
- *E. scabra*
- Equines
- *E. leuckarti*
- *Klossiella equi*

Pathogenesis

Oocysts are taken through contaminated water/ feed which germinate and liberate the sporozoites. Sporozoites infect the epithelium of intestine and forms schizonts and merozoites that causes damage to intestines leading to haemorrhage. After formation of gametes and fertilization oocysts are again formed and released through stool.

Characteristic Symptoms
- Bloody diarrhoea
- Emaciation

Macroscopic and microscopic features
- Hemorrhage in intestines
- Anemia
- Hepatic lesions and icterus in rabbits
- Coccidia in the epithelial cells of villi in mucosa of intestine.
- Eosinophilic inflammation
- Hemorrhagic enteritis

Diagnosis
- Symptoms and lesions
- Demonstration of coccidial parasites in stool, or intestinal tissue sections.

SARCOSPORIDIOSIS

Sarcosporidiosis is a protozoan parasitic disease of animals caused by several species of sarcocystis and characterized by presence of cysts in skeletal and cardiac muscles without much inflammatory reaction.

Etiology
- *Sarcocystis cruzi*- Cattle
- *S. gigantean*- Sheep
- *S. canis*- Dogs
- *S. capracanis*- Goat

Pathogenesis

On ingestion the sarcocystis enter through blood vessel by damaging the endothelial cells of arteriols and capillaries leading to hemorrhage and anemia, fever occurs during parasitemia and the parasite lodged in muscles.

Characteristic Symptoms
- Fever, emaciation, anemia
- 'Rat tail' appearance
- Muscle twitching, loss of hair in neck, rump
- Abortion

Macroscopic and microscopic features
- Sarcocyt on oesophagus, cardiac and skeletal muscle
- Loss of hairs on neck, tail
- Sarcocysts distort myofibrils in cardiac and skeletal muscle
- No or mild inflammatory reaction
- Rupture of sarcocyte may cause granulomatous inflammation

Diagnosis
- Symptoms and lesions
- Histopathological examination of muscles.

SCHISTOSOMIASIS

Schistosomiasis is a parasitic disease of animals caused by blood fluke characterized by formation of granulomatous pseudo tubercle, cercarial dermatitis and nasal granuloma.

Etiology
- *Schistosoma nasalis*
- *S. indicum*
- *S. bovis*
- *S. spindale*

Pathogenesis

When the cercariae find a suitable host, they penetrate the skin of susceptible host usually between the hair follicles and converted into metacercariae. Metacercariae enter in small peripheral veins and reach into lungs through venous circulation where they break the lung parenchyma and migrate directly to the liver. In intra hepatic portal system, the flukes grow in size then eventually migrate to the portal, mesenteric or pelvic vein where they attain their adult form.

Characteristic Symptoms
- Dyspnoea
- Epistaxis
- Dermatitis (Swimmers' itch)
- Itching

Macroscopic and microscopic features
- Granulomatous growth in nasal passage
- Dermatitis
- Hemorrhagic ulcers
- Micro abscess containing neutrophils and eosinophils surrounding ovum
- Granulomatous reaction-eggs surrounded by mononuclear cells and fibrosis
- Endarteritis, periarteritis

Diagnosis
- Symptoms and lesions
- Examination of lesion and/or blood for flood flukes.

DISTOMIASIS

Distomiasis is a trematode parasitic disease of animals caused by *Fasciola* sp. and characterized by hepatitis, cholecystitis and icterus.

Etiology
- *Fasciola hepatica*
- *Fasciola gigantica*

Pathogenesis

The ova of the parasite are disseminated through faeces, which germinate and form miracidium. The miracidium penetrates the body of snails and after several stages, it becomes cercariae which is attached to plants/ vegetation in water source. This form is called as metacercariae, which are ingested by the animals, and reaches in intestine. They penetrate the intestine and migrate to liver to eventually develop in bile ducts and gall bladder.

Characteristic Symptoms
- Anemia, emaciation
- Icterus, diarrhoea/ constipation
- Edema in lower parts of body

Macroscopic and microscopic features
- Necrotic channels in liver
- Abscess formation
- Presence of parasites in bile duct/ gall bladder
- Infiltration of eosinophils, lymphocytes and mononuclear macrophages
- Fibrosis/ cirrhosis of liver

Diagnosis
- Symptoms and lesions
- Faecal examination
- Liver/ gall bladder examination during necropsy for the presence of adult flukes
- Demonstration of parasitic antigens in faeces, milk and/ or serum using ELISA

CRYPTOSPORIDIOSIS

Cryptosporidiosis is a protozoan parasitic disease of animals characterized by chronic diarrhoea in calves, villous atrophy and infiltration of lymphocytes in mucosa of intestine.

Etiology
- *Cryptosporidium bovis*
- Protozoan parasite just like coccidia

Pathogenesis

Oocysts of cryptosporidia enter in body through faecal-oral route and establish in mucosa of intestine. The merozoites penetrate villous epithelium causing chronic diarrhoea.

Characteristic Symptoms
- Inapparent signs
- Chronic diarrhoea

Macroscopic and microscopic features
- Congestion of intestines
- Enlargement of mesenteric lymph nodes
- Villous atrophy
- Infiltration of lymphocyte, plasma cells
- Intracellular parasite- basophilic
- Necrosis

Diagnosis
- Symptoms and lesions
- Microscopic examination of faecal samples and intestinal scrapings
- Demonstration of parasites in intestinal tissue sections

ASCARIASIS

Ascariasis is a parasitic disease of animals caused by Ascarid worms and characterized by diarrhoea, jaundice, and obstruction of bile duct, peritonitis and obstruction of intestinal lumen.

Etiology
- *Ascaris lumbricoides*- Pig
- *Toxocara canis*- Dog
- *T. cati*- Cats, dog
- *Neoascaris vitulorum*- Cattle
- *Parascaris equorum*- Horse

Pathogenesis
The eggs or larvae are ingested through feed/ water. Larvae invade the intestine and pass through liver to the lungs, enter in bronchi and trachea and then are swallowed to develop adult parasite in intestinal lumen. In cattle larvae may also reach to the foetus through prenatal or trans mammary passage.

Characteristic Symptoms
- Diarrhoea
- Fever
- Constipation
- Jaundice

Macroscopic and microscopic features
- Presence of adult worms in intestinal lumen
- Hepatitis with sub-capsular fibrosis
- Granulomatous nodules in kidneys, liver, lung, myocardium and lymph nodes
- Larvae may migrate in abnormal host - *visceral larva migrans* in man
- Caseous hepatitis with fibrosis
- Eosinophilic enteritis
- Hemorrhage in intestines and lungs

Diagnosis
- Symptoms and lesions
- Faecal examination for the presence of parasitic ova
- Presence of parasites in intestines during necropsy

ANCHYLOSTOMIASIS

Anchylostomiasis is a parasitic disease of animals characterized by dermatitis creeping eruptions, anemia, diarrhoea and progressive emaciation. This is also known as *hook worm disease*.

Etiology
- *Anchylostoma caninum*- Dog
- *Bunostomum phlebotomum*- Cattle
- *B. trigonocephalum*- Sheep, goat
- *Globecephalus urosubulatus*- Pig

Pathogenesis
Eggs are released in faeces, which hatch under suitable conditions into larvae that infect the host through skin penetration or ingestion. Larvae migrate to the lungs and finally reaches in intestine through cough swallowing. During migration, they may penetrate placenta and infect foetus or may appear in milk to infect suckling neonates.

Characteristic Symptoms
- Dermatitis
- Itching on skin
- Coughing
- Anemia, melena
- Progressive weakness

Macroscopic and microscopic features
- Anemia
- Lobular pneumonia
- Hemorrhage in intestines
- Fibrotic nodules in intestines
- Dermatitis
- Placentitis
- Hemorrhage in intestine

- Blunting and fusion of villi
- Fibrosis in intestine
- Leucocytic infiltration in lungs and intestines

Diagnosis
- Symptoms and lesions
- Faecal examination for the present of ova
- In intestine adult worms are seen during necropsy
- Demonstration of parasite in tissue sections

TRICHOSTRONGYLOSIS

Trichostrongylosis is a parasitic disease of animals characterized by melena, emaciation, progressive weakness, anemia and death.

Etiology
- *Hemonchus contortus*- stomach worm
- *H. placei*- stomach worm
- *Ostertagia ostertagi*- brown stomach worm
- *Trichostrongylus axei*- hair like worm
- *T. colubriformis*- hair like worm
- *Cooperia punctata*- stomach worm

Pathogenesis

Larvae are ingested through feed or water, which penetrate the abomasum and attach with mucosa. They take the blood of host and become mature within 18-19 days. Adult worms live free in lumen but suck blood from the wall of abomasum. Some may pierce the mucosa deep to remain in the wall for longer period that leads to formation of small nodules.

Characteristic Symptoms
- Diarrhoea
- Melena
- Anemia

Macroscopic and microscopic features
- Nodules in gastric wall
- Hemorrhage in gastric mucosa
- Blood mixed intestinal contents
- Anemia
- Edema in subcutis
- Abomasum may have large number of worms
- Mucosa of abomasum becomes haemorrhagic and atrophic
- Infiltration of leucocytes specially of eosinophils

Diagnosis
- Symptoms and lesions
- Faecal examination
- Identification of parasites from stomach during necropsy

OESOPHAGOSTOMIASIS

Oesophagostomiasis is a parasitic disease of animals characterized by diarrhoea, anemia, emaciation, cachexia, prostration and death.

Etiology
- *Oesophagostomum radiatum*
- *O. columbianum*
- These are known as **nodule worms**

Pathogenesis

Eggs pass through faeces and germinate into larvae in soil. Larvae through contaminated feed/ water reaches in gut of animal. The larvae penetrate the intestinal mucosa, moult in sub mucosa and return to the lumen for maturation to become adult worm.

Characteristic Symptoms
- Diarrhoea
- Anemia, emaciation, cachexia

- Prostration and death

Macroscopic and microscopic features
- Catarrhal enteritis
- Hemorrhage in intestines
- Anemia
- Nodules in sub mucosa
- Parasites in intestines
- Catarrhal, haemorrhagic and eosinophilic enteritis
- Infiltration of lymphocytes, macrophages and giant cells

Diagnosis
- Symptoms and lesions
- Faecal examination
- Demonstration of parasite in intestinal wall/ lumen

CESTODIASIS

Cestodiasis is a tapeworm parasitic disease of animals characterized by anemia, haemorrhagic enteritis, abdominal pain, emaciation and diarrhoea. This is also known as *tapeworm disease* or *taeniasis*.

Etiology
- *Anoplocephala magna*- horse
- *Moniezia expansa*- sheep, goat, cattle, buffaloes
- *M. benedeni*- sheep, goat, cattle, buffaloes
- *Avitellina centripunctata*- sheep, goat, cattle, buffaloes
- *Diphyllobothrium latum*- pigs, dogs
- *Mesocestoides lineatus*- dogs
- *Dipylidium caninum*- dogs
- *Taenia pisiformis*- dogs

Pathogenesis

Adult tapeworms suck the blood from mucosa of intestines through suckers and hooks causing enteritis and anemia.

Characteristic Symptoms
- Anemia
- Blood mixed faeces, diarrhoea
- Emaciation, progressive weakness
- Jaundice
- Abdominal pain

Macroscopic and microscopic features
- Haemorrhagic enteritis
- Presence of parasites in intestines
- Blood mixed intestinal contents
- Anemic musculature
- Hemosiderin in liver and spleen
- Fatty degeneration of brain tissue
- Hemorrhagic enteritis

Diagnosis
- Symptoms and lesions
- Faecal examination
- Presence of parasitic segments in intestine of host

CYSTICERCOSIS

Cysticercosis is a parasitic disease of animals characterized by the presence of cysts in different organs of body. This is caused by larval stages of the tapeworms and is also known as *bladder worm disease*.

Etiology
- *Cysticercus cellulosae* – larvae of *Taenia solium*
- *C. bovis* – larvae of *T. saginata*
- *Coenurus cerebralis* – larvae of *Multiceps multiceps*

Pathogenesis

Cysticercosis is caused by the larval stages of tapeworms, which forms cysts like bladder in different organs including muscles, liver, heart etc.

Parasitic Diseases

Characteristic Symptoms
- No characteristic symptoms
- Paralysis of affected organs such as tongue
- Convulsions
- In sheep- this disease is known as *Gid*

Macroscopic and microscopic features
- Pressure atrophy due to cyst in adjoining tissue/ organ
- Presence of cysts up to several millimeter diameter in muscle, heart, liver, tongue, lungs, brain etc.
- Measly beef or pork
- Presence of bladder with scolex and hooks in tissue sections surrounded by connective tissue capsules.
- Eosinophilic infiltration

Diagnosis
- Symptoms and lesions
- Presence of cysts in different organs during necropsy

ECHINOCOCCOSIS

Echinococcsis is a parasitic disease of animals characterized by presence of cysts in different organs. This is also known as *hydated cyst disease*, which is caused by the intermediate stage of tapeworm echinococcus.

Etiology
- *Echinococcus granulosus*
- *E. multilocularis*

Pathogenesis

The cysts may affect organ/ tissue which depends on the size of the hydated cyst.

Characteristic Symptoms
- No characteristic symptoms
- Depends on organ involved

- Anaphylactic shock, allergic reaction
- Dyspnoea, diarrhoea, blindness, paralysis

Macroscopic and microscopic features
- Presence of cysts up to several centimeter in diameter
- Atrophy of adjoining tissue/ organ
- Calcified nodules
- Cysts are surrounded by inflammatory reaction with eosinophils, giant cells and fibrous connective tissue

Diagnosis
- Presence of cysts in different organs/ tissue during necropsy
- CFT, DTH, HA test
- Histopathology

DIROFILARIASIS

Dirofilariasis is a nematode parasitic disease of animals characterized by presence of parasites in blood, heart and arteries causing emboli, ascites, hypertrophy of right ventricle and granulomatous inflammation in visceral organs. This is also kwon as *"Heart worm disease"* or *canine filariasis"*

Etiology
- *Dirofilaria immitis* - dogs
- *D. repens*- dogs
- *Setaria cervi*- cattle
- *S. equina*- Horses
- *Dioctophyma renale*- Pig, dog

Pathogenesis

Transmission of microfilarial worms occurs by biting mosquitoes, in which after some developmental stages, infective larvae enters in body tissues of susceptible hosts. It further develops in muscles, subcutaneous tissue and reaches up to few cm in length and enters in circulation to reach in heart.

Characteristic Symptoms
- Ascites
- Hemoptysis
- Dyspnoea with short breathing
- Weakness

Macroscopic and microscopic features
- Enlargement of right ventricle
- Presence of worms in heart
- Congestion of lung, liver and spleen
- Ascities
- Pulmonary emboli due to parasite
- Microfilariae in eyes of horse
- Microfilariae in blood
- Microfilariae in tissue sections with granulomatous inflammatory reaction in kidney
- Cystitis

Diagnosis
- Symptoms and lesions
- Blood examination
- Demonstration of parasite in tissue sections
- Immunodiagnostic tests for detection of parasitic antigen

DRACUNCULOSIS

Dracunculosis is a nematode parasitic disease of animals characterized by urticarial rashes, low-grade fever, abscess involving subcutaneous tissue of abdominal wall and legs. It is also known as *guinea worm disease*.

Etiology
- *Dracunculus medinensis*
- *D. insignis*

Pathogenesis

Infection occurs after ingestion of Cyclops (intermediate host) in water that leads to release of larvae in intestine. They migrate to the connective tissue of abdominal wall, where they become adult and lay eggs, which forms papule and causes itching and oedema.

Characteristic Symptoms
- Intense pruritus, itching in legs and abdominal wall
- Edema
- Urticaria
- Low grade fever

Macroscopic and microscopic features
- Edema
- Papular eruptions on abdominal wall, legs,
- Urticarial swellings
- Subcutaneous nodules
- Parasites in blood
- Neutrophilic infiltration
- Congestion, oedema in subcutaneous tissue and abdominal wall

Diagnosis
- Symptoms and lesions
- Blood examination
- Demonstration of parasite in tissue sections

PULMONARY NEMATODIASIS

Pulmonary nematodiasis is a nematode parasitic disease of animals characterized by dyspnoea, coughing, diarrhoea, stunted growth and nodules in lungs. It is also known as *lungworm disease* or *verminous pneumonia* or *dictyocauliasis*.

Etiology
- *Dictyocaulus viviparus*- cattle lung worm

- *D. filaria*- cattle lung worm
- *Filaroides osleri*- dog lung worm
- *F. milksi*- dog lung worm
- *Dictyocaulus arnfieldi*- horse lung worm

Pathogenesis

Adult parasites remain in trachea, bronchi and bronchioles and embedded in mucosa. Eggs are laid and swallowed with cough in the gut. The eggs hatch to produce larvae that come with faeces. The third stage larvae are ingested by susceptible animal and penetrate the intestinal wall and migrate to lymph nodes, where they develop 4th stage larvae. By way of lymphatics and pulmonary artery, they enter in bronchioles and bronchi to cause lung lesions.

Characteristic Symptoms
- Hacking cough with dyspnoea
- Diarrhoea
- Retarded growth

Macroscopic and microscopic features
- Nodules in lungs
- Hemorrhage in bronchiole and alveoli
- Granulomatous pneumonia
- Presence of worms in trachea/ bronchiole
- Presence of parasitic sections in lung tissue
- Eosinophilic infiltration
- Atelectasis and emphysema

Diagnosis
- Symptoms and lesions
- Faecal examination
- Parasite in trachea/ bronchiole
- Demonstration of parasitic sections in lung tissue

EQUINE STRONGYLOIDOSIS

Equine strongyloidosis is a nematode parasitic disease of equines characterized by verminous arthritis, aneurysm, saddle thrombi, anemia and intestinal infarction.

Etiology
- *Strongylus vulgaris*
- *S. equinus*

Pathogenesis

Eggs of parasite pass through faeces; first stage larvae hatched out and develop up to 3rd stage, which are ingested through feed/ water. These larvae penetrate intestine, moult in sub mucosa and reach in anterior mesenteric artery. After maturation, the adult parasites return to the intestine particularly in caecum.

Characteristic Symptoms
- Diarrhoea with melena
- Abdominal pain
- Weakness of the legs
- Anemia

Macroscopic and microscopic features
- Parasites in blood vessel
- Intestinal hemorrhage
- Aneurysm
- Arteritis
- Thrombosis and embolism
- Parasitic arteritis infiltrated by eosinophils and mononuclear cells
- Infarction
- Proliferation of intima and endothelium
- Hemorrhage

Diagnosis
- Symptoms and lesions
- Demonstration of parasites in blood vessel
- Eggs in faeces- faecal examination
- Histopathological examination

SPIROCERCOSIS

Spirocercosis is a nematode parasitic disease of animals characterized by vomiting, oesophageal obstruction and presence of tumour like nodule in aortic wall. This is also known as *oesophageal worm disease.*

Etiology
- *Spirocerca lupi* in dogs

Pathogenesis
Eggs are released in faeces of infected animal and are taken up by beetles in which they hatch to produce larvae. If eaten by the host, the larvae penetrate the stomach or intestinal wall and following the course of arteries migrating through tunica adventitia and media, the larvae reaches in the wall of aorta and localizes in adventitia of aorta in upper thoracic portion. From here, it can migrate to adjacent oesophagus and penetrate its wall to develop cystic nodule.

Characteristic Symptoms
- Vomiting
- Oesophageal obstruction
- Sudden death

Macroscopic and microscopic features
- Tumour like nodule in aorta, oesophagus (near cardia)
- Aneurysm in aorta
- Hemorrhage due to aneurysm
- Sometimes nodule in stomach and lungs
- Worm in tunica adventitia or media of aorta
- Leucocytic infiltration

- Necrotic tract in aorta

Diagnosis
- Symptoms and lesions
- Faecal examination
- Presence of parasite in nodule of oesophagus and aorta

CEREBROSPINAL NEMATODIASIS

Cerebrospinal nematodiasis is a nematode parasitic disease of animals characterized by loss of balance, incoordination, paresis of limbs, drooping of ears or eyelid and eosinophilic encephalitis. It is also known as *neurofilariasis, setariasis* and *lumbar paralysis* and in horses *"Kumri"*.

Etiology
- *Setaria digitata*- sheep, goat, cervids
- *Pneumostrongylus tenuis*- sheep, goat, cervids
- *Micronema deletrix*- horse

Pathogenesis
Adult parasites are harmless while the immature forms occur in brain and spinal cord of sheep, goat and horses.

Characteristic Symptoms
- Paralysis of limbs
- Incoordination of limbs
- Loss of balance

Macroscopic and microscopic features
- Not well known
- Encephalomyelomalacia
- Presence of parasite in lesion
- Encephalomyelomalacia
- Eosinophilic infiltration in brain and spinal cord
- Degenerative and necrotic lesions in brain and spinal cord
- Perivascular cuffing of lymphocytes
- Parasite in tissue sections

Diagnosis
- Symptoms and lesions
- Microscopic examination of brain and spinal cord

TRICHURIASIS

Trichuriasis is a nematode parasitic disease of animals characterized by catarrhal, hemorrhagic or necrotizing typhlitis and colitis. It is also known as *whipworm disease*.

Etiology
- *Trichuris ovis*- cattle, sheep, goat
- *Trichuris suis*- pig

Pathogenesis

Eggs of parasite are ingested through feed/ water, which hatch in intestine and liberate larvae that penetrate the mucosa of caecum and colon.

Characteristic Symptoms
- Diarrhoea with melena
- Weakness and emaciation

Macroscopic and microscopic features
- Catarrhal/ hemorrhagic inflammation of caecum and colon.
- Presence of worms in caecum
- Catarrhal, haemorrhagic and/or necrotizing typhlitis and colitis
- Parasite in tissue sections
- Eosinophilic infiltration

Diagnosis
- Symptoms and lesions
- Faecal examination
- Histopathological examination of caecum and colon for demonstration of parasitic section

TRICHINOSIS

Trichinosis is a nematode parasitic disease of animals characterized by muscular pain, nausea, vomiting, diarrhoea, fever, oedema of face, urticarial skin eruptions and enteritis. It is also known as *trichinelliasis*.

Etiology
- *Trichinella spiralis*

Pathogenesis
Uncooked or raw pork products are the source of infection. Infective larvae released from meat and mature in intestine. It enters in intestinal mucosa and through blood stream it reaches in muscles (cardiac, skeletal)

Characteristic Symptoms
- Muscular pain and fever
- Nausea, vomiting and diarrhoea
- Edema of face
- Urticarial skin eruptions
- Paralysis

Macroscopic and microscopic features
- Catarrhal enteritis
- Nodule in muscles containing parasite with calcified area
- Parasitic nodules in cardiac muscles
- Leucocytosis with eosinophilia
- Catarrhal enteritis
- Chalk coloured streaks in skeletal muscles
- Parasite in muscle section

Diagnosis
- Symptoms and lesions
- Parasites or ova in faeces
- Parasitic demonstration in muscles

STEPHANOFILARIASIS

Stephanofilariasis is a parasitic disease of animals characterized by dermatitis, hyperkeratosis and scab formation. This is also known as *hump sore* or *ear sore*.

Etiology
- *Stephanofilaria dedosi*
- *S. assamensis*- hump sore
- *S. zaheeri*- ear sore

Pathogenesis

Transmission of parasite occurs through flies. Poor condition of animal and high rainfall are predisposing factors in causation of disease. Disease starts with papular lesions on skin along with itching.

Characteristic Symptoms
- Intense itching
- Rubbing with hard object leading to haemorrhage and abraded wounds
- Hump sore
- Ear sore

Macroscopic and microscopic features
- This is verminous dermatitis also known as *'Cascado'*
- Papular eruptions, abrasion wounds
- Parasite in epithelial layer of skin
- Hyperkeratosis and parakeratosis
- Presence of parasites in tissue sections of skin surrounded by inflammatory cells i.e. eosinophils, lymphocytes and giant cells
- Hyperkeratosis and parakeratosis

Diagnosis
- Symptoms and lesions
- Demonstration of parasite in skin

MANGE

Mange is a skin disease caused by arthropod parasite mite and characterized by intense pruritus, loss of hairs, hyperkeratosis and thickening of skin.

Etiology
- Mites- arthropod parasite
- *Sarcoptes* sp.
- *Psoroptes* sp.
- *Demodectes* sp.
- *Chorioptes* sp.

Pathogenesis

Disease spreads through contact, fomites and rubbing brushes etc. The mites penetrate the stratum corneum layer of skin and forms tunnels in epidermis leading to hyperkeratosis and inflammatory reaction.

Characteristic Symptoms
- Intense itching
- Red papular eruptions or abrasion wounds in skin
- Loss of hairs

Macroscopic and microscopic features
- Thickening of skin
- Loss of shining of skin and hairs
- Hyperkeratosis
- Scratch wounds
- Eosinophilic dermatitis
- Presence of mites in skin sections
- Hyperkeratosis and parakeratosis

Diagnosis
- Symptoms and lesions
- Microscopic examination of skin scrapings/ tissue

Chapter 32
Avian Inflammation

Inflammation is a process which begins following a sublethal injury to tissue and ends with complete healing or death. It is characterized by five cardinal signs. Cardinal signs of inflammation are:
- Redness
- Heat
- Swelling
- Pain
- Loss of function
- Inflammation is beneficial in most of cases except
  - In prolonged or unending process
  - In inflammation of immunological origin i.e. hypersensitivity and autoimmunity.
- It provides basic foundation of pathogenesis and pathology.
- It is now said that immunity is the resistance of body, while inflammation is the process by which the immune mechanism are implemented.
- The basis of inflammation remains same be it mammal or birds. For details, one can refer the chapter inflammation. However, there are some differences in reaction in birds which are briefly listed below:
1. Adult bird has greater capacity to react in comparison to embryos and chicks
2. In birds, there is increased permeability in venules. While in mammals it occurs in capillary/ arterioles.

3. In poultry, Heterophils are the first line of defence and comes first in inflammation followed by mononuclear cells. However, in mammals the sequence is not clear.
4. In poultry, Basophils are seen in significant numbers at the site in early stage of inflammation. These cells degranulate to release histamine. However, in mammals basophils are rarely seen.
5. Formation of perivascular foci due to infiltration of lymphoid cells causing cuffing around blood vessels. This is very common in avian inflammatory reaction. However, in mammals it has been seen only in some specific inflammations of brain.
6. Giant cells are the feature of avian inflammation and are observed in acute and chronic inflammation while in mammals these are seen only in chronic inflammation.
7. In birds, thrombocytes act as phagocytic cells.
8. Biphasic vascular permeability response occurs in chicken. First reaction is mediated by histamine while another reaction is mediated by unknown factors. It has been proved by treatment with antihistaminic drugs which did not stop the inflammatory reaction.
9. In chicken, inflammation caused by phytohaemagglutinin or concanavalin-A (Con-A) is characterized by skin response with infiltration of heterophils, monocytes and basophils. While in mammals, there are no neutrophils and basophils in such reactions.

Chapter **33**

Pathology of Nutritional Disorders

Pathology of nutritional deficiency diseases are described in chapter 2 etiology of the book "Illustrated Veterinary Pathology". However, specific deficiency of nutrition that leads to development of clinical signs and lesions in poultry are summarized as under:

VITAMIN DEFICIENCY

1. **Hypovitaminosis A**
- Vitamin A is considered infection resisting vitamin because it facilitates the proper development of bursa, immunity and epithelium on mucosal and skin surfaces.
- Deficiency of vitamin A leads to swollen glands in oesophagus i.e. nutritional roup.

2. **Hypovitaminosis D**
- Rickets
- Cage layer paralysis
- Deformed rib junctions

3. **Hypovitaminosis E**
- Encephalomalacia
- Chicks push their head beneath the breast *"Crazy Chick Disease"*
- Muscular dystrophy with white necrotic areas on muscles
- Distortion of hock joint

4. **Hypovitaminosis K**
- Increased blood clotting time
- Blood tinged droppings
- Pale bone marrow
- Haemorrhage in breast and thigh muscles

5. **Hypovitaminosis C**
- Case layer fatigue

6. **Hypovitaminosis B_1**
- Star grazing in chicks
- Atrophy of testes
- Atrophy of ovary

7. **Hypovitaminosis B_2**
- Curled toe paralysis

8. **Nicotinic acid/ niacin deficiency**
- Enlargement of joints
- Legs bend outwards

9. **Pentothenic acid deficiency**
- Nodular hyperplasia and cracks at foot pad.
- Scabs at commissures of the mouth; eyelids and toes
- Stunted growth
- Hypoplasia of spleen

10. **Pyridoxine (B_6) deficiency**
- Stunted growth
- Encephalomalacia
- Jerking movements

11. **Folic acid deficiency**
- Anemia
- Retardation of growth
- Perosis

Pathology of Nutritional Disorders

12. Biotin deficiency
- Dermatitis
- Perosis
- Embryonic death
- Distorted limbs
- Big web between 3rd and 4th phalanges

13. Choline deficiency
- Perosis (Slipped tendon)
- Deformity in tibio-tarsal joint
- Fatty liver syndrome

14. Vitamin B_{12} deficiency
- Stunted growth
- Reduced hatchability
- Atrophic leg muscles
- Hemorrhage

MINERAL DEFICIENCY

1. Calcium deficiency
- Rickets
- Nodular swelling at costocondral junctions of ribs
- Bending of legs

2. Phosphorus deficiency
- Pica

3. Manganese deficiency
- Perosis
- Defective growth of bone (osteodystrophy and chondrodystrophy)
- Parrot beak

4. Zinc deficiency
- Perosis

- Scaly limb disease
- Immunosuppression

5. Copper deficiency
- Anemia
- Improper bone growth

6. Magnesium deficiency
- Stunted growth

7. Selenium deficiency
- Muscular degeneration
- Deformity in embryos (absence of beak, eye or limb)

8. Nickel deficiency
- Enlargement of hock joints

9. Iodine deficiency
- Stunted growth

10. Fluorosis/ excess of fluorine
- Retarded growth
- Drop in egg production
- Deformity in bones

Chapter 34
Viral Diseases

RANIKHET DISEASE

Ranikhet disease is a contagious viral disease of poultry characterized by high mortality petechial hemorrhage in proventriculus, ulcers and hemorrhage at caecal tonsils and pneumoencephalitis. It is also known as *Newcastle disease*.

Etiology
- Paramyxovirus
- RNA virus-3 types
- Lentogenic- mild virulent
- Mesogenic- moderate virulent
- Velogenic- highly virulent

Pathogenesis

The birds showing respiratory disease shed the virus in air in the form of droplets of mucus which is inhaled by susceptible birds. The virus also transmitted through ingestion of contaminated food and water and reaches in intestines where its replication occurs. The virus is attached to cells with receptors mediated by the hemagglutinin glycoprotein. Then the virus membrane fuses with cell membrane with fusion glycoproteins. Thus nucleocapsid complex enters in the cell. During replication glycoprotein is cleaved for the progeny virus particle to be infective. The virulent viruses invade and replicate in many tissues and organs resulting in the production of infective virus throughout the body and cause development of lesions.

Characteristic symptoms
- Yellowish/ greenish diarrhoea
- Twitching of neck
- Heavy mortality
- Early chick mortality
- Paralysis
- Respiratory distress
- Prostration and mortality

Macroscopic and microscopic features

Velogenic form
- Petechial hemorrhage on the tip of the proventriculus papillae.
- Hemorrhagic ulcers in intestines particularly at ileocaecal junction (caecal tonsils).
- Petechial hemorrhage on serosal surfaces of visceral organs.

Mesogenic form
- Congestion of lungs and brain
- Pneumoencephalitis
- Mottling of spleen

Lentogenic form
- Haemorrhagic lesions are few or absent and low mortality.
- Drop in egg production with congestion of ovaries.
- Proliferation of endothelial cells of blood vessels in brain.
- Cytoplasmic vacuolation in neurons.
- Proliferation of glial cells.
- Thrombosis in blood vessels of intestine.
- Necrosis of mucosa leading to ulcer formation in intestines specially at caecal tonsils.

Viral Diseases

- Proliferation of Kuffer cells in liver.
- Congestion in lungs.
- Congestion of ovaries and oviduct.

Diagnosis

- Symptoms and lesions
- Demonstration of antigen in brain tissue
- Immunological tests such ELISA, AGPT, CIEP for detection antigen/ antibody.

AVIAN INFLUENZA

Avian influenza is a highly contagious viral disease of poultry characterized by high morbidity and mortality, serofibrinosis pericarditis, air sacculitis, pneumonia, sinusitis and caseous exudate in upper respiratory tract. This disease is also known as *fowl plague* and occurs in pandemic form.

Etiology

- Orthomyxovirus, HPAI- H5N1
- RNA virus
- Several subtypes based on Hemagglutinin (H) and Neuraminidase (N) antigens.

Pathogenesis

The source of infection is infected bird which excretes virus from respiratory tract, conjunctiva and faeces. The faecal/ oral route is the main mode of transmission. The avian influenza virus adsorbs to glycoprotein receptors on the cell surface. The virus then enters in the cell by receptor mediated endocytosis. The tissue tropism of virus is involved in its pathogenicity which is receptor specific. Pathogenicity of virus is due to hemogglutinin molecule which is cleaved by host proteases and the cleaved hemagglutinin is deciding factor for viral replication and for production of infective virion particles. Due to presence of proteases the virus invades and replicates in tissues and organs resulting in generalized disease and death.

Characteristic symptoms
- Cyanosis of comb and wattle
- Edema of face
- Respiratory distress
- Convulsions, blindness and paralysis

Macroscopic and microscopic features
- Oedema of face.
- Hemorrhage on epicardium, breast muscles and inner surface of sternum.
- Necrotic foci in spleen, liver, kidneys, intestine and pancreas.
- Visceral gout and nephrosis with swollen kidneys.
- Sinusitis with caseous or mucopurulent exudate.
- Caseous exudates in air sacs.
- Perivascular cuffing by lymphocytes in brain, heart, spleen and lungs.
- Coagulative necrosis in kidneys, spleen, lungs, pancreas and liver.
- Edema in myocardium and lungs.
- Dialated tubules in kidneys with urate crystalline casts.

Diagnosis
- High morbidity and mortality.
- Symptoms and lesions
- Perivascular cuffing in brain which is absent in Ranikhet disease.
- Demonstration of H and N antigens using HA/ HI test.

MAREK'S DISEASE

Marek's disease is a highly contagious disease of poultry mainly affecting young birds and characterized by thickening of nerves and malignant lymphoma in gonads and other visceral organs.

Viral Diseases

Etiology
- DNA virus
- Herpes virus
- Cell associated virus
- Produces a tumour specific antigen on the cell membrane MATSA (Marek's associated tumour surface antigen).

Pathogenesis
Feather follicle cells are the most important source of infection to the susceptible birds. However, other sources include poultry house dust and litter. Air borne spread and respiratory tract infection is most important route of infection. The virus enters through respiratory tract and it is picked up by the phagocytic cells that leads to four phase of infection.
- *Early productive* infection causes mainly degenerative changes i.e. cytolytic changes.
- *Latent infection* which coincides with the development of immune responses. Mostly T-cell are infected in latency although B-cells may also involved.
- *Second-phase* of cytolytic productive restrictive infection coinciding with permanent immunosuppression.
- *Proliferative phase* involving non-productively infected lymphoid cells which may progress to lymphoma formation. The lymphoproliferative changes constitute the final responses and may progress to tumour development.

Characteristic symptoms
- Lameness, paralysis and hanging wings
- Torticollis
- Head turns upside down
- Tumours on skin

Macroscopic and microscopic features
- Thickening of nerves (Sciatic, brachial, vagus) with loss of cross striations.

- Tumours of malignant lymphoma in ovary/ testes, liver, spleen, lungs, muscles, heart, kidneys, proventriculus and intestines.
- Tumours on skin.
- Lymphocytic infiltration in nerves.
- Lymphofollicular reaction in visceral organs like gonads, liver, spleen, lungs and heart.
- Lymphocytes are immature and pleomorphic showing characteristic anaplastic changes.

Diagnosis
- Symptoms and lesions
- Sexually immature birds mostly affected
- Demonstration of MATSA in cells
- AGPT using feather follicles as source of viral antigen.

AVIAN LEUCOSIS

Avian leucosis is a cancerous viral disease of poultry characterized by tumourous growth of blood cells in liver, spleen, lungs, ovary, kidneys and other visceral organs. Disease occurs sporadically in adult birds also known as *big liver disease*.

Etiology
- Avian leucosis virus is a RNA virus of retroviridae family
- Virus has reverse transcriptase enzyme to convert viral RNA to DNA which incorporated in cellular DNA.

Pathogenesis

The avian leucosis virus is transmitted vertically from hen to chicks through eggs as well as horizontally through direct and indirect contact. It is a malignancy of the bursa-dependent lymphoid system. The target cells are transformed in the bursa of most birds, only few birds develop lymphoid leucosis most of tumours regress and only few enlarges and their cells enter into vascular system and produce metastatic foci in other visceral organs.

Characteristic symptoms
- Pale comb
- Enlarged abdomen
- Profuse haemorrhage from feather follicles
- Boot like appearance of shank

Macroscopic and microscopic features
- Avian leucosis complex includes:

a) *Lymphoid leucosis*
- Tumours of lymphoblasts in liver, spleen, ovary and other organs.
- Tumours are white/ grey, raised and glistening.

b) *Erythrodblastosis*
- Immature erythrocytes in blood stream, bone marrow and liver.
- Bone marrow hypertrophied and becomes cherry red in colour.

c) *Myeloblastosis*
- Neoplastic growth of granulocytes in liver, spleen and other organs.

d) *Osteopetrosis*
- Thickening of the long bones, limbs and ribs due to overgrowth.
- Anaplastic blood cells.
- Malignant cells with mitotic figures.

Diagnosis
- Symptoms and lesions
- Big liver size with tumours.
- Sporadic occurrence in adult birds.
- Histopathological examination of affected tissue.

INFECTIOUS BURSAL DISEASE

Infectious bursal disease is an immunosuppressive disease of birds caused by birna virus and characterized by lesions in bursa of Fabricious, lack of B-lymphocytes, deposition of urates in kidneys and ureter and hemorrhagic myositis. Morbidity rate is as high as 100% and mortality is upto 80%.

Etiology
- Birna virus
- Double stranded RNA virus having two segments.
- 5 serotypes in India.
- Very stable at 60°C for 30 min.

Pathogenesis

The virus is transmitted through contaminated feed, water and droppings of the infected birds. Most common route of infection is oral route but conjunctival and respiratory routes are also important. The incubation period is 2-3 days. After infection, within hours virus is found in macrophages and lymphoid cells in the caeca, duodenum, jejunum and kupffer cells of the liver. The virus first reaches the liver then enters in the blood stream and distributed to different tissues including bursa. There is development of viraemia. The virus causes destruction of affected lymphoid cells (mainly B- cells and their precursors) in the bursa of Fabricious, spleen and caecal tonsils. Bursal depletion in early life may result in impaired immune responses which causes immunosuppression leading to lowered resistance to diseases.

Characteristic symptoms
- Symptoms vary due to immunosuppression
- Trembling of body
- Picking of vent
- Watery diarrhoea
- Prostration

Macroscopic and microscopic features
- Enlargement of bursa of Fabricious.
- Gelatinous exudate around bursa.
- Hemorrhage in bursa giving it a blackish brown colour.
- Atrophy of bursa after 5-7 days of infection.
- Urates on kidneys and in ureter with swelling.
- Echymotic hemorrhage in muscles of thigh or breast region.
- Spleen may become swollen and later on atrophied.
- May show lesions of other diseases due to immunosuppression.
- Depletion of lymphocytes in bursal follicles.
- Edema, congestion and haemorrhage in bursa.
- Hyperplasia and vacuolar degeneration of bursal epithelial cells.
- Proliferation of fibrous tissue.
- Eosinophilic casts in tubular lumen in kidneys.
- Edema, congestion, haemorrhage in muscles with necrosis.

Diagnosis
- Symptoms and lesions
- Immunodiagnostic tests such as AGPT, ELISA for detection of antigen/ antibody.
- Isolation and identification of virus.

INFECTIOUS BRONCHITIS

Infectious bronchitis is a viral disease of poultry caused by corona virus and characterized by sneezing, coughing, respiratory rales, cheesy exudates in bronchi, affections of ovary and oviduct and deposition of urates in kidneys

Etiology
- RNA virus belongs to coronaviridae family.

- Very fragile, 100 nm diameter
- May be complicated by Mycoplasma, E.coli, adenovirus and/or reovirus

Pathogenesis

The virus is transmitted through inhalation and also through direct contact from bird to bird. The incubation period of IB is 18-36 hours. After entering through airborne route, virus replicates in trachea and lungs and causes viraemia. Through blood stream, it reaches to various organs like kidneys, oviduct etc where it replicates and causes damage of kidney tubules which leads to reduced absorption of water, glucose and electrolytes causing dehydration and acidosis.

Characteristic symptoms
- Sneezing, coughing, respiratory rales and dyspnoea
- Drop in egg production
- Thin shelled eggs
- Thin and watery yolk

Macroscopic and microscopic features
- Catarrhal or cheesy exudates in trachea, bronchi.
- Gaseous plugs in bronchi where it enters in lungs.
- Cystic dilation of oviduct.
- Ova may rupture with thin, watery albumin and yolk.
- Enlarged kidneys with deposits of urates, ureters distended due to urates.
- Stones in kidneys in layers.
- Hyperplasia of epithelium in trachea.
- Congestion, hemorrhage, edema and lymphocytic infiltration in mucosa of trachea and bronchi with necrosis and desquamation of mucosal epithelium.
- Focal accumulation of lymphocytes in oviduct and kidneys.
- Lymphoid depletion in bursa.

Diagnosis
- Symptoms and lesions
- Immunological tests to demonstrate antigen in tissue/ antibody in serum
- Isolation and identification of virus

INFECTIOUS LARYNGOTRACHEITIS

Infectious laryngotracheitis is a viral disease of poultry caused by herpes virus and characterized by gasping, blood tinged nasal discharge, haemorrhage in trachea and deposition of cheesy exudates in larynx and trachea. The disease mostly occurs in adult birds.

Etiology
- DNA virus belongs to herpes virus group.
- Carrier birds may excrete virus in faeces for several months.

Pathogenesis

The disease is transmitted through ingestion and inhalation. The incubation period of disease is 6-12 days. After infection, the virus intensely replicates in upper respiratory tract without viremia. After 4-7 days of exposure virus goes to trigeminal ganglion from tracheal exposures and remains in latency. After long period activation of latent virus may occur.

Characteristic symptoms
- Watery fluid from eyes
- Dyspnoea
- Sneezing, coughing and rales
- Gasping

Macroscopic and microscopic features
- Blood tinged exudate in nostrils.
- Cheesy exudate forming plugs in trachea and larynx.
- Hemorrhage in trachea.

- Conjunctivitis and swelling of intra orbital sinus.
- Bird may become blind.
- Necrosis and desquamation of epithelium in tracheal mucosa with congestion and haemorrhage.
- Infiltration of lymphocytes in mucosa of trachea.
- Presence of eosinophilic intranuclear inclusions in tracheal epithelium.

Diagnosis
- Symptoms and lesions
- Tracheal impression smear may show inclusions in epithelial cells.
- Immunodiagnostic test to demonstrate antigen or antibody.

REOVIRUS INFECTION

1. Tenosynovitis (viral arthritis)

Tenosynovitis is a disease of adult birds of heavy breeds or parent stock caused by reovirus and characterized by swelling of hock joints, lameness and high morbidity with low mortality.

Etiology
- Reovirus, double stranded RNA virus with segmented genome having 10 segments.
- Very stable virus.
- May pass from parents to chicks through vertical transmission.

Pathogenesis

After oral infection, the virus settles in joints of the birds. It causes swelling of joint due inflammatory reaction and rupture of gastrocnemius muscle tendon.

Characteristic symptoms
- Lameness

Viral Diseases

- Swelling of hock joint
- Rupture of gastrocnemius tendon

Macroscopic and microscopic features
- Swelling of hock joints and foot pads.
- Swelling of synovial sheath of tendons.
- Rupture of gastrocnemius tendon.
- Purulent or caseous exudate in joint
- Epithelial hyperplasia in synovial sheaths.
- Follicular infiltration of lymphocytes.
- Ulcers on articular surface of joint.

Diagnosis
- Symptoms and lesions
- Demonstration of antigen in tendon/ synovial cells.
- Antibody in serum using immunodiagnostic tests.
- Isolation and identification of virus

2. Avian Stunting Syndrome

Avian stunting syndrome is a disease of birds affecting mainly broilers at the age of 2-4 week and characterized by low weight gain, pasty vent, and atrophy of pancreas.

Etiology
- Reovirus- double stranded RNA virus
- Very stable virus

Pathogenesis

After oral infection, the lesions are most pronounced in the mid jejunum. In enterocytes, small virion particles are detected in the villous epithelial cells. Virus causes necrosis of enterocytes and there is marked infiltration of macrophages and lymphocytes into the villi. Then through macrophages, virus spreads to lamina propria surrounding crypts and multiplication of virus causes necrosis and loss of crypts. There is villous atrophy leading to impaired digestion, poor growth and poor feathering. It also affects the pancreas causing fibrosis and atrophy.

Characteristic symptoms
- Diarrhoea
- Soiling of cloaca with semisolid cement like cheesy material *'Pasty vent'*
- Stunted growth of birds

Macroscopic and microscopic features
- Stunting of the birds, low weight in about 20-50 % of the birds
- Pasty cement like grey coloured deposition on and around vent.
- Undigested food material in intestine with catarrhal enteritis
- Greenish discolouration of liver with distension of gall bladder.
- Pancreas becomes atrophied.
- Necrosis and desquamation of villus epithelial cells in small intestines.
- Necrosis of pancreatic islands and proliferation of fibrous tissue.
- Infiltration of lymphocytes in intestine, pancreas, liver and gall bladder.

Diagnosis
- Symptoms and lesions
- Immunodiagnostic tests to demonstrate antigen in intestinal and pancreatic tissues.
- Isolation and identification of virus

VIRAL NEPHRITIS

Viral nephritis is caused by an enterovirus characterized by nephropathy deposition of urates, lymphofollicular reaction and poor growth in broilers particularly at the age of 1-4 weeks. It is also known as *baby chick nephropathy*.

Etiology
- RNA virus belongs to entero virus of picornaviridae family.
- Two serotypes

Pathogenesis

The disease is transmitted through ingestion of faeces contaminated materials and eggs. After ingestion, virus is detected in faeces within 2 days and maximum shedding occurs at 4-5 days. Virus is widely distributed with maximum titers in kidneys and jejunum and lower titers in bursa of Fabricious, spleen and liver. The lesions develop only in young chickens kidneys.

Characteristic symptoms
- Stunted growth of birds
- Soiling of cloaca with semisolid cheesy material and urates
- Early chick mortality

Macroscopic and microscopic features
- Deposition of urates in kidneys with their swelling
- Urates deposition on visceral organs
- Poor growth of the birds
- Catarrhal enteritis
- Interstitial nephritis with lymphofollicular reaction.
- Protein casts in tubules.
- Increased number of goblet cells in intestines.

Diagnosis
- Symptoms and lesions
- Demonstration of virus in intestinal epithelium and kidney tubules using immunodiagnostic tests.
- Detection of antibodies in serum
- Isolation and identification of virus

AVIAN ENCEPHALOMYELITIS

Avian encephalomyelitis is a disease of chicks caused by a picornavirus and characterized by muscle tremors, blindness, incoordination of movements, grayish spots in muscles of gizzard and proventriculus and proliferation of microglial cells in brain. It is also known as *epidemic tremors* and occurs as an egg borne disease.

Etiology
- RNA virus of enterovirus group in picornaviridae family.
- Affinity to nervous system.
- Only one serotype.

Pathogenesis
The virus enters through ingestion of faeces contaminated feed and water. It enters in duodenal mucosa and causes viraemia. Then the virus settles in different organs like pancreas, liver, heart, kidneys, muscle, brain and spleen. The virus multiplies in Perkinje cells and cerebellum and produces lesions.

Characteristic symptoms
- Tremors of muscles of head and neck.
- Paralysis leading to torticollis.
- Opacity leading to blindness.
- Morality 10-50%.

Macroscopic and microscopic features
- Grayish spots in muscle of gizzard and proventriculus.
- No characteristic gross lesion.
- Swelling of neurons.
- Neuronal degeneration, chromatolysis and nodular microglial proliferation.
- Perivascular lymphocytic cuffing.
- Lymphofollicular reaction in heart, liver, pancreas, proventriculus and gizzard.

Diagnosis
- Symptoms and lesions
- Demonstration of antigen/antibody using immunodiagnostic tests.
- Isolation and identification of virus

ROTAVIRAL DIARRHOEA

Rotaviral diarrhoea occurs in young birds and characterized by dehydration, enteritis and poor growth of the birds.

Etiology
- Rotavirus (serotype-7)
- Double stranded RNA virus with segmented genome (11 segments)
- Not related of mammalian rotavirus.

Pathogenesis

The virus in transmitted through faeces of infected birds through direct or indirect contact. Rotavirus infection is mainly confined to intestinal tract. The virus multiplies in the mature villus epithelial cells of small intestine. The infected epithelial cells are destroyed, resulting in villous atrophy and compensatory crypt hypertrophy. There is replacement of mature cells by immature cells deficient in digestive enzymes and in their ability to transport water and electrolytes leading to maldigestion, malabsorption and diarrhoea.

Characteristic symptoms
- Diarrhoea in chicks at 1-2 weeks of age.
- Dehydration and mortality in 5-10% birds.
- Reduced growth.

Macroscopic and microscopic features
- Catarrhal, enteritis with undigested food material in intestines.
- Atrophy of bursa.

- Intestine and caeca contain fluid and gas.
- Cracking of feet/ digits with feacal crusts.
- Reduction in size of villi with necrosis and desquamation of mucosal villous epithelial cells.
- Infiltration of lymphocytes and mononuclear cells in intestinal mucosa.

Diagnosis
- Symptoms and lesions
- Demonstration of antigen in intestinal tissue
- Isolation and identification of virus

AVIAN POX

Avian pox is a viral disease of poultry caused by a DNA virus of pox group and characterized by appearance of characteristic pock lesions on feather less parts of the body.

Etiology
- Pox virus
- Four serotypes fowl pox, canary pox, pigeon pox, turkey pox,
- Produces pock lesions on CAM of chick embryo

Pathogenesis

The virus is transmitted through direct contact. A break in the skin is required for the virus to enter the epithelial cells. The cells of mucosa of the upper respiratory tract and mouth is highly susceptible for virus. After entering in epithelial cells, it spreads from cell to cell which is helped by production of epidermal growth factor causing proliferation of cells. Some virus enters in blood circulation and causes viraemia. Through circulation it reaches to certain organs like spleen and liver. In epithelium of skin, it produces pock lesions.

Characteristic symptoms
- Nodules on feather less parts of body *i.e.* comb, wattle and face

Viral Diseases

- Yellowish cheese like material in buccal cavity
- Swelling of eyelid leading to blindness

Macroscopic and microscopic features
- Cutaneous form characterized by papule and scab on comb, wattle, face and other feather less parts of body.
- Yellowish nodules later on becomes blackish.
- In diphtheritic form, there is yellowish cheese like material on tongue, palate, laryngeal orifice.
- Proliferation of epithelium in stratum spinosum layer of epidermis
- Cells show hydropic degeneration.
- Presence of intra cytoplasmic eosinophilic inclusions in cells of epidermis.

Diagnosis
- Symptoms and lesions
- Demonstration of virus inclusions in skin epithelium.
- Immunodiagnostic tests for demonstration of antigen/antibody.

INCLUSION BODY HEPATITIS (IBH)

Inclusion body hepatitis is caused by adenovirus and characterized by anemia, necrotic and haemorrhagic lesions in liver and hemorrhage in muscles. It affects mainly growers with a mortality of about 30%. It occurs due to stress or immunosuppression in birds.

Etiology
- Aviadenovirus
- DNA virus of aviadenovirus group
- Quite resistant virus and found in all poultry rearing areas.

Pathogenesis

Not known. However, virus produces basophilic and eosinophilic intranuclear inclusion bodies in hepatocytes.

Characteristic symptoms
- Anemia
- Sudden mortality

Macroscopic and microscopic features
- Muscles and bone marrow become pale and anemic.
- Swollen and mottled liver with petechiae and necrotic foci.
- Atrophy of bursa.
- Petechiae and ecchymoses in muscles and kidneys.
- Urates in ureters.
- Hydropericardium.
- Intranuclear eosinophilic or basophilic inclusion bodies with margination of nucleus in hepatocytes.
- Necrosis and lymphocytic infiltration in liver.
- Lymphofollicular reaction in trachea.
- Depletion of lymphoid cells in spleen and bursa.

Diagnosis
- Symptoms and lesions
- Demonstration of inclusions in impression smear of liver.
- Blood examination- anemia.
- Immunodiagnostic test for antigen or antibody detection

HYDROPERICARDIUM SYNDROME

Hydropericardium syndrome in caused by adenovirus and characterized by watery straw colored fluid in pericardial sac, hepatitis and atrophy of lymphoid organs. Disease occurs in growers after immunosuppression or stress with 5-10% mortality.

Viral Diseases

Etiology
- Aviadenovirus
- DNA virus
- Present in poultry house environment
- Quite resistant virus
- Affects birds after stress

Pathogenesis
The disease spreads through both vertical and horizontal transmission. In breeding stocks, virus may remain in latent phase until onset of maturity and sheds when there is immunosuppresion or stress. The virus multiplies in intestine and through circulation reaches in various organs including pericardium and produces lesions.

Characteristic symptoms
- Enlargement of abdomen
- Anemia
- Sudden mortality

Macroscopic and microscopic features
- Straw colored fluid in pericardial sac (8-10 ml fluid).
- Atrophy of heart with petechiae on myocardium.
- Hemorrhagic and necrotic foci in liver.
- Atrophy of bursa and spleen.
- Hemorrhage in myocardium, increased distance in myofibrils due to oedema.
- Degenerative changes in myofibrils.
- Intranuclear eosinophilic or basophilic inclusions in liver cells
- Infiltration of lymphocytes in liver, heart and kidneys
- Lymphoid depletion in spleen and bursa.

Diagnosis
- Symptoms and lesions

- Fluid in pericardial sac
- Isolation and identification of virus
- Immunodiagnostic tests for detection of antigen of antibody.

EGG DROP SYNDROME

Egg drop syndrome occurs in adult laying birds caused by adenovirus and characterized by decrease in egg production, oedema in oviduct and spleenomegaly.

Etiology
- Aviadenovirus
- DNA virus

Pathogenesis

The disease is mainly transmitted through vertical transmission. After infection in laying hens, the virus grows to a limited extent in nasal mucosa followed by viremia with replication of virus in lymphoid tissues throughout body specially in spleen and thymus. Infundibulum of oviduct is consistently affected, massive viral replication occurs in the pouch shell glands which coincides with production of thin shell eggs.

Characteristic symptoms
- Drops in production of eggs by 35- 40 percent.
- Thin shelled depigmented and cracked shelled eggs.
- Diarrhoea.

Macroscopic and microscopic features
- Thin shelled, cracked or depigmented eggs.
- Oedema of oviduct, later on atrophy of oviduct.
- Spleenomegaly.
- Lymphoid aggregates in oviduct, lungs, liver and kidneys.
- Degeneration and necrosis of glandular epithelium.
- Hyaline changes in muscular layer of oviduct.
- Lymphoid hyperplasia in spleen.
- Intranuclear inclusions in epithelial cells of tubular glands.

Diagnosis
- Symptoms and lesions
- Immunodiagnostic tests for detection of antigen or antibody
- Isolation and identification of virus

CHICKEN ANEMIA

Chicken anemia is a viral disease of growers caused by DNA virus and characterized by watery blood, pale mucous membrane, reduced body weight and atrophy of bursa and thymus. It is also known as *Anemia dermatitis syndrome*. Disease occurs in birds with stress or immunosuppression. It may also be transmitted in chicks through vertical transmission.

Etiology
- DNA virus
- Chicken anemia agent (CAA)
- Smallest virus having 24-26 nm diameter

Pathogenesis

The disease is transmitted both horizontally and vertically. In vertical transmission through hatching eggs and horizontally by direct/ indirect contact usually through oral route by ingestion of infected materials. After entering in chicks, it causes functional changes in splenic thymocytes and splenic and bone marrow macrophages. The main site of viral replication are precursor T-cells in the thymic cortex and hematoblasts in bone marrow. Destruction of these cells is responsible for immunosuppression and anemia.

Characteristic symptoms
- Pale skin and mucus membrane
- Loss of weight
- 5-10% mortality
- Thin watery blood with increased PCV

Macroscopic and microscopic features
- Subcutaneous petechiae.
- Pale muscles, week emaciated carcass with reduced weight.
- Atrophy of bursa and thymus.
- Pale bone marrow.
- Depletion of erythroid and myeloid cells in bone marrow.
- Depletion of lymphoid tissue in thymus, bursa and spleen.
- Infiltration of lymphocytes in liver, heart and kidneys
- Perivascular lymphoid infiltration in liver with fibrinoid thrombi in sinusoids.

Diagnosis
- Symptoms and lesions
- Immunodiagnostic tests for detection of antigen or antibody.
- Isolation and identification of virus

Chapter 35
Bacterial Diseases

SALMONELLOSIS

Salmonellosis is caused by G -ve bacteria Salmonella and characterized by early chick mortality with necrosis and haemorrhage in liver, heart and spleen and enlarged bronze coloured liver with focal or diffuse necrosis, marbled spleen and/or oophoritis and salpingitis in adults.

Etiology
- *Salmonella enteritidis* var.Galinarum *(S. Galinarum)*.
- G-, rod, non lactose fermenter.
- White small colonies on MLA and pink on BGA.

Pathogenesis

The organism is transmitted horizontally through contaminated feed and water and vertically through ovary from hen to chicks. Its incubation period is generally 4-5 days. After entering through oral route, the bacteria adhere to intestinal epithelial cells, which is first step of disease occurrence; adherence occurs with type I fimbriae and a mannose resistant haemagglutinin. The virulence of organism depends on the initial degree of mucosal invasiveness and diarrhoea. In vertical transmission, the organism enters into the ovary and infects the eggs. When there is development of chicks, infected yolk serves as source of infection to the developing embryo and causes disease.

Characteristic symptoms
- Diarrhoea
- Soiling of cloaca with semisolid cheesy material

- Early chick mortality
- Huddling near the source of heat
- Cyanosis of comb and wattle in adults

Macroscopic and microscopic features
- *Chicks*
- Focal or diffused necrosis in liver.
- Semisolid cheesy material in cloaca.
- Unabsorbed yolk.
- *Adults*
- Copper colour enlarged liver with focal or diffuse necrosis.
- Enlarged, mottled spleen.
- Catarrhal enteritis.
- Necrotic lesions on heart.
- Ovaries/ testes congested.
- Necrotic hepatitis
- Necrosis in myocardium with infiltration of lymphocytes, heterophils and macrophages.
- Congestion in ovary, testicles and oviduct with suppuration.
- G -ve organisms demonstrable in central necrotic areas.

Diagnosis
- Symptoms and lesions
- Isolation of organism from heart blood and/or liver.
- Gram's staining of smears for demonstration of salmonella organism.

COLIBACILLOSIS

Colibacillosis is caused by *E.coli* and characterized by various syndromes like colisepticemia, air sacculitis, coligranuloma, and omphalitis in birds depending on the age and type of strain of *E.coli* involved.

Etiology
- *Escherichia coli*
- G -ve Coccobacilli
- Pink colony on MLA and white colony on BGA

1. Colisepticemia

Colisepticemia is a disease of young broilers due to bad management and stress and characterized by fibrinous pericarditis and hepatitis

Pathogenesis

Faecal contamination of the eggs may result in the penetration of *E. coli* through the shell due to creation of negative pressure inside the eggs. This is considered most important source of infection. Bacteria may be found in the litter, dust and faecal matter. Feed is often contaminated with excreta. The bacteria is normal inhabitant in digestive tract of poultry. Birds with intact defense is resistant to *E. coli* but when defense system is compromised due to bacterial, viral, parasitic infections, toxins, poor ventilation, dust conditions etc., this infection may cause disease. Exposure to dust and ammonia results in removal of cilia of upper respiratory tract which permits the bacteria to colonize and cause respiratory infection. On entry the bacteria multiply in blood and produce septicemia.

Characteristic symptoms
- Diarrhoea
- Soiling of cloaca with semisolid cheesy material
- Dyspnoea

Macroscopic and microscopic features
- Milky fluid in pericardium
- Presence of whitish pseudo membrane over pericardium.
- Fibrinous covering over liver.
- Fibrinous pericarditis with infiltration of heterophils, macrophages and lymphocytes.

- Necrosis in liver with fibrinous and purulent exudate.

2. Coligranuloma (Hjarre's Disease)

Coligranuloma is a sporadic chronic disease of adult birds characterized by the presence of nodule in intestines.

Pathogenesis

The bacteria enter in the intestines through penetration and settles there to cause chronic inflammation characterized by formation of nodules in intestines. These nodules are composed of cheesy material and fibrosis.

Characteristic symptoms
- Diarrhoea
- Soiling of cloaca with semisolid cheesy material

Macroscopic and microscopic features
- Presence of nodules on intestine.
- Small millet size or large nodule on duodenum, caecum and liver.
- Sporadic occurrence, chronic disease seen in adults or age old birds.
- Caseous necrotic area in centre covered by macrophages, lymphocytes and giant cells.
- Organisms can be demonstrated on Gram's staining in central necrotic area.

3. Air sacculitis

Air sacculitis is a disease of growers and adults and occurs along with *Mycoplasma gallisepticum* infection as Chronic Respiratory Disease.

Pathogenesis

This organism is normal inhabitant of gut and is continuously excreted in droppings which contaminate the litter and environment of the poultry house. Adverse weather conditions and accumulation of ammonia and poor ventilation with dusty environment predisposes birds for *E.coli* infection as there is loss of cilia in upper respiratory tract that facilitates the entry of organisms to cause disease.

Characteristic symptoms
- Generally occurs in birds of 5-12 weeks age
- Common in overcrowded environment
- Gasping
- Dyspnoea

Macroscopic and microscopic features
- Cloudiness in air sacs.
- Increased thickening of air sacs.
- Milky fluid in pericardium.
- Fibrinous pericarditis.
- Suppurative air sacculitis.

4. Omphalitis

Omphalitis is a disease of newly hatched chicks and characterized by thin, watery, coagulated unabsorbed yolk.

Pathogenesis

This infection is generally associated with inflammed naval or bacteria can multiply in the hatching eggs following faecal contamination of the shell. Some other bacteria also cause yolk sac infection like staphylococcus, pseudomonas, proteus and clostridia. The bacteria rapidly multiply in the intestine of newly hatched chicks and infection spreads from chick to chick in hatchery and brooders.

Characteristic symptoms
- Sleepiness
- Aggregation near the source of heat

Macroscopic and microscopic features
- Presence of unabsorbed yolk
- Yolk becomes thin and watery with precipitates

- Yolk sac membrane becomes thickened due to congestion and exudate
- Intestines congested
- Focal necrotic hepatitis.
- Congestion and infiltration of heterophils in yolk sac membrane.

Diagnosis
- Symptoms and lesions
- Isolation of *E.coli* from heart blood.
- Gram's staining of impression smears made from nodules in coligranuloma.

INFECTIOUS CORYZA

Infectious coryza is a disease of adult birds caused by *Haemophilus paragallinarum* and characterized by swollen head, foul smelling discharge from nostrils and eyes.

Etiology
- *Haemophilus paragallinarum.*
- G -ve, bipolar, filamentous, coccoid

Pathogenesis

Source of infection is infected and carrier birds. It spreads through drinking water contaminated by nasal discharge. Airborne infection or direct contact may also play role in transmission of disease. After entry organism adhere to the ciliated mucosa of upper respiratory tract. The bacteria contain the capsule and haemagglutination antigen (HA) which play an important role in colonization. During proliferation, toxic substances are released leading to development of lesions.

Characteristic symptoms
- Discharge from nostrils and eyes
- Swollen face and wattle
- Sneezing

- Dyspnoea

Macroscopic and microscopic features
- Swelling of face due to exudate in infraorbital sinuses.
- Congestion of nasal mucosa.
- Watery discharge from nostrils.
- Mucopurulent exudate in trachea.
- Fibrinopurulent cellulites
- Mesothelial hyperplasia, fibrinous exudates with oedematus thickening of air sacs.

Diagnosis
- Symptoms and lesions
- Smear from edematous fluid, stained with Gram's staining for bipolar, G -ve organisms.
- Isolation from swabs taken from infraorbital sinuses.

FOWL CHOLERA

Fowl cholera is a contagious disease of poultry caused by *Pasteurella multocida* and characterized by cyanotic comb, swelling of wattles, fibrinous air sacculitis and pneumonia.

Etiology
- *Pasteurella multocida*
- G -ve, bipolar, capsulated.

Pathogenesis

Source of infection are infected birds and rats act as reservoir. The disease mainly spreads through contaminated water and feed troughs. Birds may also be infected by oral, nasal and congenital routes. The organism enters through mucous membrane of the pharynx or upper respiratory tract. After entry organism produces sufficient quantities of endotoxin to contribute pathological processes.

Characteristic symptoms
- Cyanosis of comb and wattle
- Diarrhoea and soiling of cloaca
- Discharge from nostrils

Macroscopic and microscopic features
- Bluishness of comb and oedema of wattles.
- Petechiae on heart, gizzard muscles and intestinal serosa.
- Fibrinous air sacculitis.
- Small necrotic (pinpoint size) foci on liver.
- Focal area of necrosis in liver with suppuration.
- Congestion and heterophilic infiltration in lungs.
- Bipolar organisms can be demonstrated in lung and liver.

Diagnosis
- Symptoms and lesions
- Demonstration of bipolar organisms in blood smears/ impression smears stained by methylene blue.
- Isolation of organisms.

NECROTIC ENTERITIS

Necrotic enteritis is caused by clostridium, which commonly occurs after coccidiosis in chickens and characterized by necrotic patches in intestines, atrophy of spleen and breast muscles.

Etiology
- Alpha toxins of *Clostridium perfringens* type A, C, E and F.
- Intestine predisposed by coccidiosis, which provides anaerobic conditions to *Clostridium sp.* organisms.

Pathogenesis

The bacteria are present in faeces, soil, dust, contaminated feed and litter or intestinal contents. Contaminated feed or litter act as source of infection. The coccidial infection causes damage in the intestines to produce anaerobic conditions which predisposes the birds for clostridial infection. After entering through damaged intestines of the birds, the organism proliferates and liberates toxins which are responsible for intestinal mucosal necrosis.

Characteristic symptoms
- Drooling of saliva
- Emaciation in chronic cases
- Watery diarrhoea

Macroscopic and microscopic features
- Yellowish brown necrotic areas involving whole small intestine.
- Small necrotic patches in liver.
- Distended gall bladder.
- Atrophy of spleen, breast muscles and testes.
- Necrosis of villi of intestinal mucosa.
- Degeneration and necrosis of hepatocytes.
- Atrophy of spleen and bursa as evidenced by proliferation of connective tissue.

Diagnosis
- History- It occurs after coccidiosis
- Symptoms and lesions
- Demonstration of G$^+$ rods in the necrotic lesions of intestine and liver

CAMPYLOBACTER HEPATITIS

Campylobacter hepatitis is caused by *Campylobacter* sp. and characterized by necrotic hepatitis, hydropericardium, and catarrhal enteritis.

Etiology
- *Campylobacter jejuni*
- *C. hepaticus* and *E.coli* mixed infection
- Comma shaped, Gram negative

Pathogenesis

Transmission of disease occurs through faecal contamination of water, feed, utensils and other fomites. The organism affects the liver from where it can be isolated. It causes enlargement of liver besides necrosis and haemorrhage.

Characteristic symptoms
- Pale comb
- Drop in egg production(25-33%)

Macroscopic and microscopic features
- Liver enlarged, friable with necrotic and haemorrhagic areas.
- Rupture of liver with hematoma in abdominal cavity
- Hydropericardium
- Atrophy of ovaries/ testes
- Enlargement of spleen
- Pale and watery bone marrow.
- Necrosis of hepatocytes and infiltration of heterophils in liver.
- Necrosis of myofibrils and hemorrhage in epicardium.
- Catarrhal enteritis.
- Comma shaped, Gram-negative organisms in liver sections and impression smears.

Diagnosis
- Demonstration of comma shaped organisms in impression smears of liver, bile and intestinal mucosa.
- Isolation of causative organisms.

STAPHYLOCOCCOSIS

Staphylococcosis is caused by *Staphylococcus aureus* and characterized by haemorrhagic or gangrenous dermatitis, bumble foot, septicemia, arthritis and sternal bursitis.

Etiology
- *Staphylococcus aureus*.
- G +ve, cocci, Coagulase positive.
- Toxins - enterotoxins, leucocidin and hemolysin.

Pathogenesis

The bacteria is often found in the skin, nasal passage, on beak and foot of apparently normal chickens. When there is injury in the skin or mucus membrane, it is exposed to the infection. There is formation of abscess with swelling, heat and some pain. In bumble foot the undersurface of the foot is first affected.

Characteristic symptoms
- Inflammed and haemorrhagic skin
- Formation of gangrene- greenish/ blackish disclouration of skin
- Swelling of joints
- Hard swelling of foot pad with ulceration

Macroscopic and microscopic features
- Dermatitis and gangrene in skin of broilers
- Bumble foot characterized by hard, fibrous swelling and ulceration of foot pad.
- Arthritis and synovitis with swelling of joints, caseous mass in joints.
- Endocarditis
- Sternal bursa showed deposition of caseous mass.
- Suppurative dermatitis with areas of gangrene formation in skin.
- Demonstration of G^+, cocci organisms in caseous mass of the tissue sections.

Diagnosis
- Symptoms and lesions
- Isolation of staphylococci.

- Demonstration of organisms in impression smears/ tissue sections stained with Gram's stain.

TUBERCULOSIS

Tuberculosis is a chronic disease of birds caused by *Mycobacterium avium* and characterized by granulomatous nodules in liver, spleen, intestines, air sacs and lungs. The disease occurs sporadically in adult birds.

Etiology
- *Mycobacterium avium*
- Acid fast bacilli.
- 30 serotypes, serotype 1 and 2 are pathogenic.

Pathogenesis

The most important source of infection are infected birds which shed the causative organisms in faeces. It is transmitted through ingestion of contaminated feed and water. After ingestion, it causes delayed type hypersensitivity and the activated macrophages have an increased capacity to kill the organisms. DTH reaction is mediated by lymphocytes which release lymphokines that act to attract, immobilize and activate mononuclear cells from blood at the site where virulent bacilli or their product exists. Tumour necrosis factor (TNF) alone or along with interleukin-2 (IL-2) is associated with macrophage killing of bacteria. Activated macrophages that lack sufficient microbicidal components to kill virulent tubercle bacilli are destroyed by the intracellular growth of the organisms. The toxic lipids and factors released cause disruption of the phagosome, inhibits phagolysosome formation, interfere with release of hydrolytic enzymes from the affected lysosomes or inactivate lysosomal enzymes released into the cytoplasmic vacuoles.

Characteristic symptoms
- Weakness
- Emaciation

Macroscopic and microscopic features
- White, raised, dry and cheesy exudate containing nodules in liver, spleen, intestines, air sacs and lungs.
- Rupture of liver, haemorrhage and clot in abdominal cavity.
- Caseative necrosis infiltrated by macrophages, lymphocytes, epithelioid and giant cells.
- This tubercle is covered by proliferation of fibroblasts.
- Acid fast bacilli in the central necrosed area

Diagnosis
- Demonstration of pea size granulomatous lesions.
- Impression smear from necrotic lesion and acid fast staining to demonstrate the acid fast bacilli.
- Tuberculin testing with avian tuberculin on skin of wattle or comb. 0.2 ml I/ D tuberculin and reaction observed after 48 hrs as hot, painful swelling at the site of injection.
- Histopathological examination of affected tissue and demonstration of acid fast bacilli using special stains.

Chapter 36
Chlamydial Disease

ORNITHOSIS
Ornithosis is caused by Chlamydia and characterized by enlargement of liver and spleen, serofibrinous pericarditis, air sacculitis and enteritis. This is also known as *chlamydiosis*, *psittacosis* and is more common in parrots, pigeons and other psittacine birds.

Etiology
- *Chlamydia psittaci* group B
- Size 0.3 to 1.5 m
- Disease spreads from wild birds

Pathogenesis
The disease mainly spreads through inhalation of contaminated dust. After entering into body, the organism multiplies in the lungs, air sacs and pericardium. Through hematogenous spread, the organism reaches in the liver, spleen and kidneys where further replication occurs along with the production of reticulate and elementary bodies.

Characteristic symptoms
- Greenish diarrhoea
- Decrease in egg production
- Decreased fertility and hatchability

Macroscopic and microscopic features
- Enlargement of spleen and liver with necrotic foci.
- Serofibrinous pericarditis.

- Air sacculitis, depositions of cheesy material.
- Greenish intestinal contents with catarrhal enteritis.
- Necrosis and lymphoid aggregations in liver.
- Serofibrinous pericarditis.
- Catarrhal enteritis.

Diagnosis
- Symptoms and lesions
- Organism can be demonstrated in smears of spleen, liver, air sacs and stained with Giemsa stain
- Red coccoid elementary bodies
- Demonstration of chlamydial inclusions in liver cells in impression smear or tissue sections using special stain.

Chapter 37
Mycoplasmal Diseases

Chronic Respiratory Disease (CRD)

Chronic respiratory disease is caused by *Mycoplasma gallisepticum* and *E.coli* in birds under poor management and characterized by cloudy air sacs with thickening of their wall, accumulation of cheesy material in air sacs and lungs.

Etiology
- *Mycoplasma gallisepticum*
- *E. coli*
- Bad management like poor ventilation and inclement weather conditions
- Disease occurs more during winter and rainy season.

Pathogenesis

The disease is transmitted through direct contact of susceptible birds with infected carrier birds. It spreads through contaminated air, dust, droplets or feathers. It can also spread through infected eggs. The organism itself is not pathogenic but due to other pathogens like viruses of Ranikhet disease, Infectious bronchitis and Infectious bursal disease and the pathogenic strains of *E.coli* and *Haemophilus paragallinarum* may predispose the birds and make them susceptible for mycoplasma infection. Other factors include nutritional deficiency, excessive environmental dust and ammonia leads to the development of clinical signs and lesions.

Characteristic symptoms
- Gasping

- Gargling sound during respiration
- Frothy exudate in eyes with conjunctivitis

Macroscopic and microscopic features
- Congestion of trachea in conjunction with cloudiness in air sacs and bronchial mucosa.
- Hemorrhage in trachea.
- Elongation of tracheal glands.

Diagnosis
- Symptoms and circumstantial evidences
- Lesions in air sacs and lungs.
- Immunological tests such as ELISA, tube agglutination plate agglutination test.
- Isolation of causative organisms
- Demonstration of organisms in tissue sections using special stains.

INFECTIOUS SYNOVITIS

Infectious synovitis is a disease of adult birds caused by *Mycoplasma synoviae* and characterized by the presence of thick, creamy or cheesy material in synovial sac of hock joint, foot pad, keel bone and in air sacs.

Etiology
- *Mycoplasma synoviae*
- Some times complicated by *Pasteurella gallinarum*

Pathogenesis

It is transmitted through direct contact or through contaminated air, dust, droplets or feathers. After entry the organism causes mild respiratory disease and through hematogenous route, it reaches to different articular parts and respiratory tissues causing arthritis, respiratory distress, anemia and vasculitis.

Characteristic symptoms
- Swelling of foot pad and joints

- Pale comb
- Sulfur colour faeces

Macroscopic and microscopic features
- Thick cheesy material in synovial sac of hock joints, foot pad, keel bone and air sacs.
- Greenish discoloration of liver.
- Hydropericardium
- Lymphoid aggregation in synovial membrane, liver and air sacs.
- Catarrhal enteritis in duodenum.

Diagnosis
- Symptoms and lesions
- Demonstration of mycoplasma in synovial exudate.
- Isolation of mycoplasma and other causative organisms
- Immunological tests such as ELISA and plate agglutination test

Chapter 38
Spirochaetal Disease

SPIROCHETOSIS

Spirochetosis is caused by a spiral shaped organism *Borrelia anserina* and characterized by greenish diarrhoea, enlarged and mottled spleen, small necrotic patches on liver and linear hemorrhage in proventriculus. This disease is transmitted by a tick *Argas persicus* and thus also known as *"tick fever"* or *"tick paralysis"*.

Etiology
- Spirochete *Borrelia anserina*
- Spiral shape 8-24m long and 0.2 to 0.3 m wide microorganism having 8-11 spirals.
- Stained with aniline dyes

Pathogenesis
Soft ticks of genus Argas are the main reservoir of the organism. *Borrelia anserina* can survive for long period either in birds or in environment. Birds become infected from saliva introduced by the tick on bite. After entry, the spirochaete reaches in blood circulation and cause septicemia with an abrupt and marked elevation of body temperature.

Characteristic symptoms
- Greenish diarrhoea
- Cyanosis of comb
- Jaundice

Macroscopic and microscopic features
- Greenish diarrhoea with greenish intestinal contents.
- Cyanosis of comb.
- Enlargement of spleen with mottling.
- Enlargement of liver with small necrotic foci.
- Linear hemorrhage in proventriculus.
- Presence of ticks on skin/ feather follicles.
- Necrosis of hepatocytes.
- Necrosis and depletion of lymphoid tissue in spleen and hemosiderosis.
- Catarrhal enteritis.
- Perivascular gliosis in brain.
- Hemorrhagic dermatitis.
- Organism can be seen in liver sections by silver stain.

Diagnosis
- Symptoms and lesions
- Demonstration of spirochete in blood smears.
- Demonstration of ticks on skin during external examination.
- Demonstration of ticks in poultry house or on neighbouring plants.

Chapter 39
Fungal Diseases

ASPERGILLOSIS

Aspergillosis is a fungal disease of poultry caused by different species of *Aspergillus sp* and characterized by granulomatous nodules in lungs, thickening of air sacs and presence of fungal growth in lungs and air sacs in early age of chicks. It is also known as **Brooders pneumonia**.

Etiology
- *Aspergillus fumigatus*
- *A. flavus*
- *A. nidulans*
- *A. glaucus*
- *A. niger*
- *A. candidus*

Pathogenesis

The disease is transmitted through inhalation of spores. The spores are deposited on conjunctiva, nasal and tracheal mucosa, lungs and air sacs and cause granuloma formation. Through hematogenous route it reaches in brain, pericardium, bone marrow, kidneys and other tissues. In brain, it produces lesions in meninges causing large superficial white plaques leading to ophthalmitis and iridocyclitis.

Characteristic symptoms
- Dyspnoea
- Accumulation of cheesy material in eye lids
- Mortality vary from 2-50%

Macroscopic and microscopic features
- Lesions in chicks 5-7 days of age.
- Raised, pinhead size yellowish nodules in lungs.
- Thickening of air sacs.
- Growth of fungus in lungs and air sacs.
- Necrotic foci in liver, spleen, kidneys and proventriculus.
- Granulomatous lesion in lungs.
- Presence of fungus in lungs and air sacs on microscopic examination.

Diagnosis
- Symptoms and lesions
- Demonstration of fungus in impression smear of lungs
- Cultures of fungus on SDA and its identification.
- Demonstration of fungus in lung tissue sections using special stains

FAVUS

Favus is a fungal disease of birds caused by *Trichophyton* sp. and characterized by deposition of thin, white flour like material on comb and skin of other featherless parts of body. It is also known as *while comb disease*.

Etiology
- *Trichophyton magnini*

Pathogenesis

The disease is transmitted through contact or through contact with fomites. After superficial invasion of stratum corneum by hyphae, it causes epidermal hyperplasia and hyperkeratosis.

Characteristic symptoms
- Thin white flour like material deposits on comb
- Thickening of skin

Macroscopic and microscopic features
- White, flour like material deposits on comb and skin
- Necrotic foci on trachea and oesophagus.
- Scab formation on skin.
- Fungus in skin scab and scrapings of skin
- Granulomatous lesions in skin.

Diagnosis
- Symptoms and lesions
- Presence of fungus and its identification.
- Isolation and identification of fungus

CANDIDIASIS

Candidiasis is a fungal disease of poultry which occurs sporadically and caused by *Candida* sp. and characterized by Turkish towel like appearance of crop, oesophagus and ulcers in mouth and oesophagus. It is also known as ***thrush***.

Etiology
- *Candida albicans*
- *Monilia albicans*

Pathogenesis

The fungus is acquired by ingestion of contaminated materials. Then the fungus becomes part of normal flora of mouth, oesophagus and crop. When there is immunosuppression, the fungus proliferates and penetrates epithelial surface leading to the stimulation of the epithelial hyperplasia and diphtheritic membrane formation.

Characteristic symptoms
- Stunted growth of birds
- Ruffled feathers

Macroscopic and microscopic features
- Turkish towel like lesions in crop and/or oesophagus.
- Congestion in proventriculus.

- Ulcers in mouth and esophagus.
- Granulomatous lesions in crop and esophagus.
- Fungal colony in tissues.

Diagnosis
- Symptoms and lesions
- Fungus in impression smears of affected organ/ tissue.
- Isolation and identification of fungus.

HISTOPLASMOSIS

Histoplasmosis is a sporadic fungal disease of birds caused by *Histoplasma* sp. and characterized by granulomatous lesions in liver and other parts of body.

Etiology
- *Histoplasma capsulatum*

Pathogenesis

Infection spreads through inhalation of spores present in soil or dusty environment of the poultry house. The fungus settles in lungs and proliferates within the macrophages and spreads in other visceral organs.

Characteristic symptoms
- Diarrhoea
- Soiling of cloaca with semisolid cheesy material

Macroscopic and microscopic features
- Presence of round, raised, rough granulomatous lesions on liver, spleen and other organs.
- Granulomatous lesions in liver.
- Presence of round or oval yeast like fungal spores in tissues.

Diagnosis
- Symptoms and lesions
- Isolation and identification of fungus.

- Demonstration of fungus in affected tissue using special stains

AFLATOXICOSIS

Aflatoxicosis is a toxic condition of poultry widely prevalent in all parts of the country caused by fungal toxins and characterized by hepatic lesions, immunosuppression and cancer.

Etiology
- Fungal toxins of *Aspergillus flavus* and *Penicillium puberlum* and several other fungi.
- Aflatoxin B_1, B_2, G_1, G_2.

Pathogenesis

After ingestion aflatoxin, under goes biotransformation into highly reactive metabolites which binds with nucleic acids and reduce protein synthesis and causes immunosuppression. These metabolic alterations cause enlargement of liver, spleen and kidneys and atrophy of bursa of Fabricious, thymus and testicular tissues.

Characteristic symptoms
- Enlargement of abdomen
- Anemia
- Drop in egg production
- Spasms of neck muscles and arched back
- Retarded growth of birds

Macroscopic and microscopic features
- Enlargement of liver
- Necrotic foci in liver.
- Congestion and hemorrhage in liver.
- Tumourous nodules in liver.
- Atrophy of spleen.
- Hemorrhage in muscles.
- Loose attachment of mucosa of Gizzard.

- Loss of production of eggs.
- Necrosis in hepatic parenchyma.
- Proliferation of bile duct epithelium.
- Fibrosis in liver.
- Hemorrhage in muscles and myocardium.

Diagnosis
- Symptoms and lesions
- Detection of toxins in poultry feed/ tissues of affected birds using TLC or flurotoxinometer.
- Immunodiagnostic tests for detection of aflatoxins in feed and tissues- ELISA, DIA

OCHRATOXICOSIS

Ochratoxicosis is a toxic condition of poultry caused by a fungal toxin and characterized by nephrosis, visceral gout, pale bone marrow and haemorrhage in intestines.

Etiology
- Ochratoxins produced by *Aspergillus ochraceous* and several other species of *Aspergillus* and *Penicillium* sp.

Pathogenesis

Ochratoxin is found in maize and in most of the small grains contaminated with moulds. It inhibits protein synthesis, produces acute proximal tubular epithelial necrosis in kidneys and inhibits normal renal uric acid excretion.

Characteristic symptoms
- Anemia
- Increased clotting time
- Loss of pigmentation

Macroscopic and microscopic features
- Enlargement of kidneys
- Deposition of urates on kidneys

Fungal Diseases

- Hemorrhage in kidneys
- Ureters distended due to accumulation of urates.
- Haemorrhage in duodenum.
- Anemia
- Pale bone marrow.
- Atrophy of lymphoid organs
- Ascites
- Nephrosis, deposition of urates.
- Infiltration of heterophils and fibrosis.
- Hemorrhage in intestinal wall.
- Lymphoid depletion in bursa, thymus and spleen.

Diagnosis
- Symptoms and lesions
- Detection of ochratoxin in poultry feed/ tissues using TLC/ HPLC methods.
- Immunodiagnostic tests for detection of toxins in feed- ELISA, DIA

Chapter 40
Parasitic Diseases

ROUNDWORMS (NEMATODES)

1. *Ascaridia galli*

A. galli is the common roundworm of poultry seen in intestines at the time of necropsy. This parasite may cause retardation of growth, loss of egg production, catarrhal enteritis and sometimes mortality due to obstruction of gut.

Etiology
- *A. galli* parasites are grey, thread like 5-10 cm in length.
- Eggs are elliptical with thick and shiny wall.

Pathogenesis

Transmission occurs through faecal - oral route. The eggs may survive for several months in litter and they take at least 10-15 days to develop the infective stage. The eggs of parasites hatch in proventriculus or intestine to develop fully grown parasite within 40-50 days.

Characteristic symptoms
- Growth retardation
- Anemia
- Decreased egg production

Macroscopic and microscopic features
- Anemia
- Emaciation
- Presence of *A. galli* in intestines
- Catarrhal enteritis

- Presence of parasitic section in the lumen of intestine
- Catarrhal enteritis
- Eosinophilic infiltration in mucosa and sub mucosa

Diagnosis
- Symptoms and lesions
- Presence of parasites in gut at necropsy
- Examination of droppings for parasitic ova.

2. *Syngamus trachea*
- Affects growers
- Causes emaciation
- 'Y' shape red worms present in trachea

3. *Gongylonema ingluvicola*
- Worms in crop under mucosa
- Causes emaciation and retardation of growth

4. *Dispharynx nasuta* and *Tetrameres pattersoni*
- Diarrhoea, emaciation
- Hemorrhage in proventriculus
- Worms in proventricular glands

5. *Cheilospirura hamulosa*
- Emaciation
- Necrotic nodules in gizzard, presence of worms
- Hemorrhage in gizzard

6. *Heterakis gallinarum*
- Emaciation
- Typhlitis
- Presence of worms in caeca

7. *Capillaria* sp. in intestine

TAPE WORMS (CESTODES)

Avian cestodes are thin, white tape worms present in gut causing enteritis and melena leading to retardation of growth.

Etiology
- *Davainea proglottina* (3 mm in length)
- *Choanotaenia infundibulum, Raillietina tetragona* and *R. echinobothrida* (25-30 cm in length)

Pathogenesis

Transmission occurs through slugs, flies and ants infected with segments of parasites. It penetrates mucosa of intestine to cause hemorrhagic enteritis and forms nodules visible from out side of the intestines.

Characteristic symptoms
- Emaciation
- Weakness
- Red droppings due to mixing of blood

Macroscopic and microscopic features
- Catarrhal and haemorrhagic enteritis
- Granulomatous nodules in wall of intestine
- Catarrhal and haemorrhagic enteritis

Diagnosis
- Symptoms and lesions
- Presence of parasite in gut at necropsy
- Presence of parasitic segments in droppings

FLAT WORMS (TREMATODES)

Trematodes are flat worms rarely found in birds. Some of the important flat worms are:
1. *Prosthogonymus macrorchis*
2. *Echinostoma revolutum*

3. *Echinoparyphium recurvatum*
4. *Prosthogonymus indicus*
5. *Catatropis indica*

Ectoparasites

Common ectoparasites including ticks, mites and lice of poultry are:

1. Ticks
   a. *Argas persicus*
   b. *Aegyptianella pullorum*
2. Mites
   a. *Dermanyssus gallinae*- Red mite
   b. *Syringophilus bipectinatus*- Feather mite
   c. *Knemidocotes gallinae*- Feather mite
   d. *K. mutans*- Scaly leg mite
   e. *Cytodites nudus*- Air sac mite

Protozoan parasites

1. Coccidiosis

Coccidiosis is caused by protozoan parasites of *Eiemeria* sp. and characterized by hemorrhagic enteritis and mortality in chickens.

Etiology
- Intestinal form
- *Eimeria acervulina*
- *E. necatrix*
- *E. maxima*
- *E. brunetti*
- *E. preacox*
- *E. mitis*
- *E. hagani*
- *E. mivati*

- Caecal coccidiosis
- *E. tenella*

Pathogenesis

Oocysts with sporozoites are ingested by birds through contaminated feed, water or litter. The sporozoites are released and penetrate epithelial cells of villi and develop into round bodies (trophozoites). It then grows to form first generation schizont, nuclei of which have sickle shape and known as merozoites. The merozoites after breaking schizonts can start second cycle to form second generation schizonts. After 2-3 cycle, the merozoites develop sexual phase to form male (micro gametocytes) and female (macro gametocytes) cells. The micro gametes penetrate and fuse with macro gametes resulting in fertilization and formation of oocysts which are liberated in intestinal lumen and pass out along with faeces. A single ingested oocyst can develop into millions of oocysts in a bird.

Characteristic symptoms

- Emaciation and anemia
- Retarded growth
- Blood mixed droppings
- Mortality upto 50%

Macroscopic and microscopic features

- Haemorrhagic enteritis
- Typhlitis
- Thickening of intestinal wall
- Catarrhal and hemorrhagic enteritis
- Presence of coccidia in intestinal sections

Diagnosis

- Symptoms and lesions
- Examination of droppings or intestinal scrapings for the presence of coccidia.

HISTOMONIASIS

Histomoniasis is a disease of growers caused by protozoan parasite *Histomonas* sp. and characterized by necrotic ulcers in caeca and necrotic foci in liver. It is also known as **black head** disease.

Etiology
- *Histomonas meleagredis*
- Round, vacuolated cytoplasm with single nucleus.

Pathogenesis
Transmission of protozoan parasite occurs through faecal contamination of feed and water or through earthworm, flies and eggs of *Heterakis gallinarum*. Parasite enters in wall of caeca and causes lesions.

Characteristic symptoms
- Diarrhoea with sulphur colour faeces
- Icterus

Macroscopic and microscopic features
- Necrotic ulcers in caeca
- Circular, concave, green necrotic foci (1 cm diameter) in liver
- Necrosis in liver
- Presence of protozoan parasite (unicellular 8-13 µl, with four flagella)

Diagnosis
- Symptoms and lesions
- Microscopic examination of caecal contents/ scrapings.

TRICHOMONOSIS

Trichomonosis is a protozoan parasitic disease characterized by formation of yellow round nodules in esophagus and crop of pigeons.

Etiology
- *Trichomonas gallinae*

Pathogenesis

Organism is transmitted directly from infected birds to newly hatched pigeons. Small yellowish necrotic lesions develop in oral cavity specially on soft palate after 3-14 days of infection which further spreads to esophagus, crop, proventriculus, liver, lungs and intestines.

Characteristic symptoms
- Emaciation
- Accumulation of greenish fluid or cheesy material in mouth and crop
- Pendulous crop

Macroscopic and microscopic features
- Yellow, button shaped necrotic foci in mouth, oesophagus and crop
- Necrosis
- Presence of protozoan parasites in sections of oesophagus and crop

Diagnosis
- Symptoms and lesions
- Microscopic examination of nodules through smears or sections.

HEXAMITIASIS

Hexamitiasis is a protozoan parasitic disease of turkey poults of about 4-6 weeks characterized by diarrhoea and mortality.

Etiology
- *Hexamita meleagridis*
- Almond shaped parasite

Pathogenesis

The source of infection is adult carrier birds. On ingestion it produces catarrhal enteritis with bulbous areas containing watery contents on duodenum and jejunum.

Characteristic symptoms
- Diarrhoea
- Loss of weight and death

Macroscopic and microscopic features
- Bulbous nodules in intestine
- Presence of protozoan parasites in cecum, duodenum and bursa

Diagnosis
- Symptoms and lesions
- Microscopic examination of lesion/ caeca for parasites

Chapter 41

Vices and Miscellaneous Disease Conditions

CANNIBALISM

Cannibalism is a bad habit of birds in which the birds attack their fellow birds and eat their flesh. It is done through sharp end of beak, which causes deep wounds specially on vent. Sometimes the wounds are so deep that leads to death of affected bird. Two types of cannibalism vices are common i.e. vent pecking and feather pecking.

Cause/ Predisposing Factors
- Over crowding
- Genetic predisposition
- Hemorrhage in external genitalia
- Protein deficiency (arginine and methionine deficiency)
- Loss of feathers
- Wounds
- Prolapse of cloaca

Egg Eating: Sometimes a bird develops habit of eating its own eggs. This problem may start with the presence of broken eggs in poultry house and birds develop a taste for it.

Pica: Birds eat non food items such as feathers, litter material, threads, mud, bangle etc. It may occur due to phosphorus deficiency, parasitic load in gut, new litter material or poor managemental conditions.

Heat Stroke: The presence of thick layers of feathers on body of bird and absence of sweat glands on skin makes the birds more susceptible to heat stroke in summer season. Inadequate water supply, absence of trees/ vegetation around poultry houses, overcrowding, poor ventilation, etc. may predispose the birds for heat stroke which is characterized by open beak; panting, paralysis, congestion and hemorrhage in brain along with dehydration.

Prolapse of Cloaca: The prolapse of cloaca has been observed due to fusariotoxins which increases the peristalsis in layers. It may enhance the cannibalism in birds.

Impaction of Crop: Sometimes birds may eat litter material, grass, feathers, fibrous food, nails, pieces of sticks, stumps of feathers which causes impaction in crop. If the nail having sharp edge, it may penetrate and cause ingluvitis and/or proventriculitis.

Egg Bound Condition: Egg bound condition is inability of a layer bird to expel a normal egg. It may occur in new laying hens due to paralysis of nerves of oviduct or its inflammation that leads to prolapse. The egg remains in oviduct and death occurs in such birds. Sometimes, eggs from ovary do not reach in oviduct and drops in peritoneal cavity leading to egg borne peritonitis.

Toxic Fat Syndrome: In this condition, birds show accumulation of water in abdominal cavity, pericardial sac and in subcutaneous tissue giving jelly like appearance. This is also known as *"chick oedema disease"* or *"water belly"*. It may be associated with phosphorus deficient soybean diet, toxic factor associated with fat in feed and carbon monoxide, dioxin or salt poisoning.

Gout: Gout is deposition of uric acid and urates in kidneys, heart, ureters and other internal organs. It may occur due to excess of protein, deficiency of vitamin A, infectious bursal disease, infectious bronchitis, aflatoxicosis, orchratoxicosis and other diseases involving kidneys. In this conditions, one may find chalky/ sandy material on touch on the surface of the organs.

Fatty Liver and Kidney Syndrome: Fatty liver and kidney syndrome (FLKS) is characterized by pale or yellowish liver with petechiae, pale heart and kidneys and hydropericardium. It may occur due to biotin deficiency, inadequate feeding, protein deficiency and stress as a result of noise, excessive cold or heat, power failure etc.

Fatty Liver Syndrome: It is characterized by enlarged, yellowish, friable liver with rupture and internal hemorrhage. This condition is associated with faulty diet or stress of high egg production.

Blue comb Disease: This is also known as avian monocytosis and is characterized by bluish colour of comb, increased number of monocytes in blood, deposition of urates in kidneys, and atrophy of spleen. The exact cause is not known but supposedly occurs due to some nutritional factors or viral etiology.

Chapter 42
Pathology of Diseases of Wild and Zoo Animals

The pathology of diseases of wild and zoo animals is almost similar to that occur in domestic animals due to same etiological agent. It is, therefore, only name, cause of disease and a brief description is given here. For details of the pathological alterations, readers are requested to consult the diseases described elsewhere in this book. Some of the important clinical manifestations and pathological lesions of bacterial, viral, parasitic and non-infectious diseases of wild and zoo animals are listed below:

1. **Theileriosis in Gaur (*Bos gaurus*)**
   - Fever
   - Clay coloured faeces
   - Champing of jaws
   - Blood positive for *Theileria* sp.

2. **Babesiosis in tiger**
   - Fever
   - Constipation
   - Blood positive for *Babesia* sp.
   - Red colour urine

3. **Babesiosis in leopard**
   - Edema in lungs
   - Icterus
   - Enlargement of spleen
   - Hemoglobinuria

- Babesia in blood smear

4. **Anaplasmosis in leopard and white tiger**
   - *Anaplasma marginale*
   - Leucocytosis
   - Muscle tremors
   - Staggering gait
   - Fever and depression

5. **Trypanosomiasis in tiger, jaguars, wild cats, lion, jackal, sambar and wolf**
   - Convulsions, pyrexia and opacity
   - Congestion in lungs, liver, kidneys and brain
   - Blood positive for trypanosomes
   - Hemorrhage in liver, kidneys and lungs

6. **Amoebiasis in non-human primates and lion**
   - *Entamoeba histolytica*
   - Mucous mixed faeces
   - Melena

7. **Balantidiosis in monkeys and rhinos**
   - *Balantidium coli*
   - Diarrhoea, dysentery and melena

8. **Coccidiosis in Indian vulture**
   - *Isospora gypsi*

9. **Coccidiosis in Bulbul**
   - *Isospora pyenonotae*
   - *I. pyenonotus*

10. **Sarcosystosis in Gaur**
    - Sarcosysts in cardiac and skeletal muscle

11. Trichomoniasis in birds

12. **Gastrointestinal parasites in wild animals**
    - Strongyle, Trichuris, Ascaris, Moniezia, Toxocara, Anchylostoma, Oesophagostomum, Hymenolep, *Paragonimus* sp., Cooperia *Diphylobothrium* sp., Fasciola, Paramphistomum, Strongyloids, Bunostomum, Dicrocoelium, Mullerius
    - Schystosoma, Murshidia, Thelazia, Grammocephalus (hookworm), Anchylostoma
    - *Syphacia* and *Aspicularis* are pin worms of squirrel
13. Microfilariasis in wild birds (Myna, Koel)
14. **Ectoparasites**
    - *Melophagus ovinus* in hog deer
    - *Ctenocephalides felis* in leopard
    - Hematomyzus in elephants
    - Psoroptic mange in rabbit
15. Hydatidosis in Bison
16. Diabetes
17. Dystocia in elephant, Giraffe and Hyaena
18. **Tumours**
    - Fibroscarcoma in panther
    - Fibrolipoma in elephant
    - Histiocytic cell sarcoma in gnu
    - Squamous cell carcinoma in tiger
    - Malignant mesothelioma in lion
    - Fibroma in rhino and monkey
    - Adenocarcinoma in hog deer, sloth bear and monkey
    - Seminoma in monkeys
    - Adenoma in monkeys
19. Amyloidosis- Swan
20. Pneumonia- Wild buffalo bull
21. Leucosis- zoo birds
22. Colisepticemia, cannibalism and tuberculosis in pheasants

23. Suppurative pericarditis in monkeys
24. Intussusception in elephant
25. Traumatic reticulopericarditis in deer
26. Pneumoconiasis wild mammals
27. Enterolith in tiger and zebra
28. Tuberculosis in wild ruminants, rhino, tiger and pheasants
29. Johne's Disease in wild ruminants, rhino and tiger
30. Necrobacillosis in sambar
31. Botryomycosis in zebra
32. Salmonellosis in rhino and ostrich
33. Pasteurellosis in beer, hippopotami and pigeon
34. Clostridial infection in bear
35. Hematuria in wolf
36. Anthrax in rhino
37. Pox in chimpanzee
38. FMD in gaur
39. Rabies in wild ass
40. Malignant catarrhal fever in hangul
41. Feline leukemia in lion
42. Aspergillosis and candidiasis in peacocks, wild herbivores, black beer
43. Pneumomycosis in flamingo
44. Dermatophytosis in bear
45. Aflatoxicosis in ducks
46. Chronic metritis in elephant
47. Enteritis in elephant
48. Tetanus in elephant
49. Dropsy in elephant
50. Ulcerative keratitis in rhino
51. Cataract in captive pheasants
52. Ascites in panther
53. Phytobezoars in deers

Chapter 43
Pathology of Diseases of Laboratory Animals

The laboratory animal diseases are having special significance as many veterinarians are employed in laboratory animal houses of public institutions or pharmaceutical companies. Else, the Veterinary Scientists must be aware of the diseases of laboratory animals so that they can screen the animals before start of their experiment. Mainly the laboratory animals include rabbits, mice, guinea pigs, rats, etc. The special features of pathological alterations in specific diseases are described in the following text but only names of common disease are given which were described earlier elsewhere in this book or in Illustrated Veterinary Pathology.

RABBIT DISEASES

I. PARASITIC DISEASES

1. Coccidiosis

a. Intestinal- *E. megna, E. media*
- Diarrhoea
- Presence of oocysts in faeces

b. Hepatic
- *Eimeria stiedae*
- Common in weaners below 5-7 weeks of age. Angora weanlings are more susceptible.
- Enlarged liver
- Presence of oocysts in faeces

2. Mange

a. Psoroptic or sarcoptic mange
- Alopecia
- Severe pruritus
- Poor body weight gain
- Poor fur quality
- Poor reproduction

b. Otoacariasis/ ear cancer
- Caused by *Psoroptes cuniculi*
- Shaking of head frequently
- Intense pruritus and exudation in affected ear
- Spread rapidly from one rabbit to other

3. Tape worm
- *Taenia pisiformes*
- Weight loss, enteritis

4. Toxoplasmosis
- *T. gondii*
- Fever, respiratory distress and paralysis
- Death

II. BACTERIAL DISEASE

1. Pasteurellosis
- *Pasteurella multocida*
- Snuffers- Sneezing yellowish discharge from eyes and nose.
- Conjunctivitis
- Pneumonia
- Otitis media (middle ear)
- Septicemia

2. Tyzzer's disease
- Caused by *Clostridium piliformis*
- Diarrhoea and bledding from anus

- Leucopenia and elevation of serum enzymes (SGPT)
- Multifocal necrosis in liver and myocardium

3. Rabbit Syphilis (Vent disease)
- Caused by *Treponema cuniculi*
- Infertility, scab formation, small blisters, seeping ulcers with continuous discharge.
- Loss of hairs around vulva and penis
- In advance causes lesions on lips, nose and eyelids

4. Enteritis

a. Simple enteritis (weanling diarrhoea)
- Most common in age group of 5-10 weeks
- Caused by sudden change in type and composition of feed, stress and transportation.

b. Mucoid enteritis
- Etiology not known
- Indiscriminate feeding of antibiotics

c. Enterotoxaemia
- *Clostridium* spp.
- Carbohydrate overload
- Death is due to dehydration as a result of diarrhoea.

5. Mastitis
- Caused by *Staphylococcus* sp. and *Streptococcus* sp.
- Red swollen mammary glands
- Lactating animal may die if not treated properly.

III. VIRAL DISEASES

1. Pox
- Pock lesions on ears, legs, tongue, hairless parts of the body

2. Myxomatosis (big head/ Mosquito disease)
- Highly infectious transmitted by mosquitoes

- Edema of head, ears, mucopurulent discharge from eyes
- In severe cases pneumonic symptoms
- Subcutaneous swelling may be observed containing mucoid gelatinous mass
- Death within a week

IV. FUNGAL DISEASES

Dermatomycosis (Ringworm)

a. In indoor cages
- *Microsporum* sp.
- *Epidermatophyton* sp.

b. Out door cages
- *Trichophyton* sp.
- Circular raised patches in grey yellow on nose, face, ear and feet

V. MANAGEMENTAL DISEASES

a. Sore pad/ sore hock/ sore feet
- Due to dirty wet cages and rough hutch floor.

b. Hind quarter paralysis
- Due to sudden jerkey movements, mishandling of rabbit
- Affected animals have no control on defaecation and urination

c. Hair ball
- Due to habit of licking/ chewing of own hairs or fur
- Develop when animal has infection of mange, dermatophyte or just before kindling
- Ingested hair get accumulated in stomach and may block normal passage of food
- Severe pain

d. Wool shedding
- Unusual shedding of hairs/ wool due to deficiency of vitamin A, Mg, Zn and Cu.

- Baldness

e. Heat stroke
- In summer when temperature rises more than 36°C
- Dehydration and death

PATHOLOGY OF MOUSE DISEASES

BACTERIAL DISEASES

1. **Salmonellosis**
- Caused by *Salmonella enteritidis* var. Typhimurium
- Necrotic patches on liver and spleen

2. **Tyzzer's disease**
- Caused by *Bacillus piliformis*
- Diarrhoea

3. **Arthritis**
- Caused by *Streptobacillus moniliformis*

VIRAL DISEASES

1. **Mouse pox**
2. **Epizootic diarrhoea of infant mice (infantile diarrhoea)**
    - **Rotavirus**
    - **In 7-10 days old**
3. **Reovirus-3 infection**
    - Jaundice and emaciation

PATHOLOGY OF RAT DISEASES

1. **Labyrinthitis**
    - *Streptobacillus* sp.
    - *Mycoplasma* sp.

2. **Salmonellosis**
    - Hepatitis

3. *Leptospria icterohaemorrhagie*

- Icterus
- Nephritis

4. Tularemia- *Pasteurella tularensis*
5. CRD (Rat and Mice)
   - Caused by *Mycoplasma pulmosis* sp., *Pasteurella* sp. and *Pseumococcus* sp.
   - Pneumonia

PATHOLOGY OF HAMSTER DISEASES
- Relatively free from infection

1. Wet tail
- Most severe disease
- Severe diarrhoea
- Caused by *E.coli*

PATHOLOGY OF GUINEA PIGS DISEASES
1. Salmonellosis- *Salmonella enteritidis* var. Typhimureum, *S.* Dublin, *S.* Enteritidis
2. Pseudotuberculosis- *Yersinia pseudotuberculosis*
3. Pasteurellosis- *P. pneumotropica, P. multocida, Manheimia haemolytica*
4. *Brodetella bronchisepitca*- Acute pneumonic symptoms
5. Streptococcal pneumonia

Fungal Diseases
Ringworm caused by *Microsporum gypseum* and/or *Trichophyton* sp.

Viral Diseases
1. Lymphocytic choriomeningitis virus
2. Salivary gland virus
3. Adenovirus
4. Sendai virus

Chapter 44
Cytopathology

Cytopathology deals with interpretation of cells from animal body that either exfoliate/ desquamate spontaneously from epithelial surface or are obtained from organs/ tissues through biopsy. Histopathology is based on interpretation of distortions in tissue architecture, and the cytopathologic diagnosis rests upon alterations in morphology of a single or group of cells.

Scope

Cytopathologic diagnosis has numerous applications in diagnosis of animal diseases.

1.   Diagnosis and prognosis of neoplasms: Cytopathologic interpretations are helpful is diagnosis and prognosis of cancers in animals specially in urinary tract neoplasms, lymphoma, ovarian cancer, mammary gland tumour horn cancer and tumour of reproductive tract.

2.   Identification of benign neoplasms: With the help of imprint smears or exfoliative cells, one may diagnose and identify the extent of alterations in tumour cells e.g. fibroadenoma verses carcinoma of eyes.

3.   Diagnosis of infectious diseases: It is helpful in diagnosis of various infectious diseases of animals including bacterial and viral disease e.g. rotavirus infection in calves. One can demonstrate rotavirus antigen in desquamated cells in faeces.

Cytopathologic diagnosis can be performed through two method viz., exfoliative and interventional cytopathology.

1. Exfoliative cytopathology

In includes the examination and interpretation of cells shed off from epithelial surfaces in body cavities or body fluids, cells obtained through scraping, brushing and/or washing of mucosal surfaces are also included in exfoliative cytopathologic diagnosis. Exfoliative cytopathology is based on the fact that the rate of exfoliation is enhanced in disease state thereby yielding a larger number of cells for study. Samples from different organs that can be obtained exfoliative cytopathological diagnosis are listed in Table.

Table. Types of samples from different organs/ body sites for exfoliative cytopathologic diagnosis in animals

Site	Sample
1. Urinary tract	– Urinary sediment
	– Bladder washing
	– Prostatic massage-secretions in dogs
2. Gastrointestinal tract	– Endoscopic lavage
	– Fecal sediment
	– Rectal washings
	– Rectal pintch
	– Buccal smears
3. Respiratory tract	– Sputum
	– Bronchial washing
4. Female genital tract	– Vaginal smears
	– Cervical smears
	– Vaginal discharges
	– Endometrial washings
5. Male genital tract	– Prepucial washings
6. Body fluids	– Cerebrospinal fluid
	– Synovial fluid

- Amniotic fluid
- Seminal fluid

2. Interventional cytopathology

Interventional cytopathology includes the samples obtained from aspiration or surgical biopsy. In veterinary sciences, however, there is limited scope of aspiration interventional cytopathology except in few diseases such as in theileriosis lymph node aspirate is useful in diagnosis. But surgical biopsy is comparatively common in the diagnosis of tumours in animals. It includes fine needle aspiration cytology (FNAC) and imprint cytology.

A. Fine Needle Aspiration Cytology: Fine needle aspiration cytologic procedures are useful in palpable lesions in animals e.g. enlargement and hardness of superficial lymph nodes The FNAC technique is quick, safe and painless and carried out without any anesthesia. However, it should be performed by a trained personnel otherwise multiple attempts or repeated procedure cause inconvenience and pain to animal. This method of diagnosis is cost effective and provides first hand information to the veterinary clinician. Fine needle ranges from 25 (0.6 mm) to 20 (0.9 mm) gauge with a length of 25 mm may be used. Needles of upto 200 mm length are used for aspiration from internal organs Syringes of 10-20 ml capacity are suitable but the grip of syringe and needle should be such that it does not leak during aspiration. The needle is inserted into the targeted organ through skin puncture. On reaching the lesions, the plunger of syringe is retracted and at least 10 ml of suction is applied while moving the needle back and forth in the lesions. The direction angle of the needle may be changed to access different areas of the lesions. Aspiration is terminated when aspirated material or blood visible at the base/ hub of the needle are more than adequate. Material drawn into the barrel syringe is sometimes not recoverable and thus becomes useless for cytopathological diagnosis. Aspirated material is recovered by detaching the needle from syringe and filling the syringe with air. The syringe and needle are then reconnected and the aspirate is placed on one end of a glass slide. Aspirate deposits on the slide are inspected with naked eyes. Semisolid particulate aspirates are crush-smeared by pressing between two glass slides. Other material may be pulled just like blood smears on to slide. These smears are either wet fixed or air dried. Most cytopathologists use both type of smears. Wet fixation in done in 95% ethanol for 10-15 min and then transported to laboratory while air dried smears are wrapped and directly sent to laboratory.

B. Imprint cytology: In this touch preparations from cut surfaces of superficial cut/ excised lesions are prepared. Imprints are also prepared from draining sinuses and/or ulcerated areas. The main advantage of imprint smear examination is that the cell distribution reflects the tissue architecture thus aiding in interpretation. It is useful in quick diagnosis of several animal and poultry diseases.

C. Crush smear cytology: Crush smear preparations of particulate tissue material are helpful in diagnosis of tumours. It provides the recognition of tissue architecture in addition to better cytological details.

Chapter 45
Appendices

Appendix I

TECHNIQUES OF POST-MORTEM EXAMINATION (NECROPSY)

Necropsy is examination of animal after death. It helps in diagnosis of diseases and their control. It is said that "Necropsy is a message of wisdom from dead to living". Necropsy include systemic examination of dead animal, recording of pathological lesions, their interpretation to make diagnosis of disease. Sometimes it is difficult to arrive any conclusion merely based on gross examination of dead animal. Then one should seek the help of laboratory examinations such as Histopathology, Microbiology, Immunology and Toxicology for confirmation.

Necropsy examination is an integral part of disease investigation. Therefore, veterinarian must have the knowledge of the techniques of post-mortem examination, recording of lesions, collection of proper material for laboratory and most importantly their correlation to arrive at conclusive diagnosis. The technique of post-mortem examination is as under:

POST-MORTEM EXAMINATION OF LARGE ANIMAL

- Place animal on left side (Ruminants).
- Place horse on right side and dog on vertebral column.
- Make midventral incision with knife from chin to anus.
- Surround the prepuce, scrotum/ mammary gland.
- Remove skin dorsoventrally. Remove skin at face, neck, thorax and abdomen.
- Cut the muscles and fascia in between scapula and body; remove fore legs.

- Raise hind legs, cut the coxofemoral ligament.
- Examine s/c tissue, muscles, superficial lymphnodes- prescapular, prefemoral supramammary, etc.
- Open abdominal cavity by cutting muscles and peritoneum.
- Open thoracic cavity by cutting xiphoid cartilage at sternum; lift ribs and press them to break at joints with vertebral column.
- Examine the visceral organs in both cavities:

Thorax	:	Heart, Lungs, Trachea, Oesophagus, Mediastinal lymphnodes, Diaphragm
Abdominal cavity	:	
Ruminants	:	Rumen, Reticulum, Omasum, Abomasum
Other animals	:	Stomach
In all animals	:	Liver, Pancreas, Intestines, Mesenteric lymphnodes, Spleen, Kidneys, Ureter
Pelvic cavity	:	Urinary bladder, uterus

POST-MORTEM EXAMINATION (POULTRY)

- Dip the dead bird in antiseptic solution or in water; to avoid feather contamination.
- Keep the bird on post-mortem table at vertebral column and look for any lesion or parasite on skin.
- Examine the eyes, face and vent.
- Remove skin through a cut with knife and with the help of fingers. Expose thymus, trachea, esophagus in neck.
- Break the coxofemoral joint by lifting the legs. Examine the chest and thigh muscles.
- Cut on lateral side of chest muscles. Lift the chest muscle dorsally and break bones at joints with thorax. Cut bones

at both sides and remove muscles, bones to expose thorax, abdomen.
- Examine different organs.
- Cut proventriculus and pull the organs of digestive tract out. Separate liver, spleen, intestines, cecum, proventriculus, gizzard, etc.
- Expose bursa just beneath the cloaca.
- Cut beak at joint, examine mouth cavity and expose esophagus and trachea.
- Remove skin of head and make a square cut on skull to expose brain.
- Take a forceps and place in between thigh muscles, remove fascia and expose the sciatic nerve.
- Separate each organ, examine them for the presence of lesion.

Appendix II

STEPS IN POST-MORTEM EXAMINATION

Post-mortem examination should be conducted only after receiving of a formal request from the owner of animal having details of anamnesis and date and time of death. Without formal written request, one should not do post-mortem examination of animal. The post-mortem record includes the aspects of animal identification, illness, therapeutic and preventive measures adopted and date and time of death. This information provided by the owner or person requesting post-mortem, which helps in post-mortem examination and recording of lesions to make a conclusive diagnosis.

Various steps in post-mortem examination are as under:

1. External examination

Animal should be examined externally before opening the body for the presence of lesions on body surface. Eyes, ear, anus, vulva, mouth, nares etc. should be specifically examined for the presence of blood and any other lesion. If the blood is coming out from natural orifices, it should be examined for the presence of anthrax bacilli and such carcasses must not be opened for post-mortem examination. Following points should be taken into consideration while conducting external examination.

- Trauma, wound, fracture, cuts, etc.
- Fungal infection *e.g.* ringworm
- Parasitic infestation *e.g.* mange, lice, ticks
- Side of animal is lying down on earth.
- Discharges from openings.
- Burn, ulcers, erosions etc.

2. Subcutaneous tissue and musculature

Examine the subcutaneous tissue and musculature after removal of skin for the presence of lesions such as:

- Congestion, hemorrhage, oedema, nodule, anemia, icterus.

- Fat deposits
- Necrosis on muscles, hardening, calcification.

3. Abdominal and thoracic cavity

Just after opening the carcass, one should observe the presence of any lesion in abdominal and thoracic cavity and following points must be kept in mind.

- Accumulation of fluid (serus, serosanguinous, blood, pus etc.)
- Fibrinous or fibrous adhesions.
- Parasites
- Abscess, tumor etc.

4. Respiratory system

Organs/ tissues to be examined

External nares, nasal passage, larynx, trachea, bronchi, lungs, air sacs (poultry) mediastinal lymphnodes.

Lesions to be observed

- Discharge from external nares.
- Growth (granuloma/ polyp) in nasal passage if there is blood mixed nasal discharge.
- *Trachea and Bronchi-* Congestion, haemorrhage, presence of caseous exudate, frothy exudate etc.
- *Lungs-* Congestion, consolidation, nodules, presence of exudate on cut surfaces, edema, atelectasis, emphysema, hemorrhage, necrosis.
- *Mediastinal lymphnodes-* Edema, hardening, calcification, congestion, haemorrhage.

5. Cardiovascular system

Organs/ tissues to be examined

- Heart, aorta, arteries, veins and lymphatics

Lesions to be observed

- Fluid, blood, pus etc. in pericardial sac
- Adhesions, fibrin, fibrosis
- Congestion, haemorrhage, necrotic foci
- Hardening of blood vessel, obstruction, thrombi
- Presence of parasites
- Post-mortem clot/ thrombi.

6. Digestive system

Organs/ tissue to be examined

Mouth cavity, esophagus, crop, proventriculus, gizzard (poultry), rumen reticulum, omasum, abomasum (ruminants), stomach, intestine (duodenum, jejunum, ileum, cecum, colon, rectum), cloaca, vent (poultry), anus, liver, pancreas, gall bladder, mesenteric lymphnodes etc.

Lesions to be observed

- Erosions, ulcers, vesicles
- Congestion, hemorrhage, oedema
- Necrosis
- Icterus
- Abscess/ pus
- Perforation, needles or hard objects in reticulum.
- Intussusception, torsion, volvulus
- Parasites
- Atrophy, hardening, nodules
- Contents, catarrhal, blood mixed, digested/ undigested feed material, thickening of wall of intestines.
- Cut surface of liver for parasites, lesions in bile duct.

7. Cardiovascular system

Organs/ tissue to be examined
- Kidneys, ureter, urinary bladder, urethra

Lesions to be observed
- Congestion, haemorrhage, infarction, oedema.

- Necrosis, hardening, nodules
- Deposition of salts, calculi
- Obstruction

8. Genital system

Organs/ tissue (female)
- Ovaries, oviduct, uterus, cervix, vagina

Male
- Testicles, Epididymis, penis, prepuce

Lesions to be observed
- Cysts in ovary
- Congestion, haemorrhage, oedema
- Foetus in uterus, pus, fluid
- Necrosis, overgrowth, nodules
- Atrophy, adhesions, granularity

9. Immune system

Organs/ tissue to be examined
- Spleen, lymphnodes, bursa and thymus (poultry), bone marrow
- Peyer's patches, GALT, RALT

Lesions to be observed
- Size, shape, atrophy, hardening.
- Edema, congestion, haemorrhage

10. Nervous system

Organs/ tissue to be examined
- Brain, spinal cord, nerves, meninges

Lesions to be observed
- Congestion, hemorrhage, hematoma
- Oedema, swelling
- Abscess
- Hypoplasia

11. Miscellaneous observation
- Adhesions in pleural/ peritoneal cavity
- Any other left over information pertinent to post-mortem examination/ diagnosis

12. Post-mortem diagnosis
- Diagnosis should be made on the basis of above findings which involve any system or organ. The most involved organ based diagnosis should be written with suggestion of etiological factors or etiology based diagnosis.

Appendix III

WRITING OF POST-MORTEM REPORT

Post-mortem report consists of two parts post-mortem record and post-mortem examination as given in the format on next page. The first part *i.e.* post-mortem record is having information related to animal and is supplied by the owner or person requesting post-mortem examination. Actually, it is a part of request form of the case for post-mortem examination. This is necessary for the identification of animal. It should be filled in before conducting post-mortem examination. The proper record will be helpful in establishing accurate diagnosis based on post-mortem examination.

POST-MORTEM RECORD

1. **Species:** Here one should write the species of animal such as bovine, porcine, equine, poultry, etc.

2. **Date:** Date of the post-mortem examination.

3. **Case no.:** The serial number of your post-mortem book. It shows cumulatively how many animals are examined by you in necropsy.

4. **Breed:** Mention the breed of animal, if known or supplied in the request form, such as Murrah buffalo, Jersey cattle, etc.

5. **Age/ Born:** Age of animal or its date of birth. In case the exact age is not known then mention young, adult or chick, grower, adult in case of poultry.

6. **Sex:** Sex of animal (male or female).

7. **Identification number/ mark:** It must be filled with utmost care; the number (tattoo number or brand number) should be the same as on animal. If the identification number is not available/ illegible then write the characteristic mark of animal.

8. **Owner:** Here, the name of owner with complete address must be filled clearly. The address should be complete enough so that the report can reach the owner through post also.

9. Referred by: In this column, the name of Veterinary Officer/ any other officer who referred the case for post-mortem examination should be written. Sometimes owner himself/ herself is interested in post-mortem examination of animal; in such case the name of owner should be written.

10. History of the case: This includes the clinical illness of animal, duration of illness, epidemiological data, tentative diagnosis, therapeutic and preventive measures adopted. This is very important and information of this column has an important role in making the diagnosis.

11. Reported date and time of death: It should have the exact date and time of death of animal. Sometimes, it is difficult to note the exact time then one can write morning, noon, evening, midnight etc. to approximate the timings of death of animal. In some large farms, it is very difficult to record information with regard to each individual animal/ bird so here one can write "previous night" as time of death.

12. Date and time of post-mortem examination: Pathologist conducting post-mortem examination should write here the exact time and date of the post-mortem examination.

The above information is very important to arrive any conclusive diagnosis. The correct information enhances the specificity of post-mortem diagnosis. Some points might be looking like insignificant but one should not overlook them and write as correct as information he/ she can gather from the owner's request letter/ form.

POST-MORTEM REPORT

POST-MORTEM RECORD

1. Species: 2. Date: 3. Case No.:
4. Breed: 5. Age/ Born: 6. Sex:
7. Identification No.:
8. Owner with address: 9. Referred by:
10. History of the case: 11. Reported date & Time of Death:

12. Date and Time of post-mortem examination:

POST-MORTEM EXAMINATION
1. External appearance:
2. Subcutaneous tissue and musculature:
3. General observations after opening the carcass:
4. Respiratory system:
5. Cardiovascular system:
6. Digestive system:
7. Urinary system:
8. Genital system:
9. Immune system:
10. Nervous system:
11. Miscellaneous observations:
12. Post-mortem diagnosis:

Date:

Place: Signature of officer conducting post-mortem

POST-MORTEM EXAMINATION

It includes the observations made by the pathologist conducting post-mortem examination. This part of report should be filled in as soon as possible after the post-mortem examination. It is advisable that one should record some points on a small paper or diary during post-mortem examination and fill them in report after the conduct of post-mortem examination.

1. External appearance: Record the lesions observed in intact animal before its opening. One should place on record the side of animal lying down, lesions on skin, external parasites, trauma etc.

2. Subcutaneous tissue and musculature: The observations made after removal of skin, on subcutaneous tissue and muscle should be included in this column.

3. General observations after opening the carcass: It contains the general information or lesions present in abdominal and thoracic cavity such as accumulation of fluid, pus, blood, clot of blood, post-mortem changes such as pseudomelanosis, etc.

4. **Respiratory system:** Record the lesions observed in respiratory system right from external nares, nasal passage, trachea, bronchi and lungs alongwith mediastinal lymphnodes.

5. **Cardiovascular system:** Record the lesions present in heart, aorta, arteries, veins and lymphatics.

6. **Digestive system:** Record the lesions observed in digestive tract from month cavity, esophagus, crop, proventriculus, gizzard (poultry), rumen, reticulum, omasum abomasum (ruminants), stomach, intestines, rectum, anus, cloaca, vent (poultry), liver, pancreas, gall bladder etc.

7. **Urinary system:** Place on record the lesions present on kidneys, ureter and urethra.

8. **Genital system:** Record the lesions present in ovaries, uterus, oviduct, cervix and vagina in females and testes, penis etc. in males. Be careful in recording lesions in this column as it should match with the sex of animal written in post-mortem record section.

9. **Immune system:** Record the lesions present in spleen, bursa, thymus, lymphnodes, respiratory associated lymphoid tissue (RALT), gut associated lymphoid tissue (GALT) etc. Careful recording of lesions in these organs will be helpful in diagnosis.

10. **Nervous system:** Place on record the lesions present in brain, spinal cord and nerves. Most of the pathologists overlook this system and often not taken pain to examine the brain. It should not be done and every effort should be made to examine and place on record the lesions present in this system.

11. **Miscellaneous observations:** Here one can record any missing observation which has not been covered above.

12. **Post-mortem diagnosis:** This is very important. Based on the history and lesions present in different systems, pathologists by using his experience and conscience conclude the diagnosis.

Appendices

He/she may also write suggestions alongwith diagnosis or some points to suggest the diagnosis and/or contain the disease in other animals.

13. Signature of officer conducting post-mortem: Each and every report must be signed by the officer doing post-mortem examination. Without signature of competent officer, it has no validity.

14. Place and date: The person signing the post-mortem report must also write date and place of post-mortem examination.

Appendix IV

COLLECTION, PRESERVATION AND DISPATCH OF SPECIMENS FOR LABORATORY DIAGNOSIS

Tissue samples are collected from dead or live animals for laboratory examination to confirm the tentative diagnosis.

Purpose
- Diagnosis of disease or for identification of new disease.
- Confirmation of tentative diagnosis.
- Prognosis
- To observe the effect of treatment and give directions for future therapy.

Precautions
- Collect the tissues as early as possible after death of animal.
- Representative tissue/ sample should be collected.
- Sharp knife should be used for cutting
- Collect the tissues directly in fixative.
- Size of tissue should not be more than 1 cm for histopathology in 10% formalin.
- Hollow organs should be taken on paper to avoid shrinkage.
- Hard organs like liver, kidneys etc. should be collected along with capsule.

COLLECTION OF SPECIMENS FOR BACTERIOLOGICAL EXAMINATION
- Collect the tissues under sterile condition.
- Sterilize knife/ scalpel/ spatula on flame or in boiling water.
- Surface sterilized by hot spatula
- Cut with knife and collect sample from inner tissue.
- Body fluids/ blood should be collected in sterilized sy-

ringe or in Pasteur pipette.
- Specimens should be collected directly in media (liquid media-nutrient broth, peptone water, tetrathionate broth or even in normal saline solution/ phosphate buffer saline).
- Seal, pack and transport the collected material to laboratory in ice/ under refrigeration conditions.

BACTERIAL DISEASES

Abscesses
- Swab in sterile conditions/ pus in vials
- Collect material from margin of abscess

Actinobacillosis/ Actinomycosis
- Tissues from affected parts in 10% formalin.
- Pus in sterile test tube/ from edge of lesion
- Slides from Pus for sulphur granules.

Anthrax
- Blood smear from tip of the ear
- Blood for cultural examination
- Muzzle piece for biological test.
- Mark the specimen as *"Anthrax suspect"*

Black Quarter/ Black leg
- Smear from swelling
- Affected muscle piece in ice.

Brucellosis
- Serum after 3 weeks of abortion
- Foetal stomach tied off
- Swabs from uterine discharge
- 5 to 10 ml milk in ice

Glanders
- Smear from discharge
- Lung, liver and spleen in 10% formalin
- Serum

Johne's disease
- Bowel washings in sterile bottle
- Smear from rectal mucosa
- Mesenteric lymphnode in 10% formol saline

Leptospirosis
- Serum 21 days after abortion
- Milk/ urine in vials (1 drop of formalin in 20 ml)
- Liver, kidney tissue in 10% formalin

Listeriosis
- Half brain in ice
- Half brain in 10% formalin

Mastitis
- 10 ml milk in sterile vial in ice

Pasteurellosis
- Heart blood
- Lung, spleen and mediastinal lymphnodes in ice.
- Affected tissues in 10% formalin.

Salmonellosis
- Liver, spleen, kidney and intestine tied off in ice.

Strangles
- Smear, swab of pus in ice.

Erysipelas
- Blood
- Spleen, kidney, liver in ice.

Vibriosis/ Campylobacteriosis
- Foetal stomach tied off
- Vaginal mucosa in ice.
- In pig, intestine and liver in 10% formalin.

Colibacillosis
- Heart blood in sterile vial.
- Tissues from intestine and lymphnodes in 10% formol saline.

Tuberculosis
- Lungs, mediastinal and bronchial lymphnodes in ice and in 10% formalin.

COLLECTION OF SPECIMENS FOR VIROLOGICAL EXAMINATION
- Collect tissue under sterilized condition
- Body fluids/ blood in sterilized syringe or in Pasteur pipette
- Tissues in buffered glycerin
- PBS pH 7.2- 50%
- Glycerin- 50%
- Avoid samples in glycerin from sensitive viruses *e.g.* Rinderpest, canine distemper
- Seal and mark the specimen bottle and transport to laboratory.

VIRAL DISEASES

Foot and mouth disease
- Tongue epithelium, vesicular fluid, saliva, pancreas in 50% buffered glycerine
- Serum

Hog cholera/ swine fever
- Serum under refrigeration

- Spleen, liver, kidney in 50% glycerin/ ice
- Tissues from intestine, mesenteric lymphnode and half of the brain stem in 10% formol saline.

Infectious Canine Hepatitis
- Several pieces of liver, gall bladder and kidney in 10% formol saline.

Pox
- Scabs in ice and in 10% formol saline.

Rabies
- Intact head should be soaked in 1% carbolic acid.
- Fracture the skull with hammer.
- Remove skin and bones
- Half brain in 10% formalin
- Half brain in 50% neutral glycerin.
- Tissues from cerebellum and hippocampus in Zenker's fluid for 20 hrs, wash in tape water for 24 hr and keep in 80% ethyl alcohol for Negri bodies.

Ranikhet disease
- Liver, spleen in 50% neutral glycerin
- Proventriculus in 10% formalin
- Brain in ice.

Rotaviral enteritis
- Faecal sample
- Interstinal tissue in 10% formol saline.

Gumboro disease
- Bursa of Fabricious, kidney, muscles in 10% formol saline.
- Bursa, kidney in 50% buffered glycerine.

SYSTEMIC DISEASES

Diarrhoea/ Enteritis
- Fecal sample in sterile vial
- Serum
- Tissues of intestine, mesenteric lymphnodes in 10% formol saline.

Abortion/ Metritis
- Fetal stomach content tide off or in sterile vials.
- Serum of dam after 21 days of abortion.
- Vaginal discharges in sterile conditions.
- Tissues of placenta, fetal liver, stomach, kidney in 10% formol saline.

Pneumonia
- Nasal discharge/ nasal swabs.
- Lung tissue/ pieces in sterile vials.
- Lung tissue and mediastinal lymphnode in 10% formol saline.

Dermatitis
- Skin scrapings in 10% KOH.
- Skin tissue in 10% formol saline.

Encephalitis
- Cerebrospinal fluid in heparinised vials.
- Brain tissue in 10% formol saline.
- Brain tissue in 50% glycerol.

Nephritis
- Urine sample in sterile vial.
- Kidney tissue in 10% formol saline.

COLLECTION OF SPECIMENS FOR TOXICOLOGICAL EXAMINATION
- Stomach/ intestinal contents
- Liver, kidneys, heart blood
- Urine
- In clean glass jars
- In ice/ refrigeration without any preservative
- Seal, label, transport to laboratory.
- In veterolegal cases all specimens must be collected in presence of police.
- Type of poison suspected along with detailed history, signs, lesions/ treatment etc. should be written on letter with specimens.

TOXICOSIS/ POISONING
- Heavy metal Poisoning
- Hg, Pb, Bi, Ag
- Liver, kidney, stomach content in ice in separate containers.

Alkaloids
- Liver, stomach contents and brain tissue in ice.
- Nitrate
- Fodder
- Stomach contents, blood in ice

Strychnine poisoning
- Stomach contents, intestinal contents, urine, liver, kidney in ice.

Hydrocyanic acid
- Plants
- Stomach contents, blood, liver
- Preserved in 1% solution of mercuric chloride.

Pesticides
- Fatty tissue, liver, stomach contents, blood in ice.
- Subcutaneous, omental, mesenteric fat.

COLLECTION OF SPECIMENS FOR IMMUNOLOGICAL EXAMINATION
- Heart blood in syringe/ Pasteur pipette
- CSF/ Synovial fluid/ peritonial fluid
- Tissues in formol sublimate or in buffered formalin
- Blood/ serum/ others should be sent to laboratory under refrigeration conditions.
- Add one drop of 1:10000 merthiolate in 5 ml serum as preservative.

DISPATCH OF MATERIAL
Following points must be kept in mind while dispatching the material to laboratory for diagnosis.
1. Describe the clinical signs, lesions, tentative diagnosis and treatment given to animal in your letter. Also mention the type of test you want with your tentative diagnosis.
2. Write correct address on letter as well as on the parcel preferably with pin code, if the material is sent through post.
3. Mark the parcel 'Biological Material', 'Handle with care', 'Glass material', 'Fragile' etc. in order to avoid damage in parcel. Also mark the side to be kept on upper side with arrows.
4. Seal the container so that it should not leak in transit.
5. Try to send the material as soon as after its collection from animal.
6. Keep one copy of cover letter inside the parcel and send another copy by hand or post in a separate cover.
7. Keep adequate material like thermocol etc. in the parcel which will save the material from outside pressures/ jerks.
8. Use dry ice, if available otherwise use ice in sealed containers.

Appendix V

HISTOPATHOLOGICAL TECHNIQUES

Histopathology is the branch of pathology which concerns with the demonstration of minute structural alterations in tissues as a result of disease. Most of histopathological techniques simulating to those of applied for study the normal histological structures. For the demonstration of minute histological changes, the tissue must be processed in such a manner that it will provide maximum information. The histopathological diagnosis is an overlooked area specially in Veterinary Sciences. Many times it has been observed that the procedures are not properly followed or the qualified person trained for histopathology is not available, which in turn affects the interpretation and/or diagnosis. Histopathological procedures are described for the benefit of readers which will help them in diagnostic laboratory.

Scope

Though the histopathological techniques are labour intensive, cumbersome and time consuming, particularly when there are automation equipments are not available; however, their use in diagnosis of diseases is unequivocal. Some of the areas where histopathological diagnosis is helpful are described as follows:

- This is useful in establishing the pathogenesis and pathology of any disease caused by bacteria, virus, chlamydia, rickettsia, mycoplasma, parasite, toxin, poisons etc.
- There are certain diseases in which histopathological examination of tissues is the only alternative to diagnose the disease. *e.g.* Bovine spongiform encephalopathy. The agent of this disease takes a very long incubation period and very difficult to isolate and there is no immune response and inflammation in animal. Therefore, histopathology remains the only alternative for confirmatory diagnosis.
- In some cases, the tissues from dead animals are only available material for laboratory diagnosis. This may occur either due to lack of time or due to negligence for not collecting the material for serological tests or isolation stud-

ies. Sometimes the transportation of material from remote areas destroys the other material and the tissues fixed in formalin only remains for making diagnosis. In all such cases the histopathological examination has its pivotal role.

- The histopathological procedures produce permanent slides, which can be stored for a longer period and one cannot manipulate the findings; therefore, it is considered best reliable technique.

- The histopathological techniques are useful in carrying out the retrospective studies. The unstained slides and blocks can be stored for indefinite period; which can be examined even after many years for further studies.

- The presence of causative agents can also be demonstrated in tissue sections using routine histopathological techniques or special stainings. In this Gram's staining procedures are used for demonstration of bacteria while viral inclusions are demonstrated using hematoxylin and eoxin or other staining techniques like Macchiavello's stain or Mann's methylene blue eosin method. The Negri bodies are demonstrated by Seller's stain in case of rabies in animals. In such cases, the isolation of causative agent or their serological examination does not require; since the presence of causal agent in infected tissues gives a confirmatory diagnosis.

- The detection of chemicals in tissues like enzymes, lipids etc. is included in histochemical examination; which not only describe the structural changes but also gives idea about the functional status of the organ.

Histopathological procedures

The microscopic examination of tissues or organs can be achieved by their smears or using vital staining or by sectioning; the latter method being more commonly used in histopathological laboratories.

Smears

The microscopic examination using smears of any organ/ tissue/ cells is very rapid method which gives the results within hrs. A drop of blood is placed on clean glass slide and with the help of another slide, the smear is prepared. In this the tissue pieces from organs are cut using a sharp knife and the cut surface is mildly touched with clean glass slides with some gentle pressure. Which gives an impression on the slide. This is also known as impression smear; generally 2-5 smears are prepared on a slide. If the collected tissue material is too less then it is being pressed between two slides and the impression thus obtained on both the slides are used for study. The wet smears are fixed with methanol and can be stored or transported to laboratory for examination. The impression smears of hippocampus, cerebellum and cerebrum of brain are very useful for demonstration of Negri bodies in rabid animals for diagnosis of rabies. The impression smears are stained with seller's stain for few seconds, washed and, air dried and examined under oil immersion microscope for the presence of inclusion bodies also known as Negri bodies. These inclusions are characterized by intracytoplasmic, eosinophillic appearance with basophilic granules and round to oval in shape with a clear hallo.

In case of pox infection in animals, the impression smears are prepared from scabe or pustule for demonstration of intracytoplasmic inclusions. Sometimes the viral inoculum is inoculated on chorioallantoic membrane (CAM) of embryonated eggs; the impression smears of CAM may yield the viral inclusions. In certain bacterial diseases like haemorrhagic septicemia and enterotoxemia, it becomes very difficult to demonstrate the organism in blood or in tissues. For confirmatory diagnosis, the material is inoculated in laboratory animals like mice, guinea pigs etc. The impression smears are then prepared from liver, spleen and other relevant organs of laboratory animals for demonstration of the organism.

Vital Staining

Vital staining procedures are not much in use directly in the diagnosis. However, for detection of phagocytic cells in body the vital stains are used. In the living animals when vital staining procedures are used for localization of phagocytic cells, these are known as *intravital*. *In vitro* use of vital stains is called as *spravital staining* which is being done for the live and dead lymphocyte count in leucocyte migration inhibition test (LMIT), lymphocyte stimulation test (LST), macrophage migration inhibition test (MMIT) and macrophage function tests (MFT).

Routine Histopathological Techniques of sectioning

The tissue pieces from morbid animals should be collected properly and fixed in a suitable fixative. Then these are processed and sections of 4-5 microns are cut and taken on slides. These sections are stained and mounted to make the permanent preparations of slides. The different steps required for making the tissue slides are described briefly as follows.

1. Collection of tissue

The collection of tissues is an important step, which is many times not given proper attention. The whole diagnostic process depends upon the collection of tissue pieces. A representative tissue should have been collected carefully and should have the normal as well as abnormal (lesion) part. The tissues must be collected by qualified person after a thorough examination of each organ/ system. Some times it has been observed that the collection of tissues is performed by attendants or rudely by the qualified persons and proper attention is not paid. It should be kept in mind that a representative tissue sample will only give the correct diagnosis which cannot be remedied/ altered afterwards. At the time of tissue collection following points must be kept in mind which will be beneficial for making a correct diagnosis.

- The tissue pieces from morbid animal should be collected as early as possible after the death of animal. Once the autolytic changes started in the dead body; it will not give true picture of microscopic lesions due to autolysis.
- At the time of tissue collection, it should be kept in mind that the representative tissue piece should include the part of lesion and a part of normal tissue, which facilitates the identification of organ/ tissue at the time of microscopic examination.

- The tissue pieces should be cut with sharp knife and using only one stroke. Blunt edge knife may require many attempts for cutting, which destroys the normal architecture of tissues.
- Tissue pieces for histopathological examination should be collected from all the organs. Some times it has been noticed that the tissue sample is taken from those part of body which shows gross lesions; merely absence of gross lesion does not mean that there will not be microscopic alteration. In many disease conditions only microscopic changes occur which do not exhibited grossly. Such selective collection of tissues gives a biased interpretation, so it is better to have tissues from all the organs for proper interpretation and unbiased conclusions of histopathological studies.
- Tissues should be collected directly in the fixative and not in any other pot or water. Sometimes it has been observed that at the time of post-mortem examination, the tissue samples are collected in petridishes or in bottle and bring to the laboratory, then fixative is added. This seems to be a wrong practice. The tissue bottles filled with 2/3 fixative must be available at the time of necropsy and tissue pieces should be collected directly in the fixative.
- The size of tissue piece should not be more than 5 mm; it facilitate the homogenous and smooth fixation. Large size tissues do not get fixed properly and in the middle, the tissue gets autolysed.
- The tissue pieces from hollow organs like intestines, oviduct etc should be cut transversely and placed on a hard paper, then it should be cut longitudinally in such a way that the serosal layer sticks to paper and mucosal layer gets free. Thereafter, it should be placed in fixative along with paper. This allows a good fixation and avoids the shrinkage and folding of tissue.
- At the time of post-mortem examination, it has been noticed that the faecal matter is removed from the intestines by pressing/ squeezing them or after opening the lumen

by sharp objects like knife, slides etc.; which causes damage in the mucosal layer. The representative tissue should not be collected from such damaged portions.
- The tissues from encapsulated organs should be collected alongwith capsule or covering. like brain should be collected alongwith meninges; kidneys and liver should be collected with their capsules. The coverings of such organs also yield useful information on histopathological examination.

2. Fixation

The fixation of tissues is required for preventing the post-mortem changes like autolysis and putrefaction by saprophytes, preservation of cellular constituents in life like manner and for hardening of tissues by way of conversion of semisolids to solid material. For a proper histopathological preparation and their interpretation, the role of fixative is very crucial. Any faulty fixation cannot be remedied at any later stage. An ideal fixative should be one that fixes the tissues quickly and should not interfere with the refractive index of the tissue components.

The choice of fixative depends on the type of investigation required, the formol saline (10% formaldehyde in 0.85% sodium chloride solution) is considered best fixative for routine histopathological studies. The buffered formalin has certain advantages over formol saline and now a days it is recommended for routine use in histopathological laboratories. The buffered formalin can also be used for immunopathological studies. Buffered formalin is widely used and preferred because of its tolerance; tissues can be left for longer period without excessive hardening or damage and sectioned easily. Since it has neutral pH, the formalin pigment is also not formed in the tissues. However, for immunopathological studies like immunoperoxidase staining techniques the fixative of choice is formol sublimate. But in the absence of that buffered formalin may also be used. The time required for proper fixation is 6-12 hrs for 5 mm thick block of tissue.

3. Washing

The tissue pieces after 6-12 hr fixation are taken out from fixative and cut into 2-3 small pieces of 2-3 mm size blocks. These blocks are, then, kept in tissue capsules or in a gauge tied off with the help of thread. The identification marks written by copying pencil are also kept along with tissues. These capsules/ gauge-containing tissues should be kept in running tape water overnight for at least 12 hrs.

4. Dehydration

In routine practice, the dehydration is done in ascending series of graded ethanol. The tissue blocks are kept in 50% ethanol and then in 70%, 80%, 90%, 95% absolute ethanol I and absolute ethanol II for one hour each. These ethanol graded series should be kept in tight glass stoppered bottle or in screw cap jars to prevent the evaporation. In last bottle of ethanol II sometimes the copper sulfate is layered in the bottom, covered with filter paper, which increases the life of ethanol as it absorbs the water from alcohol. But the care should be taken, as soon as the copper sulfate begins bluish due to absorption of water, the ethanol should be changed.

To increase the process of dehydration, the tissue blocks should be agitated either mechanically in an automatic tissue processor or by shaking the container periodically. The volume of alcohol should be at least 50 times more than the tissue placed for dehydration.

5. Clearing

Usually the clearing of tissue blocks is done in xylene. Like ethanol, xylene should also be kept in tightly stoppered bottle to prevent the evaporation. After dehydration the tissue blocks should be kept in ethanol and xylene (1:1) mixture for one hr, then the blocks are transferred to xylene I and xylene II for one hr each. If xylene is not available then benzene may be used for 3 hr as its action of clearing is slower than xylene. On complete clearing, the tissue becomes transparent, then they should be transferred in paraffin wax for impregnation.

6. Impregnation

For the impregnation of tissue blocks, the paraffin wax in used either in paraffin embedding bath or in oven fixed at 60-62°C temperature. Both the oven and embedding bath are electrically operated with thermostat to adjust the desired temperature. At the time of transfer of tissue blocks from xylene II, the paraffin wax must be kept at 60-62°C in liquid form for impregnation. Three changes are given in paraffin wax; each of one hr duration. The paraffin wax should be free from dust or other gross impurities; which can be removed by filtration through muslin cloth.

7. Casting of blocks

After 3 hr impregnation of tissue blocks in paraffin wax, the blocks are formed in moulds using molten wax. The tissues are placed in moulds in such a way that desired surface should remain down ward, which should be on the base of mould. The sections are cut from this surface, so care must be taken to keep the tissue in a proper manner which should be cut into sections homogenously. The mould is then filled with molten paraffin wax and then the blocks are cooled either at room temperature or in cold water. Various types of moulds like 'L' shaped or ring shaped can be used. If the moulds are not available, the blocks can be prepared in glass petri-dishes or in empty slide boxes. But care should be taken to lubricate the surface of such petri-dishes and other moulds with liquid paraffin or glycerine which facilitates the easy removal of blocks after cooling and hardening of paraffin wax.

8. Trimming

The blocks are removed from the moulds and are cut so as to give the one tissue per block and the wax is trimmed by knife or by rubbing on a hot plate in order to remove the extra wax on the either side of tissue. The tissue is exposed, which facilitate the side determination on which the section is to be cut. The identification of tissue should by fixed on one side of the block by touching the block with the small paper kept on it with hot forcep or knife, which bears the number. Then the blocks are fixed on block holder. Care should be taken that the number of marking of block should be kept on upper side at the time of trimming of the block on microtome to remove the extra wax and expose the whole surface of tissue. The trimming of blocks is done at 10-15µ and a separate knife should be used for trimming and section cutting.

9. Section cutting

Before the sectioning, the tissue blocks are cooled on ice or by keeping them in refrigerator. The tissue floatation bath should be cleaned and filled with water having a temperature of about 60-70°C. The blocks along with block holders are fixed in the microtome in such a way that the marking number will be on upper side, giving the similar position to the blocks as it was during trimming. Usually the sections are cut at 4-6µ thickness on rotary microtome using a plain edge knife. The knife should be sharp enough that it should cut the desired thickness sections in the form of a ribbon and will not cause damage to the tissue. By using a brush and forceps, the ribbon of tissue sections are placed in tissue floatation bath. The tissue sections will spread here due to melting of paraffin wax and will take the shape similar to the tissue of that block. One can make out the selection here; the best looking sections 1-5 can be lifted on a sticky glass slide, which should be kept in a tray at an angle so that the water is removed. The glass slides are made sticky by applying a sticky material on clean glass slides, which consists egg white and glycerine in 1:1 (V/V) ratio. The sticky material facilitate the sticking of sections on slides, which will not be damaged or removed during further processing of staining. Generally, 4-5 slides are made from each block and air dried in incubator or at room temperature. The following precautions should be taken at the time of section cutting:

Appendices

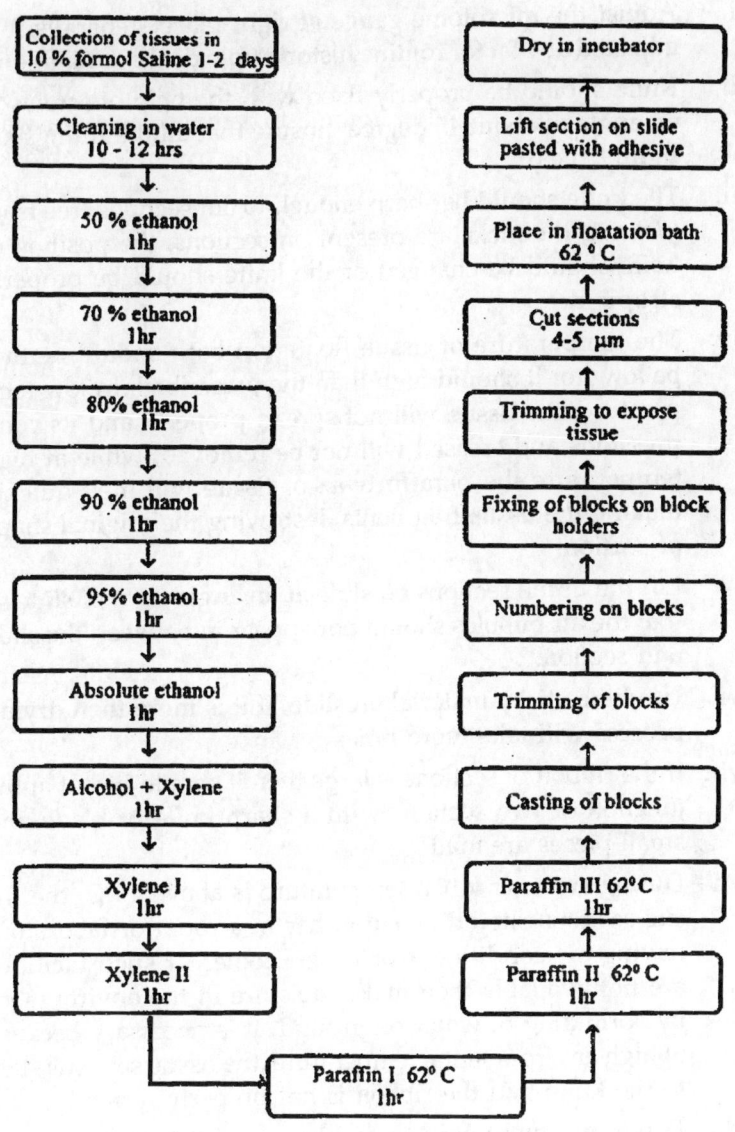

Flow Chart Showing Processing of Tissue for Histopathology

i. Adjust the microtome gauge at right place, generally it is adjusted at 4-5µ for routine histopathological examinations.
ii. Knife should be properly fixed with the help of screws at an angle of about 45 degree. Ensure that all the fittings are tightly fixed.
iii. The knife should be sharp enough to cut sections free from *nicks*. If the nicks are present on sections, the position of knife should be changed or the knife should be properly stropped.
iv. The temperature of tissue floatation bath should neither be low nor it should high than the prescribed. In low temperature, the tissue will not spread properly and its compressions and creased will not be removed, while at high temperature the paraffin wax of tissue will melt quickly making the tissue fragments destroying the original shape of section.
v. Lift the tissue sections on slide at an angle (45°) of slide so that the air bubbles should not appear in between the slide and section.
vi. Use little sticky material on slide, if it is more then drying process will take more time.
vii. If the ribbon of sections is large then it should be cut at the junction of two sections with a sharp knife or blade and small pieces are made.
viii. During summer when temperature is above 40°C, the tissue sections should be cut either in a room or laboratory having air conditioner or desert cooler. If such facilities are not available then make moisture in the environment by sprinkling of water on ground. It is necessary because at high environmental temperature, the tissue sections stick to the knife and the ribbon is not properly formed.
ix. Drive the microtome smoothly in a regular speed; jerks should not be given.
x. For marking the slides, use the diamond pencil and marking should be done at the time of section cutting itself.

10. Staining

(A) Routine procedure

After drying the slides are kept in slide cabinets. One slide of each block is selected for staining using the following procedures.

(a) *Removal of paraffin:*

The slides are slightly warmed either in incubator or at the flame of a spirit lamp and are placed in jar having xylene. Replace the xylene after 10-15 min with fresh xylene for another 10-15 min. This removes the paraffin from the tissue sections.

(b) *Rehydration*

After removal of paraffin, the slides are kept in descending series of alcohol. For this first they should be kept in absolute ethanol and xylene (1:1) mixture for 5 min; then in absolute ethanol, 95%, 90%, 80%, 70%, 50% ethanol for 5-6 min in each dilution. After that the slides are taken in water.

(c) *Cleaning of slides*

With the help of muslin cloth, clean the slides from both the sides. Leave only 1 or 2 section on a slide and remove the extra sections and/or paraffin wax. Wash the slides in running tape water.

(d) *Staining in hematoxylin*

Place the slides in Harris hematoxylin or Meyer's hematoxylin for 10-15 min. Shake the slides 2-3 times for proper staining. Remove the hematoxylin solution and wash the slides in running tape water, then dip in acid alcohol for few seconds, which helps in differentiation. Wash in tape water and place the slides in ammonia water for few seconds for blueing and place in running tape water in order to remove the ammonia.

(e) *Staining in eosin*

Place the slides in 2% aqueous eosin or alcoholic eosin for 2-5 min. After staining in eosin, quickly proceed for dehydration.

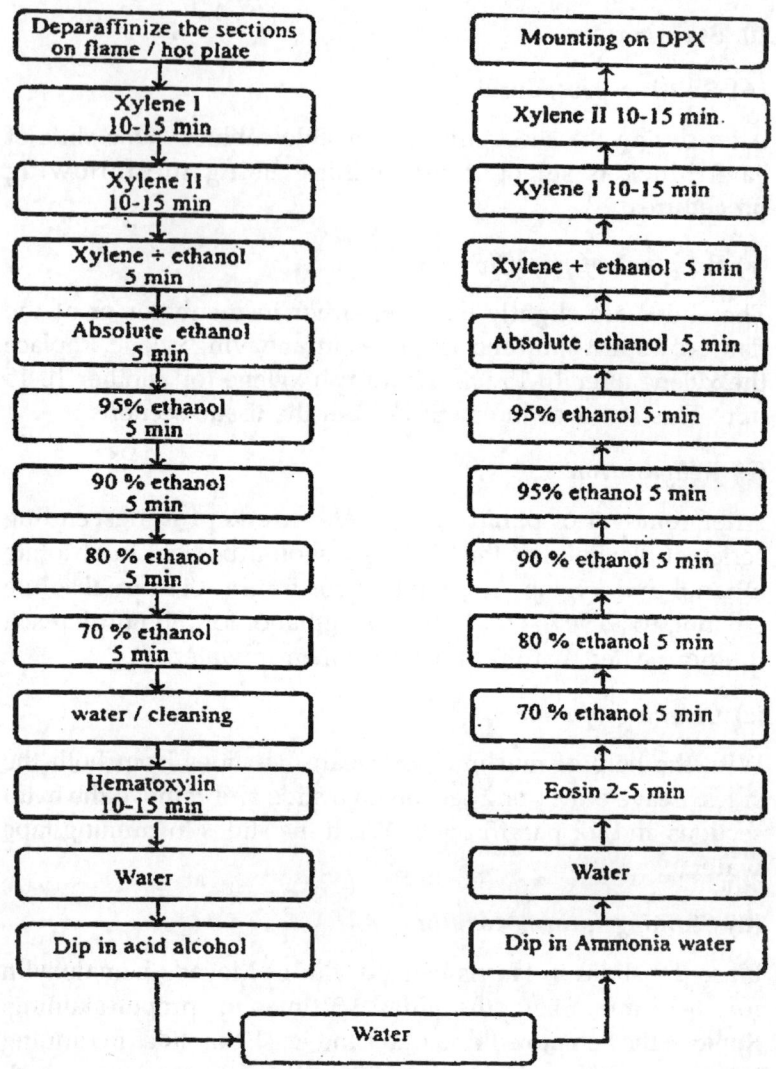

Flow Chart Showing Staining Procedure

(f) Dehydration

The slides are placed in 70%, 80%, 90% 95% Absolute ethanol for dehydration atleast for 5 min in each solution; then place them in absolute ethanol: xylene mixture (1:1) for 5 min.

(g) Clearing

Clear the sections in xylene and give 2 changes at least for 10-15 min each. The clearing in xylene II can be extended for even upto one hour.

(h) Mounting

Mount the slides with coverslip using Canada balsam or DPX mountant. For this the cover slips of desired size and shape are kept on filter paper and one or two drop of mountant is placed on coverslip. Takeout the slides from xylene and place on coverslip in such a way that the section is touched with mountant, press gently and lift the slide. Remove air bubble, if any, by pressing the coverslip with fine forcep and keep the slides in horizontal position in a tray for drying.

(i) Cleaning and labelling

After drying, clean the slides with muslin cloth and xylene. Remove the extra moutant using a blade. Label the slide with a piece of paper and stick it on one corner of slide using gum or other adhesive. At the time of examination, the histopathologist should put the name of organ, main changes in sections/ disease condition with other remarks on this label for future identification of the slide.

(j) Examination

On hematoxylin and eosin staining, the nuclei of the cells take blue stain while the cytoplasm is pink or red. Examine the tissue section using 10 x objective and if required then in high power or oil immersion. Precautions and important tips which should be considered at the time of staining:

i. Check the sections for staining after blueing in ammonia water for hematoxylin stain and after dehydration for eosin stain. If under stained then repeat the process or in case of overstained, the sections can be differentiated for some more time in acid alcohol to remove the excess hematoxylin and in ethanol for removing the excess eosin.

ii. Clean the slides thoroughly in water and remove all patches/ spots of paraffin; which gives a good look to slides.

iii. If on clearing in xylene, the cloudiness appears then repeat the dehydration process in absolute ethanol for 10-15 min. The cloudiness appears due to presence of water in the sections which reacts with xylene.

iv. At the time of mounting, ensure that the tissue section is not get dried. So to eliminate the chance of drying, proceed fast. Ensure the proper mounting of section on slides. Sometimes the opposite side of the section is mounted and section becomes dry. To ensure the proper mounting, one should feel/ touch the diamond pencil marking present on the same surface, then mount the sections. This can also be checked by touching the slide on reverse side for the presence/ absence of tissue sections.

v. Labelling with paper should be done on same side, at which the section is present; which will be helpful at the time of examination.

(B) Special procedures

In histopathological techniques, one can demonstrate bacteria, fungus, chlamydia, rickettsia or viral inclusions in the tissue sections by using special staining procedures. These special staining techniques, however, requires specific expertise but can be used in diagnostic laboratory as routine methods. Some important special staining techniques are described as under:

I. Staining for acid fast bacilli

The acid-fast bacilli are demonstrated in tuberculosis or Johne's disease in animals. The tissues are collected in formol saline or buffered formalin and processed in same manner as for routine histopathological techniques. For special staining of acid fast bacilli following procedures are followed:

Appendices

1. Deparaffinize the sections and hydrate in descending series of ethanol as described earlier.
2. Clean the slides in water and give a wash in distilled water for 5 min
3. Place the slides in carbol fuchsin solution and keep the chamber of slides in a water bath at 56°C for 1 hr.
4. Thereafter, remove the slides from water bath and keep at room temperature for few min, wash in running tape water. Dip in acid alcohol for differentiation till the colour of tissue become pale pink.
5. Wash in running tape water.
6. Place the slides in methylene blue working solution for few seconds, wash in tape water till the colour of sections becomes pale blue.
7. Dehydrate in ascending series of ethanol, clear in xylene and mount in and dPX as described earlier in histopathological procedures. Examine the slides under oil immersion. The acid fast bacilli will be of bright red in colour with a light blue back ground.
8. Precautions
(a) Care should be taken that at 56°C for 1 hr, the stain may get dry so it is always advisable to keep it in a covered jar in water bath to prevent drying.
(b) Differentiation with acid alcohol is very crucial step and should be controlled carefully; it depends on experience of a histopathologists to stain the slides properly.

II. Demonstration of Gram positive/ gram negative bacteria in tissue sections

    i. Deparaffinize and hydrate the sections to water, clean them.
    ii. Stain the slides with crystal violet for 2 min.
    iii. Wash in distilled water.
    iv. Keep the slides in Gram's iodine solution for 5 min.
    v. Wash in distilled water.

vi. Differentiate in cellosolve (Ethylene glycol monomethyl ether) until blue colour is no longer comes out from sections.

vii. Wash in distilled water and Place in basic fuchsin for 5 min and wash in distilled water.

viii. Place the slides in differentiating solution for 5 min., wash in distilled water and blot dry.

ix. Dip the slides in tetrazine for few seconds.

x. Place the slides in cellosolve 3 changes of 6 dip in each.

xi. Clear in xylene I and II for 15 min each.

xii. Mount in DPX

xiii. Examine the slides under oil immersion. The Gram positive bacteria will be of blue colour while gram negative will take a red colour against a yellow backgrounds.

III. Demonstration of spirochaetes

1. During post-mortem examination, cut about 1 mm thick slice of tissues from several sites of an organ and fix it in 10% buffered formalin for 24hrs, wash in running tape water overnight and place in 95% alcohol for 24hr.

2. Transfer the tissues in distilled water and keep till the tissues sinks to bottom.

3. Stain in silver nitrate at 37^0C in dark for 3-5 days and change the solution daily.

4. Wash in distilled water and place the tissues in reducing solution for 1-3 days.

5. Rinse in distilled water and dehydrate in ascending series of ethanol.

6. Clear in cedar wood oil for 2 hrs.

7. Impregnation/ embedding is done in paraffin wax as in case of routine histopathology, cut sections at 4-5µ, dry and deparaffinise in xylene (3 changes of 5 min each)

8. Clean the slides, remove artifacts and spots of paraffin wax

9. Mount 1-2 sections per slide with DPX
10. Examination is done under microscope; the spirochaete will be of black colour with yellow to light brown background.

IV. Demonstration of Fungi

1. Collect the tissues in formol saline or buffered formalin and process the samples in a same way as in routine histopathology and cut the section at 4-5µ, deparaffinize and hydrate to water.
2. Place the slides in 4% chromic acid for 1 hr.
3. Wash in running tape water and keep the slides in 1% sodium bisulfite solution for 3-5 min.
4. Wash in running tape water and then in distilled water.
5. Stain with methanamine-silver nitrate working solution at 60°C in water bath till sections become yellowish brown.
6. Wash in distilled water and place in gold chloride solution for 5 min.
7. Wash in distilled water and place in sodium thiosulfate solution for 5 min and wash in running tape water.
8. Stain with light green for 1 min, wash in water; dehydrate in ascending series of ethanol, clear in xylene and mount in DPX.
9. Examine the sections under microscope, the fungi will take a black colour, mycelia and hyphae will be of rose coloured with a pale green back ground.

V. Demonstration of rickettsia

1. Tissues are fixed in formol saline or buffered formalin and processed in same manner, sections of 4-5µ thick are cut, dried, deparaffinize and hydrated to water.
2. Place in methylene blue solution for overnight and decolourize in 95% ethanol for few seconds or till blue colour is lost.
3. Wash in distilled water and place the slides in basic fuchsin solution for 30 min.

4. Decolourize in citric acid solution for 1-2 sec.
5. Differentiate in absolute ethanol for few min, clear in xylene and mount in DPX.

Examine the slides, the rickettsia will be of bright red colour and nucleus of the cell will take blue colour.

Appendix VI

POST-MORTEM EXAMINATION OF VETEROLEGAL CASES

The post-mortem examination of veterolegal cases is performed as described in pervious sections. However, following points must be kept in mind while doing post-mortem examination and preparing the report.

1. For veterolegal cases, post-mortem request should be signed by a police officer not below the rank of inspector or by magistrate; without which no post-mortem examination should be done.
2. Always collect maximum information on history, date and time of death of animal and treatment given. Use self knowledge and experience to determine the time of death such as rigor morits, autolysis, putrefaction, pseudomelanosis etc.
3. Animal identification including species, breed, age and number or mark must be clearly established before conduct of post-mortem examination. It is specially necessary in insured animals as well as in religiously disputed cases.
4. All the lesions present on skin surface should be clearly defined as laceration, wound, trauma, incision, erosion, vesicle, ulcer and if there is suspected sharp edge wound or bullet injury also state its depth and width (diameter) as the case may be. Also mention the side on which the animal is lying down (ventral portion touching earth).
5. In case of dispute over still birth and calf born alive, a piece of lung should be placed in water. The lung piece will sink in water in case of atelectasis neonatum while it will float if the calf born alive.
6. If the case is suspected for toxic condition/ poisoning, try to mention the type of poison in your report. This will help the police authorities to establish/ confirm the type of toxin/ poison in forensic laboratory.
7. The post-mortem examination of wild animals should be conducted as a special case. One should conduct the post-

mortem examination only when DFO or higher officer is making request for post-mortem examination. It should be noted on the report that all the viscera including skin, bones, teeth, etc. are returned to the person requested for the necropsy and no item should be left behind.

8. Fill the post-mortem report clearly with neat hand writing and in clear language and avoid ambiguity in presentation. Avoid to write general sentences. Be specific to your findings and conclusions. Sign the report with date and must keep a copy of that with you for record and future evidences in the court of law.

9. Post-mortem examination should be conducted in day light. In darkness where the pathologist is not able to recognize the lesions, the post-mortem examination should not be conducted.

10. At the time of post-mortem examination outsiders should not be allowed. To avoid them and wild birds and animals, post-mortem examination should be done in close premises.

Appendix VII

COLLECTION, PRESERVATION AND DISPATCH OF MATERIAL TO FORENSIC LABORATORY

The collection, preservation and dispatch of different tissues/organs, fluids and viscera should be done as described in section 4 of appendix. However, in veterolegal cases, these materials should be sent to forensic laboratory under sealed packings.

1. In the suspected cases of toxic condition or poisoning, the stomach and intestinal contents should be sent after proper ligation at both the ends and sent it in ice to avoid putrefaction. Besides, samples of blood, liver, spleen and kidneys should be sent in separate container.
2. All the materials should be collected in leak proof glass or plastic bottles.
3. Tissues for histopathology must be collected in 10% formalin or formol saline, this can be sent to laboratory under normal temperature.
4. The materials suspected for toxicity should be sent in ice without adding any preservative.
5. The bottles or containers should be sealed and labelled properly indicating the name of owner, identification of animal (number, name, mark etc.), type of tissue collected and preservative used. The examination requested and disease or poisoning suspected should also be written.
6. A copy with details of post-mortem report and containing above information should be sent separately under separate cover.
7. The address of the forensic laboratory should be clearly written.
8. All the containers should be packed with cloth and sealed with sealing wax and should preferably be sent through person in order to avoid any breakage in transit.
9. One copy of the forwarding letter should be kept in file for future reference and one copy should accompany the material and one copy should be sent by post. The for-

warding letter bearing number and date should have the information about materials sent, type of preservative used, type of examination requested and identification of animals including other details of owner.

Appendix VIII

EXAMINATION OF BLOOD, URINE AND FAECES

BLOOD EXAMINATION

TOTAL ERYTHROCYTE COUNT

- Clean Neubauer's counting chamber/ hemocytometer and place clean coverslip on ruled areas.
- Suck fresh or anticoagulant mixed blood in RBC diluting pipette (red ball in bulb) upto 0.5 mark and fill the pipette with RBC diluting fluid upto 101 mark.
- Hold pipette in horizontal position and remove rubber tube. Mix the contents by rotating the pipette in between palms.
- Discard first few drops from pipette and then place a drop near the edge of cover slip to fill the space between cover slip and counting chamber.
- Keep counting chamber 1-2 min for settling of the cells.
- Count the cells under high power of the light microscope.
- Cells are counted in 5 medium squares of the central large square or 80 tertiary squares.
- Cells on top of square or left side are included in count.
- Calculate RBC per µl of blood by multiplying 10,000 to the total number of cells counted in 80 tertiary squares. It can be converted into ml by further multiplying with 1000 and in liter by 10,00,000.

TOTAL LEUCOCYTE COUNT

- Clean the New Bauer's chamber/ hemocytometer. Put the cover slip on the area demarcated for counting.
- Suck fresh/ anticoagulant mixed blood in WBC diluting pipette (white ball in bulb) upto 0.5 mark and fill the pipette with WBC diluting fluid upto 11 mark.
- Hold the pipette in horizontal position and remove rubber tube. Mix the contents by rotating the pipette in between palms.

- Discard first few drops from pipette and then place a drop near the edge of cover slip to fill the space between cover slip and chamber.
- Keep counting chamber 1-2 min for settling of the cells.
- Count the cells under low power in four large/ primary corner squares of the ruled area.
- Cells on top of square and left side are included in count.
- Calculate WBC per µl of blood by multiplying 50 to the total number of cells counted in 4 primary squares. It can be converted into ml by multiplying 1000 and in liter by 10,00,000.

PACKED CELL VOLUME (HEMATOCRIT VALUE)
- Clean and dry the wintrobe tube.
- With the help of a long needle (6") and syringe fill the blood in Wintrobe tube upto mark 100.
- Take precaution that there should not be any air bubble in the tube.
- Centrifuge the wintrobe tube at 3000 rpm for 30 min.
- Record the reading of packed cell volume in percent *i.e.* mass of erythrocytes settled down in tube.

ERYTHROCYTE SEDIMENTATION RATE
- Clean and dry Westergren pipette.
- Suck anticoagulant mixed blood in Westergren pipette upto mark 'O' and fix it in stand in vertical position
- Leave this for one hr at room temperature
- Record the reading on pipette, it is the mm fall of erythrocytes per hr.

HEMOGLOBIN
- It is measured by using Hellige- Sahli hemoglobinometer.
- Clean and dry the graduated tube of the hemoglobinometer.
- Take 5 drops of N/ 10 Hydrochloric acid in tube.

- Suck the anticoagulant mixed blood in pipette upto 20 marks.
- Place the pipette in tube containing N/10 HCL and transfer the blood into acid.
- Suck acid in pipette and leave in tube.
- Keep the tube for 5 min in dark.
- Add distilled water in the tube drop-by-drop using dropper, mix with stirring rod and match the colour with standard. Add water till the colour matches with standard.
- Read the scale on tube; it is the value of hemoglobin gram per 100 ml of blood.

DIFFERENTIAL LEUCOCYTE COUNT (DLC)

- Prepare a thin blood smear on clean glass slide. Place a drop of blood on one end of slide and spread as smear with the help of another slide using its edge at 45° angle.
- Dry the smear in air and mark identification number in the thick portion of smear.
- Fix the smear in methanol for at least 5 min and dry in air.
- Stain the smear with Giemsa stain diluted to 1:10 in distilled water for 30 min or with Leishman's stain without fixing the smear.
- Wash the slide, dry in air and examine under oil immersion microscope. Count at least 200 cells by battle ment/zigzag method. Cells counted are lymphocytes, neutrophils, monocytes, eosinophils and basophils. Cell count is presented in percent.

ABSOLUTE LYMPHOCYTE COUNT (ALC)

The absolute lymphocyte count is calculated by using the data of DLC and TLC through following formula:

$$\text{ALC}\left(10^3/\mu l\right) = \frac{\%\text{ Lymphocyte} \times \text{TLC}\left(10^3/\mu l\right)}{100}$$

ABSOLUTE NEUTROPHIL COUNT (ANC)

The absolute neutrophil count is calculated by using the neutrophil percentage of differential leucocyte count and total leucocyte count using following formula:

$$\text{ANC}\left(10^3/\ \mu l\right) = \frac{\%\text{Neutrophils} \times \text{TLC}\left(10^3/\ \mu l\right)}{100}$$

MEAN CORPUSCULAR VOLUME (MCV)

Mean corpuscular volume is determined by dividing the packed cell volume (PCV) by the total erythrocyte count in millions/ µl and multiplied by 10. The MCV is expressed in cubic microns.

$$\text{MCV}\ (\text{Cubic}\ \mu) = \frac{\text{PCV}}{\text{TEC}} \times 10$$

MEAN CORPUSCULAR HEMOGLOBIN CONCENTRATION (MCHC)

Mean corpuscular hemoglobin concentration is calculated by dividing the hemoglobin in grams per 100 ml of blood by the PCV and multiplied by 100. It is expressed in percent.

$$\text{MCHC}(\%) = \frac{\text{Hb}}{\text{PCV}} \times 100$$

MEAN CORPUSCULAR HEMOGLOBIN (MCH)

Mean corpuscular hemoglobin is calculated by dividing hemoglobin in gm per 100 ml by TEC in millions per µl of blood and multiply by 10.

$$\text{MCH}\left(10^{-12}\ g\right) = \frac{\text{Hb}}{\text{TEC}} \times 10$$

Appendices

ALTERATIONS IN HEMATOLOGICAL AND BIOCHEMICAL ATTRIBUTES IN VARIOUS DISEASE CONDITIONS OF ANIMALS

A. Hematological profile

1. **Erythrocytosis:** Brucellosis, Campylobacteriosis, Leptospirosis, Rinderpest, hemorrhagic septicemia.
2. **Erythropenia:** Leukemia, Haemorrhage, Aflatoxicosis, Theileriosis, Babesiosis, Anaplasmosis.
3. **Leucocytosis:** Pyogenic infections, Rabies, Tuberculosis, Strangles, Leptospirosis, Theileriosis Babesiosis, Anaplasmosis, Hemorrhagic Septicemia.
4. **Leucopenia:** Canine distemper, Infectious canine hepatitis, Swine fever, Brucellosis, Tuberculosis, Infectious bovine rhinotracheitis.
5. **Neutrophilia:** Acute inflammation, Pyogenic infections, Pyometra.
6. **Neutrophiliamth (shift to left):** Leptospirosis, metritis, Traumatic reticulopericarditis (TRP), Canine distemper, Glanders.
7. **Neutropenia:** Pasteurellosis, Infectious canine hepatitis.
8. **Lymphocytosis:** Leukemia, After vaccination, viral infections.
9. **Lymphopenia:** Canine distemper, Infectious canine hepatitis, Infectious bovine rhinotracheitis, Foot and mouth disease.
10. **Eosinophilia:** Allergy, Parasitic diseases.
11. **Hypohaemoglobinemia:** Anemia, Theileriosis, Strangles, Anaplasmosis, Degnala disease, Fasciolosis.
12. **Increased ESR:** Carcinoma, Nephritis, Chronic granulomatous infection, Tuberculosis, Canine distemper, Trypanosomiasis.
13. **Increased Hematocrit Value/ PCV:** Dehydration
14. **Decreased hematocrit Value/ PCV:** Anemia, Theileriosis, Strangles, Anaplasmosis, Blue tongue.

B. Biochemical attributes

1. **Hyperglycemia:** Diabetes mellitus, Chronic nephritis.
2. **Hypoglycemia:** Hepatic insufficiency, Ketosis.
3. **Hyperproteinemia:** Shock, Dehydration, Plasmacytoma, Infectious diseases.
4. **Hypoproteinemia:** Burn Diarrhoea, Renal dysfunction, Hepatic disorders, Tuberculosis.
5. **Hyperglobulinema:** Dehydration, Leukemia, Bacterial, Viral and parasitic infections.
6. **Hypogammaglobulinemia:** Anemia, Haemorrhage, Immunodeficiency.
7. **Hypercalcemia:** Hyperparathyroidism, bone cancer, Nephrolithiasis.
8. **Hypocalcemia:** Hypoparathyoidism, Rickets, Osteomalacia, Ketosis.
9. **Hyperphosphatemia:** Renal failure, Hypoparathyroidism, Healing of fracture.
10. **Hypophosphatemia:** Chronic diarrhoea, Pica, Rheumatism like syndrome, Hemoglobinuria. Hyperparathyroidism.
11. **Increased levels of Blood urea nitrogen:** Renal impairment, nephritis, Urinary obstruction.
12. **Decreased levels of BUN:** Acute hepatic insufficiency, nephrosis, Chronic wasting diseases
13. **Increased level of creatinine:** Severe nephritis, urinary obstruction, severe toxic nephrosis
14. **Hypermagnesemia:** Chronic infection, Oxalate poisoning
15. **Hypomagnesemia:** Grass tetany, Lactation tetany, Wheat pasture poisoning.
16. **Increased levels of SGOT:** Hepatic necrosis, Myocardial infarction, Muscular degeneration/ necrosis in dog and cat, Azoturia.
17. **Increased levels of SGPT:** Hepatic necrosis, Infectious canine hepatitis
18. **Increased levels of Alkaline phosphatase:** Obstructive

Appendices

jaundice, hepatitis, Hyperparathyroidism.
19. **Decreased level of Alkaline phosphatase:** Chronic nephritis.
20. **Increased level of Acid phosphatase:** Prostate carcinoma, Leukemia.
21. **Increased level of Lactic dehydrogenase:** Malignant lymphoma.
22. **Increased level of Serum isocitric dehydrogenase:** Hemolytic anemia in horses
23. **Increased level of Ornithine carbamyl transferase:** Liver disorders in dogs.

URINE EXAMINATION

PHYSICAL EXAMINATION

1. Colour:
- Note the colour of urine as
- Watery/ colourless
- Amber colour
- Red
- Brown
- Yellow/ Yellowish green
- Black
- Pale

2. Odour
- Record the smell of the urine
- Uremic
- Sweetish/ Fruity
- Fetid

3. Turbidity
- Look for the presence of suspended material in urine
- Clear
- Turbid +, ++, +++, +++
- Cloudy

4. Foaming
- Shake the urine in a test tube
- No/ Slight foams
- Yellow/ Green foams
- Red/ brown foams

5. Specific Gravity
- This is measured by urinometer
- Urine is filled in cylinder and urinometer is left in the urine
- Record the specific gravity in urinometer.

CHEMICAL EXAMINATION

1. Reaction
- Reaction is determined by using pH strips or pH meter.
- For this take a pH strip and dip in urine
- Read the change in colour on scale given with pH strips.

2. Glucose
- Take 0.5 ml urine in a clean and dry test tube.
- Mix 5.0 ml Benedict's reagent in the urine and keep it in boiling water bath/ flame for 5 min.
- Remove the tube and cool them on test tube stand.
- Record the changes of colour in tube as follows:
- Blue (-) No glucose
- Blue to green (+) mild glucose
- Yellow with heavy sediment (++) moderate glucose
- Orange with heavy sediment (+++) highly positive for glucose

3. Protein
- Take 2 ml of urine in a clean and dry test tube.
- Place 2 ml Robert's reagent over urine.
- If protein is present in urine, then a white ring will appear at the interjunction of two fluids. It is graded as follows:

Appendices

- No ring (-) negative
- Mild ring (+) mild positive
- A wide ring (++) moderate positive
- Heavy ring (+++) positive
- Very heavy ring (++++) highly positive

KETONE BODIES

1. Acetone

- Take 1.0 gm mixed powder of sodium nitropruside and ammonium sulfate (Sod. Nitropruside 1 part, Amm. Sulfate 100 parts) in a test tube.
- Add 5 ml urine in the salts and mix them properly.
- To this slowly overlay 20% ammonium hydroxide solution.
- Record the colour at the interjunction of two fluids.
- If it is red to purple then it is acetone positive.

2. Acetoacetic acid

- Take 10 ml urine in a clean and dry test tube.
- Add 5 drops of Lugol's iodine and 3 ml chloroform, mix them and allow to stand.
- Record the colour of urine

  Colourless   :   positive

  Red/ violet colour :   negative

3. Beta hydroxybutyric acid

- Take 20 ml urine in a small beaker and add 20 ml distilled water and few drops of acetic acid.
- Boil the contents over flame till it remains 10 ml, add distilled water to make it 20 ml and place in two test tubes 10 ml in each.
- In one test tube add 1 ml H_2O_2 and warm it for 1 min, cool it.
- Add 1 ml glacial acetic acid, 1 ml freshly prepared sodium

nitropruside solution in both tubes, mix thoroughly.
- To this overlay strong amonia water and allow to stand for 3-4 hrs.
- Record the change in colour in H_2O added tube if it is purple colour ring then it is positive.

Bile salts
- Take 4-5 ml urine in a test tube and shake it. If persistent foams are present then it is positive for bile salts.
- Add sulphur granules over surface of urine. In case of positive, sulphur granules will sink in urine.

Blood
- Take 2 ml urine in a test tube I.
- Take 1 ml saturated solution of Benzidine in test tube II. Add 1 ml 3% H_2O_2 and mix well
- Mix the contents of tube I and II.
- Record the development of colour. In positive case a green to blue colour will appear.

Hemoglobin/ Myoglobin
- Take 5 ml urine in a test tube.
- Add 2.8 gm ammonium sulfate
- Shake well and allow to stand for few min.
- If urine become clear/ watery in colour. Then it is positive for hemoglobin. If colour remains same as before the test then it is positive for myoglobin.

Microscopic examination
- Take 5-10 ml urine in a centrifuge tube and centrifuge it at 1000 rpm for 10 min.
- Discard supernatant and place a drop of sediment on clean, dry glass slide.
- Cover it with a cover slip and examine it under microscope for the followings:

- Epithelial cells
- Leucocyte
- Erythrocytes
- Microorganisms
- Casts

FAECAL EXAMINATION

GROSS EXAMINATION

- Collect feces in clean and dry petridish or in small sample bottle.
- With clean spatula and glass rod spread the faeces and note the followings:
    - Colour
    - Consistency
    - Odour
    - Presence of blood
    - Presence of parasite/ segments of parasite

MICROSCOPIC EXAMINATION

Direct Smear method

- Place a drop of distilled water on clean and dry glass slide.
- Add small amount of faeces in distilled water on slide.
- Mix with glass rod/ tooth pick/ matchstick.
- Place a cover slip on it.
- Examine under microscope for the presence of parasitic ova.

Qualitative concentration method (Simple floatation method)

- Take about 1.0 gm faeces and mix it in small amount of distilled water.
- Filter it through sieve/ muslin cloth.
- Filterate is mixed with 4-5 ml of saturated salt solution.
- Place the mixture in a tube or cylinder and fill it upto the top.

- A clean coverslip or glass slide is placed on the mouth of tube/ cylinder.
- Keep it for 30 to 60 min at room temperature.
- Remove the coverslip or slide and examine it under microscope for parasitic ova.

Qualitative concentration method (Centrifugation floatation method)

- Take about 1.0 gm faeces and mix it in small amount of distilled water.
- Mixture is filtered through fine sieve/ muslin cloth.
- Mix the filtrate with saturated salt solution (1:3) in a centrifuge tube.
- Centrifuge it at 1500 rpm for 5 min.
- Take a drop of superficial contents on a clean glass slide and examine under microscope.
- Sediment is examined for eggs of liver flukes.

Chapter **46**

Self Assessment – MCQ

Select most appropriate word(s) from the four options given with each question.

1. INTRODUCTION

1. The process of phagocytosis by macrophages was first described by...............
   (a) B. Muller   (b) E. Metchnikoff
   (c) Bittner   (d) Bichat

2. First Veterinary School was established in the year ....
   (a) 1762   (b) 1884   (c) 1889   (d) 1773

3. The Originator of modern Experimental Pathology is ....
   (a) R. Koch   (b) J. Cohnheim
   (c) John Hunter   (d) R. Virchow

4. Study of tumors is known as ....
   (a) Cytopathology   (b) Clinical Pathology
   (c) Chemical Pathology (d) Oncology

5. Study of zoonotic diseases fall under the branch of .... Pathology.
   (a) Nutritional   (b) Comparative
   (c) Experimental   (d) Systemic

6. Humoral Pathology is the study of alterations in...............in animals.
   (a) Antibodies   (b) Fibrin   (c) Urine   (d) Faeces

7. Immunodeficiency disorders of animals falls under the branch of ....
   (a) Cytopathology   (b) Humoral Pathology
   (c) Microscopic Pathology   (d) Immunopathology
8. General Pathology does not include one of the following activity
   (a) Fatty changes   (b) Embolism
   (c) Inflammation   (d) Digestive system disorders.
9. Examination of dead animals is known as ....
   (a) Necropsy   (b) Autopsy
   (c) Lethopsy   (d) Microscopy
10. Nutritional roup is an example of .... Pathology
    (a) Chemical   (b) Nutritional
    (c) Humoral   (d) Postmortem

2. ETIOLOGY

1. Hog cholera occurs in.......................
   (a) Pig   (b) Dog   (c) Horse   (d) Cow
2. Partial loss of epithelium on skin or mucous membrane is known as.................
   (a) Abrasion   (b) Erosion
   (c) Laceration   (d) Contusion
3. Burn area of skin and tissues remains sterile till..........
   (a) 12 hrs   (b) 16 hrs   (c) 20 hrs   (d) 24 hrs
4. Epidermis and dermis are destroyed leading to shock in ....burn.
   (a) I degree   (b) II degree
   (c) III degree   (d) IV degree
5. Radiation affects the dividing cells of.......
   (a) Ovary   (b) Testes
   (c) Lymphocytes (d) All of the above
6. Leptospira is a......... which causes abortions in cattle.

Self Assessment – MCQ

    (a) Bacteria   (b) Virus
    (c) Chlamydia   (d) Spirochaete

7. *Coxiella burnetti* is a...... which causes Q-fever in animals.
   (a) Mycoplasma   (b) Bacteria
   (c) Rickettsia   (d) Chlamydia

8. Ringworm is caused by a.......
   (a) Bacteria (b) Virus (c) Fungi (d) Parasite

9. Transmission of diseases from one generation to another is known as.......
   (a) Vertical   (b) Horizontal
   (c) Triangular   (d) All of the above

10. Aflatoxins are produced by..........
    (a) *Aspergillus flavus*   (b) *Asperfillus parasiticus*
    (c) *Penicillium puberlum*   (d) All of the above

11. Pesticides includes......
    (a) Insecticide   (b) Rodenticide
    (c) Weedicide   (d) All of the above

12. Acetone, b-hydroxybutyrate and acetoacetic acid are known as.......
    (a) Ochratoxins   (b) Ketone bodies
    (c) Heinze bodies   (d) Pyknotic bodies

13. Prolonged starvation leads to................... of muscles
    (a) Hypertrophy   (b) Hyperplasia
    (c) Atrophy   (d) Metaplasia

14. Deficiency of vitamin A causes....................
    (a) Nutritional roup   (b) Nyctalopia
    (c) Calculi in urethra   (d) All of the above

15. Vitamin D regulates the activity of......................
    (a) Lymphocytes   (b) Macrophages
    (c) All of the above   (d) None of the above

16. Star grazing in chicks in caused by .... deficiency

(a) Vitamin B1   (b) Vitamin B2
(c) Vitamin B6   (d) Vitamin B12
17. Curled toe Paralysis is caused by .... deficiency
    (a) Thiamine   (b) Riboflavin
    (c) Choline   (d) Biotin
18. Crazy chick disease is caused by .... deficiency
    (a) Vitamin A   (b) Vitamin C
    (c) Vitamin D   (d) Vitamin E
19. Perosis is caused by .... deficiency.
    (a) Biotin   (b) Choline
    (c) Manganeese (d) All of the above
20. Rheumatism like syndrome is caused by deficiency of ....
    (a) Calcium (b) Phosphorous (c) Copper (d) Zinc

3. GENETIC DISORDERS, DEVELOPMENTAL ANOMALIES AND MONSTERS

1. Each chromosome contains the DNA content as...................
   (a) 20%   (b) 10%   (c) 70%   (d) 30%
2. The study of karyotyping of chromosomes falls under ....
   (a) Immunogenetics   (b) Cytogenetics
   (c) Moleculer genetics (d) Nuclear genetics.
3. In heterozygous, one gene character is manifested in phenotype and such gene is called as...
   (a) Autosomal   (b) Recessive
   (c) Dominant   (d) Sex linked
4. In karyotyping, colchicine is added in culture of peripheral blood lymphocytes for arresting the cell division in ....
   (a) Telophase   (b) Meiosis
   (c) Anaphase   (d) Metaphase

Self Assessment – MCQ

5. In heteroploidy, the chromosome number will be ....in cells.
    (a) n   (b) 2n   (c) 3n   (d) All of them
6. Intersexes is the condition in animals which occurs due to ambiguity in................
    (a) Genitalia   (b) Bones   (c) Ears   (d) Eyes
7. In Turner's syndrome, mare is having karyotype as......................
    (a) XX   (b) XXX   (c) XXXX   (d) XO
8. Mules are having chromosome number as............
    (a) 61   (b) 62   (c) 63   (d) 64
9. Bovine lymphosarcoma occurs in animals having chromosome number........
    (a) 60   (b) 61   (c) 62   (d) 64.
10. Dogs are more prone to lymphoma with chromosome number.........
    (a) 76   (b) 78   (c) 77   (d) 75
11. Absence of lower jaw in foetus is known as.............
    (a) Acrania   (b) Adactylia
    (c) Agnathia   (d) Abrachia
12. Rachischisis is a cleft in ....
    (a) Spinal column   (b) Abdomen   (c) Skull   (d) Lips
13. Hare lip is due to fissure in lips and also known as..............
    (a) Palatoschisis   (b) Cranioschisis
    (c) Schistosomus   (d) Cheilioschisis
14. Fusion of eyes occurs in monsters and is known as...................
    (a) Renarcuatus   (b) Columbia
    (c) Cyclopia   (d) Anophthalmia
15. Increased number of limbs in monsters is known as ....
    (a) Polythelia   (b) Polymastia
    (c) Polymelia   (d) Polydactylia

16. Dextrocardia is transposition of heart in.............
    (a) Right thorax   (b) Left thorax
    (c) Neck   (d) Abdomen
17. Tumor arising from embryonic defect and composed of more than two tissue.....
    (a) Dermatoma   (b) Hematoma
    (c) Papilloma   (d) Teratoma
18. A monster having two separate brains with bodies separately arranged at an acute angle......
    (a) Cephalothoracopagus   (b) Dicephalus
    (c) Craniopagus   (d) Cranioschisis
19. A monster united at thorax region and with complete development as twin is known as.........
    (a) Prosopothoracopagus   (b) Thoracopagus
    (c) Dipygus   (d) Cephalothoracopagus
20. A monster having thorax and lumber portion of vertebral column united in twin is known as.....
    (a) Rachipagus   (b) Craniopagus
    (c) Thoracopagus   (d) Dipagus

4. DISTURBANCES IN GROWTH

1. Cerebral hypoplasia in calves is caused by..............
   (a) Adenovirus   (b) Rotavirus
   (c) Bovine viral diarrhoea virus   (d) Coronavirus
2. Increase in size of cells leading to size of organ is known as............
   (a) Atrophy   (b) Hyperplasia
   (c) Hypertrophy   (d) Metaplasia.
3. Fibrosis may lead to ....
   (a) Atrophy   (b) Hyperplasia
   (c) Dysplasia   (d) Hypertrophy
4. Transformation of one type of cells to another cell type is known as ....

(a) Hypoplasia   (b) Dysplasia
(c) Anaplasia   (d) Metaplasia

5. Reversion of cells towards embryonic type is known as........
   (a) Anaplasia   (b) Neoplasia
   (c) Metaplasia (d) Hypoplasia

6. Spermatozoa with defective head and tail piece is an example of ....
   (a) Dysplasia   (b) Anaplasia
   (c) Neoplasia   (d) Metaplasia

7. Hyperchromasia in cells with their enlargement is known as ....
   (a) Hyperplasia (b) Hypertrophy
   (c) Metaplasia (d) Anaplasia

8. Increased number of cells leading to increase in size and weight of organ is known as.........
   (a) Hypertrophy (b) Anaplasia
   (c) Hyperplasia (d) Metaplasia

9. Environmental pollution may lead to .... of lymphoid organs.
   (a) Atrophy (b) Aplasia (c) Agenesis   (d) Hypoplasia

10. Failure of an organ to develop its full size is known as ......
    (a) Hyperplasia (b) Aplasia
    (c) Neoplasia   (d) Hypoplasia

5. DISTURBANCES IN CIRCULATION

1. Petechial haemorrhage are of .... size.
   (a) 1 mm   (b) 2 mm   (c) 5 mm   (d) 10 mm

2. Parasitic emboli are formed in dogs due to ....
   (a) *Strongylus* spp   (b) *Dirofilaria immitis*
   (c) *Coccidia* spp.   (d) *Sarcoptes canis*

3. Metrorrhagia is haemorrhage from ....
   (a) Intestine   (b) Stomach
   (c) Oviduct   (d) Uterus
4. Septic thrombus must have........................ in it.
   (a) Virus   (b) Parasite   (c) Fungi   (d) Bacteria
5. Presence of foreign material in blood vessels is known as ....
   (a) Thrombus   (b) Emboli   (c) Ischemia   (d) Infarction
6. Accumulation of fluid in peritoneal cavity is known as..........
   (a) Anasarca   (b) Hydropericardium
   (c) Hydrothorax   (d) Ascites
7. Shock is circulatory disturbance characterized by ....
   (a) Reduced blood volume   (b) Reduced blood flow
   (c) Hemoconcentration   (d) All of the above
8. Active hyperemia is accumulation of blood in ....
   (a) Veins   (b) Lymphatics   (c) Arteries   (d) Intestines
9. Escape of all blood constituents through intact blood vessel is known as..........
   (a) Rhexis   (b) Ecchymosis
   (c) Petechiae   (d) Diapedesis
10. Erythrophagocytosis is a feature of ....
    (a) Congestion   (b) Oedema
    (c) Sludged blood   (d) Infarction

6. DISTURBANCES IN CELL METABOLISM
1. Hydropic degeneration leads to .... formation in skin.
   (a) Vesicle   (b) Pustule   (c) Scab   (d) Papule
2. Cloudy swelling is characterized by hazy cytoplasm due to swollen ....

(a) Endoplasmic reticulum (b) Golgi bodies
(c) Mitochondria (d) Nucleus
3. The mucous containing cells in mucous membranes are known as ....
   (a) Epithelial cells (b) Pearl cells
   (c) Columnar cells (d) Goblet cells
4. Mucin stains .... by H&E stain.
   (a) Blue (b) Pink (c) Yellow (d) Black
5. Sago spleen is observed in ....
   (a) Amyloid (b) Mucin (c) Hyaline (d) Pseudomucin
6. Epithelial pearl is an example of ....
   (a) Amyloid (b) Mucin (c) Hyaline (d) Cell Swelling
7. Ketosis in cow may cause...............
   (a) Hyaline degeneration (b) Fatty change
   (c) Amyloid (d) Cell swelling
8. Mucous degeneration in intestine is caused by ....
   (a) Rotavirus (b) *E. Coli* (c) Ascaris (d) All of the above
9. Corticosteroid therapy may lead to ....
   (a) Fatty changes (b) Hyaline
   (c) Glycogen (d) Cell swelling
10. Amyloid occurs in body as a result of ....
    (a) Immune complexes (b) Antigen
    (c) Antibody (d) Starch

7. NECROSIS, GANGRENE AND POST-MORTEM CHANGES

1. In liquifactive necrosis.............. cells are present
   (a) Monocytes (b) Lymphocytes
   (c) Eosinophils (d) Neutrophils
2. Programmed cell death is known as .... in living body.

(a) Apoptosis (b) Necrosis
(c) Autolysis (d) None of the above
3. Chalky white deposits are observed in .... necrosis
   (a) Coagulative (b) Liquefactive
   (c) Fat (d) Caseative
4. Gangrene in lungs is an example of .... grangrene.
   (a) Dry (b) Moist (c) Gas (d) All of the above
5. Degnala disease is an example of .... gangrene
   (a) Dry (b) Moist
   (c) Gas (d) None of the above
6. Digestion of cells/ tissues by their own enzymes is known as ....
   (a) Necrosis (b) Autolysis
   (c) Gangrene (d) Putrefaction
7. Greenish discolouration of tissues after death is also known as ....
   (a) Pseudomelanosis (b) Melanosis
   (c) Necrosis (d) Imbibition of bile
8. Algor mortis is the .... of body.
   (a) Staining with hemoglobin (b) Cooling
   (c) Hardening (d) Softening
9. Rigor mortis remains in body .... hrs
   (a) 12-15 hrs (b) 20-30 hrs
   (c) 35-48 hrs (d) 5-10 hrs
10. Lysis of chromatin material is known as ....
    (a) Karyolysis (b) Karyorhexis
    (c) Chromatolysis (d) Caseation

8. DISTURBANCES IN CALCIFICATION AND PIGMENT METABOLISM

1. Dystrophic calcification occurs in animals due to ....

Self Assessment – MCQ

   (a) Tuberculosis (b) Parasitic infection (c) Necrosis
   (d) All of the above
2. Melanosis is the brown/ black discolouration of tissue/ organ as a result of excessive accumulation of melanin due to ....
   (a) Hyperadrenalism (b) Hyperthyroidism
   (c) Hyperparathyroidism (d) Hypermelanemia
3. Hemosidern is...............colour pigment.
   (a) Green (b) Red (c) Golden Yellow (d) Blue
4. Urobilinogen is the ....form of bilirubin.
   (a) Unconjugated (b) Conjugated and reduced
   (c) Conjugated (d) Conjugated and oxidised
5. Hemolysis may give rise to............
   (a) Prehepatic icterus (b) Posthepatic icterus
   (c) Toxic icterus (d) None of the above
6. Obstructive jaundice occurs as a result of
   (a) Hemolysis (b) Liver necrosis
   (c) Cholangitis (d) Prioplasmosis
7. Indirect Van den Bergh reaction is an indication of...............
   (a) Obstructive icterus (b) Hemolytic icterus
   (c) Hepatic jaundice (d) None of the above
8. Deposition of carbon particles in lungs is known as............
   (a) Silicosis (b) Asbestosis
   (c) Pneumoconiosis (d) Anthracosis
9. Gout is the deposition of............... in tissues.
   (a) Uric acid crystals (b) Oxalate crystals
   (c) Hemosiderin (d) Urobilin
10. The absence of............... in poultry is the main cause of gout.
    (a) Trypsin (b) Lymphnodes (c) Amylase (d) Uricase

9. INFLAMMATION AND HEALING

1. Inflammation is implementation of ....
   (a) Cardinal signs (b) Blood vascular changes
   (c) Immunity   (d) Fibroplasia
2. Which one of the following is not a cardinal sign of inflammation ....
   (a) Redness (b) Pain   (c) Edema   (d) Heat
3. Inflammation of gums in known as.........
   (a) Cheilitis (b) Gingivitis   (c) Glossitis (d) Orchitis
4. Inflammation of ovary is known as ....
   (a) Uveitis   (b) Urethritis
   (c) Oophoritis   (d) Metritis
5. Primary granules of neutrophils contain.........
   (a) Lactoferin   (b) Lysozyme
   (c) Myeloperoxidase   (d) Lipase
6. Lecucocytes marginate during vasodilation and comes out from blood vessels through pseudopodia movement; the process is known as.........
   (a) Diapedesis   (b) Rhexis
   (c) Pavementation   (d) Leucopenin
7. Macrophages become elongated with marginal nuclei to kill the acid fast bacteria and are known as ....
   (a) Giant cells   (b) Epithelial cells
   (c) Epithelioid cells   (d) Plasma cells
8. Langhans type of giant cells are observed in lesions in.............
   (a) Tuberculosis   (b) Neoplasms
   (c) Leukemia   (d) Rinderpest
9. Lymphocytes modified to produce antibodies is known as ....
   (a) T- helper cells   (b) T-cytotoxic cells
   (c) Plasma cells   (d) Epithelioid cells

Self Assessment – MCQ

10. Fibroblasts proliferates in ....inflammation.
    (a) Acute   (b) Subacute
    (c) Per acute   (d) Chronic
11. C_3a, C_5a and C_4a are the complement components which are also known as .....
    (a) Anaphylotoxin   (b) Prostaglandins
    (c) Vasoactive amines   (d) None of the above
12. Cytokines are ....in action.
    (a) Autocrine   (b) Paracrine
    (c) Endocrine   (d) All of the above
13. Tumor necrosis factor or cytotoxins are produced by macrophages and T-cells and are associated with ....in tumor.
    (a) Necrosis   (b) Necrobacillosis
    (c) Degeneration   (d) Apoptosis
14. Coating of foreign particles/ bacteria by immunoglobulins to make it more readily palatable by phagocytic cells is known as ....
    (a) Opsonization   (b) Adherence
    (c) Chemotaxis   (d) Digestion
15. Catarrhal inflammation is characterized by increased number of..........
    (a) Goblet cells   (b) Neutrophils
    (c) Giant cells   (d) Epithelial cells
16. Fibrinous inflammation is characterized by the presence of ....as principal constituent of exudates.
    (a) Serum   (b) Neutrophils   (c) Fibrin   (d) Fibroblasts
17. The principal constituent of purulent exudates is ....
    (a) Serum   (b) Plasma
    (c) Neutrophils   (d) Eosinophils
18. Granulomatous inflammation is chronic in nature and is found in ....

(a) Tuberculosis (b) Rinderpest
(c) Canine distemper (d) H.S.
19. In parasitic and allergic diseases, ...inflammation is mostly seen.
   (a) Fibrinous (b) Hemorrhagic
   (c) Eosinophilic (d) Granulomatous
20. Granulation tissue is found in ....
   (a) Tuberculosis (b) Johne's disease
   (c) Repair (d) Rinderpest

10. CONCRETIONS

1. Calculi are stone like bodies which have ....origin.
   (a) Endogenous (b) Hematogenous
   (c) Exogenous (d) None of the above
2. Piliconcretions are made up of ....
   (a) Plant fibers (b) Polythenes
   (c) Hairs (d) Desquamated cells
3. Urinary calculi are formed in renal tubules and in horse they are made up of ....
   (a) Calcium carbonate (b) Calcium phosphate
   (c) Magnesium carbonate (d) All of the above
4. Choleliths may cause ....
   (a) Toxic jaundice (b) Post hepatic Jaundice
   (c) Prehapatic jaundice (d) Hemolytic jaundice
5. Sialoliths occur in ....
   (a) Pancreas (b) Salivary gland
   (c) Sinus (d) Seminal vesicle
6. Coprolith may occur in dogs due to presence of ....in food.
   (a) Sand (b) Muscles (c) Plant fibers (d) Bones
7. Cholelithiasis may lead to inflammation of ....

(a) Gall bladder (b) Intestine
(c) Stomach (d) Pancreas
8. Enteric calculi are more common in horse due to feeding of ....
(a) Grams (b) Wheat bran (c) Grass (d) Beans
9. Polyconcretions are formed due to accumulation .... in G.I. Tract.
(a) Hairs (b) Polysaccharides
(c) Polyuria (d) Polythenes
10. Vitamin .... deficiency may lead to formation of urinary calculi.
(a) A (b) B (c) D (d) K

11. IMMUNITY AND IMMUNOPATHOLOGY

1. This animal is not resistant to feline panleucopoenia virus infections
   (a) Dog (b) Cattle (c) Cat (d) Pig
2. Natural or paraspecific immunity does not include ....
   (a) Tears (b) NK Cells
   (c) Cytokines (d) Sensitized Tc cells
3. A foreign material capable of inducing the production of antibodies in animal is known as ......
   (a) Agglutinin (b) Antigen
   (c) Antipyretic (d) Antidote
4. Antibodies are chemically .... in nature
   (a) Lipopolysaccharide (b) Lipid
   (c) Glycoprotein (d) Protein
5. Which of the following is not an adjuvant
   (a) Oil (b) Wax (c) Alum (d) Glucose
6. Serum contains mainly this antibody..............
   (a) IgG (b) IgM (c) IgA (d) IgD

7. IgD is found abundantly in ....
   (a) Cow   (b) Rat   (c) Sheep   (d) Horse
8. IgE is found in very low concentration in serum which has the property to bind with receptors present on ....cells
   (a) Neutrophils   (b) Eosinophils
   (c) T- lymphocytes   (d) Mast cells
9. IgD in not found in serum due to lysis by ....during clotting
   (a) Bacteria   (b) Proteaes
   (c) Endonucleases   (d) Peroxidases
10. Processing of antigen by macrophages is comparatively less efficient due to lysis of antigen by ...
    (a) Proteases   (b) Peroxidases
    (c) Endonucleases   (d) Lipases
11. There is a latent period in antibody production on exposure to any antigen which is ....
    (a) 6 days   (b) 20 days   (c) 25 days   (d) 4 weeks
12. The peak antibody titres are found at ....
    (a) 2 days   (b) 20 days   (c) 2 weeks   (d) 4 weeks
13. The exogenous antigen are processed in dendritic cells/ macrophages and along with ....molecule it is presented to Th cells.
    (a) MHC class Ia   (b) MHC class II
    (c) MHC class III   (d) MHC class Ib
14. T-cytotoxic cells recognize ....specifically to destroys them.
    (a) Bacteria   (b) Virus
    (c) Antigen containing cells   (d) Fungi
15. Anaphylaxis is also known as ....Hypersensitivity
    (a) Type I   (b) Types II
    (c) Type III   (d) Type IV

16. Equine infectious anemia virus may cause ....hypersensitivity
    (a) Type I   (b) Types II (c) Type III   (d) Type IV
17. Reagin type of antibody is ......
    (a) IgA   (b) IgD   (c) IgM   (d) IgE
18. DTH reaction is mediated by ....
    (a) IgA   (b) IgG   (c) IgM   (d) Sensitised T –cells
19. Combined immunodeficiency syndrome occurs as a result of absence of ....
    (a) Stem cells   (b) B-cells
    (c) T-cells   (d) Macrophages
20. Autoimmunity develops in body when immune mechanisms are directed towards .... antigens.
    (a) Self (b) Foreign (c) Protein (d) Bacterial
21. In respiratory mucosa secretions, this antibody is mainly found.
    (a) IgG   (b) IgM   (c) IgA   (d) IgE
22. Corticosteroids binds with receptors present on ....cells leading to decrease in antibody production.
    (a) T- helper   (b) Macrophages
    (c) B-cells   (d) T-suppressor
23. Canine distemper virus activates the ....cells
    (a) T-helper cells   (b) T-suppressor cells
    (c) B-cells   (d) Macrophages
24. Surgery may enhance the activity of ....cells and therefore modulate the immune response.
    (a) T- helper cells   (b) T-suppressor cells
    (c) T- Cytotoxic cells   (d) Macrophges
25. Pesticides are common contaminants of environment and may induce .... in animals
    (a) Immunosuppression   (b) Autoimmunity
    (c) Hypersensitivity   (d) All of the above
26. Lead, mercury and cadmium are .... leading to immunosuppression.

(a) Immunotoxic   (b) Nephrotoxic   (c) Hepatotoxic
(d) Neurotoxic

27. Aflatoxin may cause .... in animals.
    (a) Immunopotentiation
    (b) Immunosuppression
    (c) Activation of macrophages
    (d) Reduction of complement

28. Aspirin decreases ....
    (a) Antibody production   (b) Phagocytosis
    (c) All to the above   (d) None of the above

29. Bovine viral diarrhoea virus reduces............................
    (a) T-suppressor cells   (b) IL-1
    (c) IL-2   (d) Interferon

30. Equine herpes virus (EHV-1) causes reduction in ......
    (a) B-cell   (b) T-cells   (c) Macrophages   (d) NK cells

12. PATHOLOGY OF CUTANEOUS SYSTEM

1. In congenital icthyosis, the skin of calves resembles with the skin of ....
   (a) Toad   (b) Fish   (c) Tortoise   (d) Zebra

2. Acanthosis is .... of skin epithelium.
   (a) Hypoplasia   (b) Aplasia
   (c) Hyperplasia   (d) Anaplasia

3. Vesicle formation occurs in skin as a result of ....
   (a) Cloudy swelling   (b) Hydropic degeneration
   (c) glycogen storage   (d) Fatty change

4. Acariasis is caused by ....
   (a) Bacteria   (b) Virus   (c) Chlamydia   (d) Mite

5. Enlargement of seald off hair follicle or sebaceous gland is known as ....
   (a) Acne   (b) Folliculitis   (c) Fissure   (d) Bleb

6. A break in the continuity of the epidermis exposing dermis is known as ....

(a) Erosion (b) Ulcer (c) Fissure (d) Vesicle

7. Hyperkeratosis is the thickening of ....
   (a) Prickle cell layer   (b) Stratum lucidum
   (c) Stratum corneum   (d) Dermis

8. Superficial loss of epithelium on skin or mucous membrane is known as ....
   (a) Erosion (b) Abrasion (c) Ulcer (d) Fissure

9. Papule is hyperplasia of .... Epithelium.
   (a) Stratum corneum   (b) Stratum lucidum
   (c) Stratum spinosum   (d) Dermis

10. Retention of nucleus in keratin layer of skin is known as ....
    (a) Hyperkeratosis   (b) Parakeratosis
    (c) Urticaria   (d) Acanthosis

13. PATHOLOGY OF MUSCULOSKELETAL SYSTEM

1. Equine rhabdomyolysis is also known as .... morning disease
   (a) Sunday   (b) Monday
   (c) Tuesday   (d) Wednesday

2. Accumulation of .... is responsible for hardening of muscles in azoturia.
   (a) Lactic acid   (b) Myoglobin
   (c) Haemoglobin   (d) Glycogen

3. White muscle disease is caused by .... deficiency.
   (a) Vit-A (b) Vit-D (c) Vit-C (d) Vit-E

4. Rickets is caused by deficiency of vitamin...............
   (a) A (b) D (c) C (d) E

5. Osteoporosis is caused by deficiency of ....
   (a) Copper (b) Zinc (c) Iron (d) Calcium

6. Osteopetrosis is also known as .... disease
   (a) Brittle bone   (b) Marble bone
   (c) Both a & b   (d) None

7. Fibrous osteodystrophy is characterized by .... condition
   (a) Lock jaw	(b) Rubbery jaw
   (c) Bottle jaw	(d) None
8. Osteomyelitis is inflammation of ....
   (a) Bone	(b) Bone marrow
   (c) Both a & b	(d) None
9. *Brucella* sp may cause .... in animals and man.
   (a) Pulmonary osteoarthropathy	(b) Spondylitis
   (c) Rickets	(d) Osteopetrosis
10. Rheumatoid arthritis is caused by ....
    (a) Antigen-antibody complex	(b) *E. coli*
    (c) Reovirus	(d) *Brucella* sp.

14. PATHOLOGY OF CARDIOVASCULAR SYSTEM

1. Acute heart failure is not caused by ....
   (a) Anoxia	(b) Shock
   (c) Cardiac Temponade	(d) Fever
2. Left sided heart failure is characterized by ....
   (a) Heart failure cells	(b) Pulse in jugular vein
   (c) Shock	(d) Oedema
3. "Bread and butter" appearance of heart is due to deposition of ....
   (a) Fibrin	(b) Neutrophils
   (c) Fibroblasts	(d) Collagen
4. Endocarditis is caused by ....
   (a) *Actinomyces pyogenes*	(b) Erysepalas
   (c) Staphylococci	(d) All of the above
5. Vegetative growth in heart is caused by ....
   (a) *Actinomyces pyogenes*	(b) Staphylococci
   (c) Clostridia	(d) Erysepalas
6. Arteriolosclerosis affects arterioles in ....

(a) Kidneys (b) Spleen (c) Pancreas (d) All of the above
7. Atherosclerosis is ....of blood vessels
   (a) Hardening   (b) Softening
   (c) Aneurysm   (d) Thinning
8. Arteritis is inflammation of arteries caused by ....
   (a) Equine viral arteritis (b) *E.coli*
   (c) Salmonella   (d) Rotavirus
9. Phlebitis is the inflammation of ....
   (a) Artery (b) Vein (c) Lymph vessel (d) Capillary
10. Lymphangitis is inflammation of ....
    (a) Lymph node   (b) Lymph gland
    (c) Lymph vessel (d) Lymphocytes

15. PATHOLOGY RESPIRATORY SYSTEM

1. Nasal polyps are caused by ....
   (a) *Schistosoma nasalis*   (b) *Rhinosporidium sceberi*
   (c) *E. coli*   (d) *Mycoplasma mycoides*
2. Canine tracheobronchitis is caused by...........
   (a) Adenovirus   (b) Influenza virus
   (c) Herpes virus (d) All of the above
3. Presence of caseous plugs in bronchi at the point of entrance in lungs in characteristic lesions of ....
   (a) Infectious bronchitis
   (b) Infectious laryngotracheitis
   (c) Air sacculitis
   (d) Pleuritis
4. This is not the pathologic lesion of pneumonia...........
   (a) Congestion   (b) Red hepatization
   (c) Yellow hepatization (d) Resolution
5. Infection through aerogenous route may cause ....pneumonia
   (a) Lobar   (b) Lobular
   (c) Hypersensitivity (d) Fibrinous

6. Verminous pneumonia is caused by ....
   (a) Mycoplasma (b) Chlamydia
   (c) *Dictayocaulus* sp. (d) *E.coli*
7. Langhan's type giant cell is characteristic feature of ....pneumonia
   (a) Tuberculous (b) Verminous
   (c) Broncho (d) Pulmonary adenomatosis
8. Atelectasis neonatorum is characteristic features of ....
   (a) Premature birth (b) Aborted foetus
   (c) Still birth (d) None
9. Hypersensitivity pneumonitis is caused by ....
   (a) Allergens (b) Parasites
   (c) Moldy hay (d) All of the above
10. Pneumoconiasis is characterized by ....lesions in lungs
    (a) Serus (b) Fibrinous
    (c) Hemorrhagic (d) Granulomatous

16. PATHOLOGY OF DIGESTIVE SYSTEM

1. Turkish towel like lesions are observed in ....
   (a) Candidiasis (b) Histomoniasis
   (c) Moniliasis (d) Coccidiosis
2. Vesicular stomatitis is seen in cases of ....
   (a) Rinderpest (b) Mucosal disease
   (c) Hog cholera (d) FMD
3. Choked esophagus may cause .... in ruminants.
   (a) Impaction (b) Vomition
   (c) Tympany (d) Gastritis
4. Rumen is distended due to accumulation of .... in bloat.
   (a) H_2S (b) CO_2 (c) CO (d) All of the above
5. Traumatic reticulitis may lead to ....
   (a) Pericarditis (b) Peritonitis (c) Pleurisy (d) All

Self Assessment – MCQ

of the above
6. Increase in .... cells is observed in catarrhal enteritis.
   (a) Mast cells   (b) Eosinophils
   (c) Goblet   (d) Neutrophils
7. Punched out ulcers are produced by ....
   (a) Theileria   (b) Babesia
   (c) Hog cholera   (d) *Clostridium* sp.
8. Granulomatous lesions in intestine of poultry are observed in ....
   (a) Coli granuloma (b) *E. coli* infection
   (c) Hjarre's disease (d) All of the above
9. Telescoping of intestine is also known as ....
   (a) Torsion   (b) Volvulus
   (c) Intussusception (d) None
10. *Eimeria tennella* causes .... in intestines.
    (a) Typhlitis   (b) Enteritis
    (c) Colitis   (d) Proctitis
11. Necrosis of hepatocytes at one side of central vein in liver is known as .... necrosis.
    (a) Centrilobular (b) Midzonal
    (c) Paracentral   (d) Focal
12. Parasitic cirrhosis is caused by ....
    (a) *Hemonchus* sp. (b) *Ascaris lumbricoides*
    (c) *Fasciola* sp. (d) Amphistomes
13. Cholecystitis is the inflammation of ....
    (a) Urinary bladder (b) Bile duct
    (c) Gall bladder   (d) Pancreas
14. Reovirus causes .... of pancreas.
    (a) Hypertrophy   (b) Atrophy
    (c) Hyperplasia   (d) Hypoplasia

15. 'Pearly disease' is caused by ....
    (a) Streptococci   (b) Staphylococci
    (c) *Mycobacterium* sp.   (d) None
16. Erosive stomatitis is seen in ....
    (a) Rinderpest   (b) Mucosal disease
    (c) Pox   (d) FMD
17. Ingluvitis is the inflammation of ....
    (a) Colon   (b) Rectum   (c) Jenjunum   (d) Crop
18. Sub-epithelial fibrous nodules are produced in .... esophagitis.
    (a) Traumatic   (b) Bacterial
    (c) Viral   (d) Parasitic
19. Sudden change in feed with lush green fodder is the cause of ....
    (a) Impaction   (b) Tympany
    (c) Reticulitis   (d) None
20. Acute abomasitis characterized by oedema, congestion and haemorrhage of abmasal folds is feature of ....
    (a) Enterotoxemia   (b) Black disease
    (c) Braxy   (d) Blue tongue
21. Corrugations in large intestines are observed in ....
    (a) Tuberculosis   (b) Paratuberculosis
    (c) Pseudotuberculosis (d) All of the above
22. Pica may lead to formation of ....
    (a) Piliconcretions   (b) Polybezoars
    (c) Both a & b   (d) None
23. Enterolith may cause ....in horses.
    (a) Enterotoxemia   (b) Colic
    (c) Lameness   (d) Diarrhoea
24. Frothy bloat occurs in buffaloes due to ....
    (a) Saponin   (b) Fatty acids

(c) Carbohydrate (d) None
25. Button ulcers are produced in abomasum due to ....
 (a) *Salmonella* sp. (b) Staphylococci (c) *E. coli* (d) FMD

17. PATHOLOGY OF HEMOPOITIC AND IMMUNE SYSTEM

1. Congenital defects in lymphocytes may result into ....
 (a) Lymphopenia (b) Agammaglobulinemia
 (c) Hypoplasia of spleen (d) All of the above
2. The size of RBC varies from small to large in peripheral blood and this condition is known as...
 (a) Poikilosytosis (b) Anisocytosis
 (c) Polychromatophilia (d) Heinz bodies
3. Hemolytic anemia is caused by ....
 (a) *Anaplasma* spp. (b) Coccidia
 (c) Hemonchus (d) *Proteus* sp.
4. Hematuria is an example of ....anemia
 (a) Hemolytic (b) Autoimmune
 (c) Hemorrhagic (d) Deficiency
5. Eosinophilia occurs in ....infection
 (a) Bacterial (b) Prion (c) Viroid (d) Parasitic
6. Decrease in number of all components of leucocytes is known as ....
 (a) Leucopoenia (b) Panleucopenia
 (c) Leucocytosis (d) Leukemia
7. Pesticides may cause ....
 (a) Neutropenia (b) Lymphopenia
 (c) Hypogammaglobulimia (d) All of the above
8. Depletion of lymphoid tissue from follicles of bursa ....
 (a) Gumboro disease (b) Rinderpest
 (c) Coccidiosis (d) Salmonellosis

9. Macrocytic normochromic anemia is.........
   (a) Large size RBC
   (b) Decreased Hb
   (c) Small size RBC
   (d) Large size RBC & Normal Hb
10. Erythrocytes having minute dark spots are known as ....
    (a) Heinz bodies   (b) Theleiria
    (c) Basophilic Stippling   (d) None

18. PATHOLOGY OF URINARY SYSTEM

1. C_3 component of complement is found in which type of glomerulonephritis (MPGN).
   (a) Type-I (b) Type-II (c) Type III (d) Type-IV
2. In cattle, pyelonephritis is caused by ....
   (a) *E. coli*   (b) *Proteus* spp.
   (c) *Corynebacterium renale*   (d) *Actinomyces pyogenes*
3. Nephrosclerosis is .... disease of kidney
   (a) Acute   (b) Chronic (c) Subacute   (d) Peracute
4. Hypovitaminosis ....may cause urolithiasis
   (a) A   (b) B   (c) C   (d) D
5. Ureteritis is the inflammation of ....
   (a) Uterus   (b) Uterine glands
   (c) Ureter   (d) Uterine tube
6. .... amino acid forms calculi in animal which causes obstruction in urethra.
   (a) Arginine (b) Lucine (c) Cystine (d) Gsolucine
7. Bracken fern causes ....
   (a) Hematuria   (b) Pyuria
   (c) Hemoglobinuria   (d) Anuria
8. Urethra may become infected by ....virus.
   (a) Picorna (b) Picobirna   (c) Birna   (d) Adeno
9. Hyperplasia of collecting tubes with their dilation causes ....cysts in kidneys.
   (a) Type-I (b) Type-II (c) Type-III (d) Type-IV

Self Assessment – MCQ

10. Uremia is caused by the increased level of .... in blood.
    (a) Urea (b) Uric acid
    (c) Creatinine (d) All of the above

19. PATHOLOGY OF GENITAL SYSTEM

FEMALE GENITAL SYSTEM

1. Cryptorchidism may lead to .... of testicles.
   (a) Hypoplasia (b) Aspermatogenesis
   (c) Neoplasia (d) All of the above
2. Ventral deviation of penis is known as ....
   (a) Corkscrew penis (b) Phallocampsis
   (c) Rainbow penis (d) None
3. Hydrocele is accumulation of serus fluid in ....
   (a) Oviduct (b) Testes
   (c) Mammary gland (d) Tunica vaginalis
4. Funiculitis is the inflammation of ....
   (a) Schirrhous cord (b) Seminal vesicle
   (c) Glans penis (d) Prepuce
5. Phimosis is caused by ....
   (a) Balanitis (b) Posthitis
   (c) Balanoposthitis (d) All of the above
6. Presence of follicular cysts in ovary may lead to ....
   (a) Sterility (b) Nymphomania
   (c) Continuous oestrus (d) All of the above
7. Inflammation of oviduct leads to sterility due to .... nature of the exudate to sperms.
   (a) Toxic (b) Obstructive
   (c) Penetrative (d) None
8. Mastitis is mostly caused by ....
   (a) Trauma (b) Hematogenous infection
   (c) Toxins/ poisons (d) Infection

9. Summer mastitis is caused by ....
   (a) Staphylococci (b) *Actinomyces pyogenes*
   (c) Streptococci   (d) *Candida albicans*
10. Parturition of a dead foetus on its full development and gestation is termed as ....
    (a) Abortion   (b) Still birth
    (c) Premature birth (d) Normal birth

20. PATHOLOGY OF NERVOUS SYSTEM

1. Neuritis is observed in ....
   (a) Mucosal disease   (b) Infectious bursal disease
   (c) Marek's disease   (d) ILT
2. Necrosis of brain in known as ....
   (a) Encephalomalacia (b) Polioencephalomalacia
   (c) Myelomalacia   (d) None of the above
3. Removal of dead neurons through microglial cells in known as ....
   (a) Satellitosis   (b) Neuronophagia
   (c) Perivascular cuffing (d) None
4. Increase in number of white blood cells in cerbrospinal fluid in termed as ....
   (a) Encephalitis (b) Satellitosis
   (c) Pleocytosis   (d) Leukoencephalomalacia
5. Spongiform encephalopathy is caused by ....
   (a) Virus   (b) Viroids
   (c) Prions (d) Deficiency of vit B_{12}
6. Inflammation of durameter is known as ....
   (a) Leptomeningitis (b) Pachy meningitis
   (c) Meningitis   (d) Meningoencephalitis
7. Congenitally small size brain is termed as ....
   (a) Anencephaly   (b) Hydrocephalus
   (c) Microencephaly (d) Cranioschisis

Self Assessment – MCQ

8. Phagocytic cells of brain is ....cell(s)
   (a) Astrocytes (b) Microglial
   (c) Oligodendroglial (d) All of the above
9. Increase in CSF in sub arachnoid space is known as ....
   (a) Pleocytosis (b) Hydrocephalus
   (c) Microencephaly (d) Hypoplasia
10. Hernia of meninges through craninoschisis is known as ....
    (a) Hydrocele (b) Meningocele
    (c) Meningoencephalocele (d) None

21. PATHOLOGY OF ENDOCRINE SYSTEM, EYES AND EAR

1. Metastatic calcification occurs in..................
   (a) Hyperthyroidism (b) Hyperparathyroidism
   (c) Hypothyroidism (d) Hypoparathyroidism
2. Goiter is related with..................
   (a) Hypothyroidism (b) Hyperthyroidism
   (c) Both a & b (d) None
3. Otitis media is the inflammation of middle ear including.............
   (a) Tympanic cavity (b) Eustachian tube
   (c) Both a & b (d) None
4. Disturbance in equilibrium occurs in animals with disease of ....
   (a) External ear (b) Eyes
   (c) Middle year (d) Inner ear
5. Glaucoma is caused by..................
   (a) Neoplasm (b) Trauma
   (c) Haemorrhage (d) All of above
6. *Thelazia* spp worms may cause..................
   (a) Keratocojunctivitis (b) Microphakia
   (c) Aphakia (d) Coloboma

7. Cleft in iris is known as...............
   (a) Iritis (b) Microphakia
   (c) Aphakia (d) Coloboma
8. Equine goiter is caused by...............
   (a) Iodine deficiency (b) Iodine excess
   (c) Cabbage (d) Radiation
9. Exophthalmos is a feature of............... goiter
   (a) Colloid (b) Adenomatous
   (c) Toxic (d) Familial
10. Acromegaly is caused by...............
    (a) Hyperpituitarism (b) Hypopituitarism
    (c) Hypothyroidism (d) Hyperthyroidism

22. NEOPLASMS

1. Substitution of one type of cells by another type is known as _____.
   (a) Hyperplasia (b) Anaplasia
   (c) Metaplasia (d) Aplasia
2. Reversion of cells to a more embryonic type and less differentiated is called as _____.
   (a) Hyperplasia (b) Anaplasia
   (c) Neoplasia (d) Metaplasia
3. Hyperchromasia and pleomorphism is a characteristic feature of _____.
   (a) Metaplasia (b) Hyperplasia
   (c) Anaplasia (d) None
4. Neoplasms whose cells are anaplastic, metastasize are classified as _____.
   (a) Benign (b) Malignant (c) Both (d) None
5. Obstruction of lymphatics by tumour cells disturbs lymphatic flow to facilitate metastasis at unusual site is termed as _____.
   (a) Skip metastasis (b) Retrograde metastasis
   (c) Both (d) None

Self Assessment – MCQ

6. Meningeal tumour spreads through _____.
   (a) Blood   (b) Lymph   (c) Skin   (d) CSF
7. Abnormal enzyme ATPase on cell surface promotes _____ leading to cachexia in tumour patient.
   (a) Proteolysis   (b) Glycolysis
   (c) Both   (d) None
8. Gene responsible for suppression of cell proliferation are termed as _____.
   (a) Oncogene   (b) Antioncogene
   (c) Both   (d) None
9. v-onc and c-onc are having _____.
   (a) Homology   (b) Heterology
   (c) Both   (d) None
10. Papilloma virus has _____ oncogene.
    (a) src   (b) raf   (c) myc   (d) All of above
11. Hepadna virus has _____ oncogene.
    (a) hap   (b) src   (c) raf   (d) All of above
12. Oxygen metabolites of neutrophils' respiratory burst act as _____.
    (a) Tumour initiator   (b) Tumour promoter
    (c) Both   (d) None
13. Tumour cells develop certain biochemical alterations on their surface, that is known as _____.
    (a) Tumour antigens   (b) Tumour antibodies
    (c) Anaplasia   (d) None
14. Tumour necrosis factor (TNF-) is responsible for _____ of tumours.
    (a) Promotion   (b) Initiation
    (c) Regression   (d) None
15. Tumour antigens are _____.
    (a) Fetal antigens   (b) Alphafetoproteins
    (c) Both   (d) None

16. A stage T_2, N_2 an M_2 is considered with _____ prognosis.
    (a) Good (b) Fair (c) Guarded (d) Poor
17. A cytokine secreted by tumour cells is known as _____ which is responsible for cachexia in animals.
    (a) Interleukin (b) Tumour necrosis factor
    (c) Cachectin (d) None
18. In neoplasia, hepatocytes become _____.
    (a) Hypertrophied (b) Atrophied
    (c) Hyperplastic (d) Hypoplastic
19. _____ is a feature of neoplasms.
    (a) Hypocalcemia (b) Hypercalcemia
    (c) Both (d) None
20. Liposarcoma is a _____ tumour of adipose cells.
    (a) Benign (b) Malignant
    (c) Preneoplic (d) None
21. Tumour of flat bones are known as _____.
    (a) Compact osteoma (b) Spongy osteoma
    (c) Both (d) None
22. Leiomyoma is a benign tumour of _____ muscles.
    (a) Cardiac (b) Skeletal
    (c) Smooth (d) All of above
23. Mesothelioma is a neoplasm of _____ cells.
    (a) Epithelium (b) Endothelium
    (c) Mesothelium (d) None
24. Lymphosarcoma is a malignant neoplasm of _____.
    (a) Circulating lymphocytes (b) Tissue lymphocytes
    (c) Both (d) None
25. Leukemia is a malignant neoplasia of _____.
    (a) Circulating lymphocytes (b) Tissue lymphocytes
    (c) Both (d) None

26. Squamous cell carcinoma of _____ is more common in animals in India.
    (a) Eyes (b) Lip (c) Hoof (d) Horn
27. Epithelial pearls is a feature of _____.
    (a) Papilloma (b) Adenocarcinoma
    (c) Lymphosarcoma (d) None
28. Basal cell carcinoma is also known as _____.
    (a) Horn cancer (b) Eye cancer
    (c) Hair cell carincoma (d) None
29. Cholangiocellular carcinoma is a tumour of bile duct caused by _____.
    (a) Aflatoxins (b) Liver fluke infection
    (c) Both (d) None
30. Adamantinoma is a tumour of _____.
    (a) Adipose cells (b) Enamel (c) Eye (d) Gum

23. VIRAL DISEASES

1. The cause of FMD in animals is _____.
   (a) DNA virus (b) Rotavirus
   (c) Picornavirus (d) Corona virus
2. Foot and mouth disease is characterized by the presence of _____ lesions.
   (a) Vesicular (b) Erosive
   (c) Ulcerative (d) None
3. Vesicular stomatitis is caused by _____.
   (a) Picornavirus (b) Calcivirus
   (c) Vesiculovirus (d) None
4. Sore mouth is synonymously used _____.
   (a) FMD (b) Vesicular stomatitis
   (c) Vesicular exanthema (d) All of above
5. Rinderpest virus belongs to _____ group of paramyxoviridae family.
   (a) Orbivirus (b) Pestivirus
   (c) Flavivirus (d) Morbilli virus

6. Rabies is characterized by _____.
   (a) Encephalitis (b) Negri bodies
   (c) Babes nodules (d) All of above
7. Infectious canine hepatitis is caused by _____.
   (a) Herpes virus (b) Rhabdovirus
   (c) Adenovirus (d) Coronovirus
8. Blue eye is used synonymously with _____.
   (a) Rabies (b) ICH (c) CD (d) All of above
9. In canine distemper, the inclusions are _____.
   (a) Intracytoplasmic (b) Intranuclear
   (c) Both (d) None
10. Parvoviral infection in dogs is characterized by _____.
    (a) Necrotic enteritis (b) Mycocardial necrosis
    (c) Both (d) None
11. Blue tongue is caused by _____.
    (a) Pestivirus (b) Orbivirus
    (c) Reovirus (d) None
12. Pulmonary adenomatosis is characterized by _____.
    (a) Neoplasia (b) Anaplasia
    (c) Metaplasia (d) Dysplasia
13. Maedi-Visna is caused by _____.
    (a) Orbivirus (b) Lentivirus
    (c) Pestivirus (d) None
14. PPR is characterized by _____.
    (a) Giant cell pneumonia
    (b) Broncho pneumonia
    (c) Interstitial pneumonia
    (d) Verminous pneumonia
15. Zebra markings are seen in _____.
    (a) RP (b) PPR (c) MCF (d) All of above
16. Button ulcers in large intestines are seen in _____.

(a) Swine fever   (b) Hog cholera
(c) Both a & b   (d) None

17. Equine infectious anemia is caused by _____.
    (a) Lentivirus   (b) Pesti virus
    (c) Orbivirus   (d) All of above
18. Equine encephalomyelitis is also known as _____.
    (a) Staggers   (b) Borna disease
    (c) Forage poisoning   (d) All of above
19. Ephimeral fever is caused by _____ shaped virus.
    (a) Wheel   (b) Bullet   (c) Pin   (d) None
20. Pseudorabies is also known as _____.
    (a) Rabies   (b) Mad itch
    (c) Mad cow disease   (d) None
21. Equine plague is _____.
    (a) Equine encephalomyelitis
    (b) Equine viral arteritis
    (c) African horse sickness
    (d) None
22. African horse sickness is caused by _____.
    (a) Orbivirus   (b) Pestivirus
    (c) Rotavirus   (d) None
23. Maedi-Visna is characterized by _____.
    (a) Metaplasia   (b) Gliosis
    (c) Intracytoplasmic inclusions   (d) All of above
24. PPR is caused by _____.
    (a) Morbillivirus   (b) Pestivirus
    (c) Rubivirus   (d) None
25. Canine distemper is characterized by _____.
    (a) Pustular dermatitis   (b) Broncho pneumonia
    (c) Hard pad   (d) All of above
26. Rabies is caused by _____.

(a) Lyssa virus (b) Vesiculovirus
(c) Rhabdovirus (d) None

27. Rotavirus infection in calves is characterized by _____.
    (a) Maldigestion (b) Malabsorption
    (c) Shortening of villi (d) All of above

28. Late abortions in cattle are caused by _____.
    (a) BHV-1 (b) Rotavirus
    (c) Coronavirus (d) Picornavirus

29. Camel pox is characterized by the presence of _____.
    (a) Papule (b) Vesicles (c) Pustules (d) All of above

30. Diarrhoea is manifested in _____.
    (a) Rinderpest (b) MCF
    (c) Mucosal disease (d) All of above

24. BACTERIAL DISEASES

1. Presence of tubercles on pleura and mesentry are known as _____.
   (a) Johne's diseases (b) Epithelial pearls
   (c) Pearly disease (d) None

2. In tuberculosis _____ type of giant cells are formed.
   (a) Langhan's (b) Tuton
   (c) Tumour (d) All of above

3. Johne's disease is caused by _____.
   (a) *Mycobacterium tuberculosis*
   (b) *Mycobacterium pseudotuberculosis*
   (c) *Mycobacterium avium*
   (d) *Mycobacterium paratuberculosis*

4. Presence of _____ as a result of thickening of transverse folds due to chronic inflammation is characteristic lesion of Johne's disease.
   (a) Pearl (b) Calcification (c) Tubercle (d) Rugae

5. *Brucella abortus* produces _____ lesions.

Self Assessment – MCQ

    (a) Granulomatous   (b) Suppurative
    (c) Fibrinous   (d) All of above

6. Haemorrhagic septicemia is characterized by _____.
   (a) Oedema in neck   (b) Dyspnoea
   (c) Pneumonia   (d) All of above

7. Abortion in _____ month of gestations may occur due to brucellosis.
   (a) 5-6   (b) 7-9   (c) 3-4   (d) None

8. Marbling in lungs with extensive sero-fibrinous lesions are characteristic of _____.
   (a) Colibacillosis   (b) Pasteurellosis
   (c) Black quarter   (d) All of above

9. Painful swelling in thigh muscles with crepitating sound on touch is observed in _____.
   (a) Anthrax   (b) HS   (c) Tetanus   (d) BQ

10. Gas gangrene is caused by _____.
    (a) *Fusarium* sp.   (b) *Clostridium chauvei*
    (c) *Clostridium welchii*   (d) None

11. Pulpy kidney disease in sheep is caused by _____.
    (a) *Clostridium welchii*   (b) *Clostridium tetani*
    (c) *Clostridium perfringens*   (d) All of above

12. In camels, the enterotoxaemia is caused by *Clostridium perfringens* type _____.
    (a) A   (b) B   (c) C   (d) D

13. Braxy is caused by _____.
    (a) *Clostridium perfringens*   (b) *Clostridium welchii*
    (c) *Clostridium tetani*   (d) *Clostridium septicum*

14. Lock jaw is a feature of _____.
    (a) Braxy   (b) Anthrax
    (c) Actinomycosis   (d) Tetanus

15. In tetanus death occurs due to _____.
    (a) Asphyxia   (b) Paralysis
    (c) Dehydration   (d) None

16. Diamond skin disease is also known as _____.
    (a) Swine fever   (b) Erysepalas
    (c) Pseudorabies   (d) Canine distemper
17. Swine erysepalas is characterized by _____ endocarditis.
    (a) Haemorrhagic   (b) Suppurative
    (c) Vegetative   (d) None
18. Listeriosis is characterized by _____ meningitis.
    (a) Lepto   (b) Pachy   (c) Sero-fibrinous   (d) None
19. Turkey egg appearance of kidneys are observed in _____.
    (a) Listeriosis   (b) Salmonellosis
    (c) Pasteurellosis   (d) All of above
20. Naval ill is caused by _____.
    (a) *Salmonella* sp.   (b) *E.coli*
    (c) *Pasteurella* sp.   (d) None
21. Empyema is a feature of _____.
    (a) Glanders   (b) Strangles
    (c) Babesiosis   (d) None
22. *Pseudomonas mallei* causes _____ in horses.
    (a) Lymphangitis   (b) Lymphadenitis
    (c) Farcy   (d) All of above
23. Absence of rigor mortis is a feature of _____.
    (a) Colibacillosis   (b) Pasteurellosis
    (c) Anthrax   (d) None
24. Campylobacteriosis is characterized by _____.
    (a) Early abortion   (b) Suppurative metritis
    (c) Both   (d) None
25. Actinomycosis is characterized by _____.
    (a) Wooden tongue   (b) Lumpy jaw
    (c) Lock jaw   (d) None

26. Actinobacillosis is characterized by _____.
    (a) Wooden tongue   (b) Lumpy jaw
    (c) Lock jaw   (d) All of above
27. Botryomycosis is caused by _____.
    (a) Staphylococci   (b) Streptococci
    (c) Blastomyces   (d) None
28. Bovine farcy is also known as _____.
    (a) Tuberculosis   (b) Johne's disease
    (c) Brucellosis   (d) Nocardiosis
29. Necrobacillosis is characterized by _____.
    (a) Necrosis of liver   (b) Foot rot
    (c) Diphtheria   (d) All of above
30. Tary colour blood coming out from natural openings is a feature of _____.
    (a) HS   (b) Anthrax
    (c) BQ   (d) Leptospirosis

25. CHLAMYDIAL DISEASES

1. Chlamydiosis in cattle is caused by _____.
    (a) *Chlamydia psitaci*   (b) *Chlamydia abortus*
    (c) Both   (d) None
2. Chlamydial infection in sheep is characterized by _____.
    (a) Pruiritus   (b) Myositis
    (c) Neuritis   (d) Abortion
3. In calves chlamydia causes _____.
    (a) Poly arthritis   (b) Pneumonia
    (c) Meningo-encephalitis   (d) All of above
4. Pregnant cows are aborted during _____ month of gestation due to chlamydia.
    (a) 3-5   (b) 5-7   (c) 7-9   (d) None
5. Chlamydial infection causes _____ placentitis in cattle.

(a) Lymphocytic (b) Haemorrhagic
(c) Sero-fibrinous (d) Fibrino-purulent

26. RICKETTSIAL DISEASES
1. Anaplasmosis is caused by _____.
   (a) *Anaplasma centrale* (b) *Anaplasma marginale*
   (c) Both (d) None
2. Anaplasmosis is characterized by _____.
   (a) Icterus (b) Pneumonia
   (c) Enteritis (d) All of above
3. _____ is a feature of anaplasmosis.
   (a) Anemia (b) Hyperemia
   (c) Polycythemia (d) None
4. Anaplasma infection causes _____ reaction leading to anemia.
   (a) Hyper sensitive (b) Auto immune
   (c) Both (d) None
5. Diagnosis of anaplasmosis can be done by _____ examination.
   (a) Blood smear (b) Serum
   (c) Lung tissue (d) All of above

27. MYCOPLASMAL DISEASES
1. Contagious bovine pleuropneumonia is caused by _____.
   (a) *Mycoplasma mycoides* (b) *Mycobacterium* sp.
   (c) Both (d) None
2. CCPP is characterized by _____.
   (a) Enteritis (b) Pleurisy (c) Both (d) None
3. Mycoplasmosis is characterized by _____.
   (a) Abortion (b) Nephritis
   (c) Encephalitis (d) None
4. Generally, the mycoplasma is considered as _____

pathogen.
(a) Mild (b) Virulent
(c) Opportunistic (d) None

5. _____ is a feature of mycoplasma infection in cavles.
   (a) Polyarthritis (b) Hepatitis
   (c) Both (d) None

6. Mycoplasma causes _____.
   (a) Mastitis (b) Pneumonia
   (c) Abortion (d) All of above

7. In mycoplasmosis _____ pericarditis occurs in goats.
   (a) Granulomatous (b) Fibrinous
   (c) Both (d) None

8. _____ may make animal more susceptible for mycoplasma infection.
   (a) Immunosuppression (b) Immunization
   (c) Both (d) None

9. Mycoplasma produces _____ shaped colonies on media.
   (a) Cigar (b) Club (c) Nipple (d) None

10. _____ reaction is a feature of mycoplasmosis.
    (a) Neutrophilic (b) Eosinophilic
    (c) Lymphofollicular (d) None

28. SPIROCHAETAL DISEASES

1. Leptospira multiplies in _____ and secreted in urine to cause infection in other animals.
   (a) PCT (b) DST (c) Both (d) None

2. Leptospirosis is characterized by _____.
   (a) Haemorrhages (b) Nephritis
   (c) Icterus (d) All of above

3. Leptospirosis causes _____.
   (a) Bacterimia (b) Spirochaetemia
   (c) Septicemia (d) None

4. Leptospirosis may also cause _____ in females.
   (a) Vaginitis   (b) Cervicitis
   (c) Abortion   (d) All of above
5. _____ is a feature of leptospirosis.
   (a) Hematuria   (b) Myoglobinuria
   (c) Hemoglobinuria (d) None

29. PRION DISEASES
1. Scarpie is caused by _____.
   (a) Virus   (b) Bacteria   (c) Fungus   (d) Piron
2. BSE is characterized by _____.
   (a) Circling movements   (b) Spongy brain
   (c) Valuolation in nerve cells (d) All of above
3. Incubation period of BSE is _____.
   (a) 2-5 days   (b) 2-5 months
   (c) 2-5 years   (d) None
4. The gene coding for prion protein is normally _____ in animals.
   (a) Absent   (b) Present   (c) Not known   (d) None
5. _____ is the only diagnostic tool to confirm BSE.
   (a) Histopathology   (b) ELISA
   (c) PCR   (d) None

30. FUNGAL DISEASES
1. Ringworm is caused by _____ in cattle.
   (a) *Microsporum* sp.   (b) *Trichophyton* sp.
   (c) *Candida* sp.   (d) None
2. Characteristic lesions in ringworm are _____.
   (a) Itching and hyperkeratosis
   (b) Loss of hairs and papular lesions
   (c) Ring shaped lesions with serus discharges
   (d) All of above

Self Assessment – MCQ

3. *Caudidia albicans* causes _____.
   (a) Mastitis   (b) Pneumonia
   (c) Eso~~~~~~~~~~s   (d) All of above
4. Rhinosporidiosis is characterized by _____ growth on nasal mucosa.
   (a) Hyperplastic   (b) Polypoid
   (c) Hypoplastic   (d) Atrophic
5. *Candida albicans* causes _____ inflammation.
   (a) Suppurative   (b) Serus
   (c) Fibrinous   (d) Granulomatous
6. Aspergillus enters in body through _____ grains/feed.
   (a) Clean   (b) Wet
   (c) Mouldy   (d) Sandy
7. Aspergillus is characterized by _____.
   (a) Pneumonia   (b) Abortion
   (c) Both   (d) None
8. Blastomycosis is caused by _____.
   (a) *Blastomyces dermatitidis*   (b) *Blastomyces ovis*
   (c) *Blastomyces bovis*   (d) None
9. In coccidioidomycosis lesions are found mainly in _____.
   (a) Heart   (b) Kidney   (c) Brain   (d) None
10. Cryptococcosis is characterized by _____ disorders.
    (a) Hepatic   (b) Digestive   (c) Kidney   (d) Nervous
11. Histoplastosis is characterized by _____.
    (a) Hepatomegaly   (b) Spleenomegaly
    (c) Leucopenia   (d) All of above
12. Ulcers in intestine are seen due to _____ infection.
    (a) *Eimeria* sp.   (b) *Aspergillus* sp.
    (c) *Candida* sp.   (d) *Histoplasma* sp.

13. Encephalitis is mainly occurs due _____ infection.
    (a) *Coccidioides* sp. (b) *Cryptococcus* sp.
    (c) *Candida* sp.   (d) None
14. Degnala disease is caused by _____.
    (a) Bacterial toxins   (b) Mycotoxins
    (c) Phytotoxins   (d) None
15. Dry gangrene on extremities is the characteristic feature of _____.
    (a) Aspergillosis   (b) Rhinosporidiosis
    (c) Candidiasis   (d) Mycotoxicosis

31. PARASITIC DISEASES

1. Surra is caused by _____.
   (a) *Trypanosoma evansi*   (b) *Trypanosoma felei*
   (c) Both   (d) None
2. Trypanosoma is an _____ protozoan parasite.
   (a) Intra cellular   (b) Extra cellular
   (c) Both   (d) None
3. Theileriosis is characterized by _____.
   (a) Hepatopathy   (b) Nephropathy
   (c) Lymphadenopathy (d) All of above
4. Babesiosis is caused by _____.
   (a) *Babesia bigemina*   (b) *Babesia bovis*
   (c) Both   (d) None
5. Babesiosis is transmitted by _____.
   (a) Mosquito   (b) Flies   (c) Snails   (d) Ticks
6. Babesia is an _____ cellular parasite.
   (a) Intra   (b) Extra   (c) Both   (d) None
7. *Trichomonas foetus* causes abortion in animals during _____ months of gestation.
   (a) 3-5   (b) 6-7   (c) 7-9   (d) All of above

Self Assessment – MCQ

8. Abortions due to *Trichomonas foetus* are followed by _____.
   (a) Sterility (b) Pymetra (c) Both (d) None
9. Toxoplasmosis is characterized by _____.
   (a) Encephalitis (b) Nephritis
   (c) Myositis (d) None
10. In cattle coccidiosis is caused by _____.
    (a) *Eimeria bovis* (b) *Eimeria zuernii*
    (c) Both (d) None
11. Nasal granuloma is caused by _____.
    (a) *Schistosoma bovis* (b) *Schistosoma nasalis*
    (c) Both (d) None
12. Distomiasis is caused by _____.
    (a) Amphistomes (b) Ascaris (c) Fasciola (d) Tapeworm
13. Cryptosporidiosis is characterized by _____.
    (a) Diarrhoea (b) Pneumonia
    (c) Both (d) None
14. Ascariasis is characterized by _____.
    (a) Pleurisy (b) Lameness
    (c) Peritonitis (d) None
15. Visceral larva migrans is caused by _____.
    (a) Tapeworms (b) Ascarid worms
    (c) Both (d) None
16. Anchylostomiasis is also known as _____.
    (a) Visceral larva migrans (b) Hook worm disease
    (c) Distomiasis (d) None
17. *Ostertagia ostertagi* is _____ stomach worm.
    (a) Red (b) Hair (c) Brown (d) Black
18. Nodule worms are _____.
    (a) *Oesophagostomum radiatum*
    (b) *Oesophagostomum columbianum*

(c) Both
(d) None
19. Cestodiasis is also known as _____.
    (a) Distomiasis   (b) Taeniasis
    (c) Both   (d) None
20. Cysticercosis causes _____ in sheep.
    (a) Pneumonia   (b) Enteritis
    (c) Gid   (d) None
21. Hydatid disease is caused by _____.
    (a) Echinococcus   (b) Cysticercus
    (c) Both   (d) None
22. Dirofilariasis is also known as _____.
    (a) Heart worm disease (b) Canine filariasis
    (c) Both   (d) None
23. Guinea worm disease is caused by _____.
    (a) *Fasciola* sp.   (b) *Ascaris* sp.
    (c) *Dracunculus* sp. (d) None
24. Verminous pneumonia is caused by _____ in horse.
    (a) *Dictyocaulus vivparus* (b) *Dictyocaulus filaria*
    (c) *Dictyocaulus arnfieldi* (d) None
25. Eosophageal tumour is produced by _____.
    (a) *Spiroceria lupi* (b) *Spirocerca canis*
    (c) Both   (d) None
26. Cerebrospinal nematodiasis is also known as _____.
    (a) Neurofilariasis (b) Setariasis
    (c) Kumri   (d) All of above
27. Whip worm disease is caused by _____.
    (a) *Trichuris ovis* (b) *Trichuris suis*
    (c) Both   (d) None
28. Ear sore is caused by _____.
    (a) *Stephanofilaria assamensis*

(b) *Stephanofilaria zaheeri*
(c) Both
(d) None
29. Verminous dermatitis is also known as _____.
    (a) Cascado
    (b) Ringworm disease
    (c) Both
    (d) None
30. Mange is caused by _____.
    (a) *Sarcoptes* sp.
    (b) *Psoroptes* sp.
    (c) Both of them
    (d) None of them

32. AVIAN INFLAMMATION
1. Cardinal sign of inflammation is _____.
   (a) Itching   (b) Loss of hairs   (c) Swelling   (d) None
2. _____ cells are the feature of avian inflammation.
   (a) Epithelioid   (b) Lymphoid
   (c) Heterophil   (d) Giant
3. In avian inflammation _____ cells are seen in abundance in comparison to mammals.
   (a) Eosinophils   (b) Basophils
   (c) Neutrophils   (d) None
4. Avian inflammation is characterized by increased permeability in _____.
   (a) Venules   (b) Arterioles   (c) Both   (d) None
5. Avian inflammation caused by PHA or Con A is characterized by infiltration of _____.
   (a) Heterophils   (b) Monocytes
   (c) Basophils   (d) All of above

33. PATHOLOGY OF NUTRITIONAL DISORDERS
1. Nutritional roup occurs in poultry due to deficiency of _____.
   (a) Vitamin A   (b) Vitamin B
   (c) Vitamin C   (d) Vitamin E

2. Crazy chick disease is caused by deficiency of _____.
   (a) Vitamin A   (b) Vitamin B
   (c) Vitamin C   (d) Vitamin E
3. Excess of fluorine in water may cause _____ in birds.
   (a) Retarded growth   (b) Deformity in bones
   (c) Both   (d) None
4. Star grazing condition in chicks is caused by the deficiency of _____.
   (a) Vitamin A   (b) Vitamin B_1
   (c) Vitamin C   (d) None
5. Curled toe paralysis in chicks occurs due to deficiency of _____.
   (a) Vitamin A   (b) Vitamin B_1
   (c) Vitamin C   (d) None
6. Perosis occurs in birds due to deficiency of _____.
   (a) Choline   (b) Biotin   (c) Zinc   (d) All of above
7. Pica in birds may occur as a result of _____ deficiency.
   (a) Calcium   (b) Vitamin B
   (c) Phosphorus   (d) None
8. Manganese deficiency is characterized by _____.
   (a) Perosis   (b) Osteodystrophy
   (c) Chondrodystrophy   (d) All of above
9. Selenium deficiency may cause absence of _____ in embryo.
   (a) Beak   (b) Eye   (c) Limb   (d) All of above
10. Hypovitaminosis B_1 is responsible for atrophy of _____ in birds.
    (a) Testes   (b) Ovary   (c) Both   (d) None

34. VIRAL DISEASES

1. Highly virulent Ranikhet disease virus is _____.
   (a) Lentogenic   (b) Mesogenic
   (c) Velogenic   (d) None

Self Assessment – MCQ

2. Ranikhet disease is also known as _____.
   (a) Ornithosis   (b) Degnala disease
   (c) New Castle disease (d) All of above
3. _____ is most characteristic lesion seen in Ranikhet disease.
   (a) Ulcer at caecal tonsils   (b) Pneumonia
   (c) Diarrhoea   (d) None
4. Avian influenza is caused by _____.
   (a) Myxovirus   (b) Orthomyxovirus
   (c) Paramyxovirus (d) None
5. Avian influenza is also known as _____.
   (a) Fowl cholera   (b) Fowl plague
   (c) Both   (d) None
6. Avian influenza is characterized by oedema of _____.
   (a) Head   (b) Face   (c) Leg   (d) Chest
7. Marek's disease is caused by _____.
   (a) Herpesvirus   (b) Togavirus
   (c) Poxvirus   (d) Lentivirus
8. MATSA is produced in Marek's disease as _____.
   (a) Tumour specific antigen
   (b) Tumour specific antibody
   (c) Type specific antigen
   (d) Type specific antibody
9. _____ are mostly observed in Marek's disease.
   (a) Malignant melanoma   (b) Malignant adenoma
   (c) Malignant lymphoma   (d) None
10. Avian leucosis is also known as _____ disease.
    (a) Big spleen   (b) Big liver
    (c) Big head   (d) None
11. Avian leucosis complex includes _____.
    (a) Lymphoid leucosis   (b) Osteopetrosis
    (c) Myeloblastosis   (d) All of above

12. Infectious bursal disease is also known as _____ disease.
    (a) Gumboro   (b) New Castle
    (c) Ranikhet   (d) None
13. Infectious bursal disease is caused by _____.
    (a) Reovirus   (b) Piconavirus
    (c) Birnavirus   (d) Lentivirus
14. In infectious bursal disease, bursa shows _____.
    (a) Edema   (b) Hemorrhage
    (c) Atrophy   (d) All of above
15. In infectious bronchitis, there is plugging of respirating passage by cheesy material at _____ junction.
    (a) Larynx-trachea   (b) Trachea-bronchi
    (c) Bronchi-lung   (d) All of above
16. Infectious bronchitis is characterized by _____.
    (a) Thin watery yolk (b) Misshapen eggs
    (c) Both   (d) None
17. Infectious laryngo tracheitis (ILT) is caused by _____.
    (a) Coronavirus   (b) Paramyxovirus
    (c) Reovirus   (d) Herpesvirus
18. In infectious laryngo-tracheitis, there is plugging of respirating passage by cheesy material at _____ junction.
    (a) Larynx-trachea   (b) Trachea-bronchi
    (c) Bronchi-lung   (d) All of above
19. The inclusions in infectious laryngo tracheitis are of _____ type.
    (a) Intracytoplasmic (b) Intranuclear
    (c) Both   (d) None
20. Tenosynovitis is caused by _____.
    (a) Adenovirus   (b) Reovirus
    (c) Rotavirus   (d) Herpes virus

Self Assessment – MCQ

21. In tenosynovitis there is rupture of _____ muscle tendon.
    (a) Gastrocnemious   (b) Messator
    (c) Both   (d) None
22. Avian stunting syndrome is characterized by _____.
    (a) Low weight gain   (b) Pasty vent
    (c) Atrophy of pancreas (d) All of above
23. Avian stunting syndrome is caused by _____.
    (a) Reovirus   (b) Birnavirus
    (c) Herpesvirus   (d) Orbivirus
24. Viral nephritis is also known as _____.
    (a) Baby chick nephropathy   (b) Grower nephropathy
    (c) Both   (d) None
25. Epidemic tremor disease is caused by _____.
    (a) Enterovirus   (b) Herpesvirus
    (c) Reovirus   (d) Alphavirus
26. Avian pock lesions include _____.
    (a) Papule (b) Vesicle (c) Both (d) None
27. Inclusion body hepatitis is caused by _____.
    (a) Hepdnavirus   (b) Reovirus
    (c) Adenovirus   (d) None
28. Chicken anemia agent is a _____ virus.
    (a) DNA   (b) RNA   (c) Both   (d) None
29. Egg drop syndrome is characterized by _____.
    (a) Decrease in egg production
    (b) Increase in egg production
    (c) Stopped egg production
    (d) None
30. Hydropericardium syndrome is caused by _____.
    (a) Aviadenovirus (b) Herpesvirus
    (c) Calcivirus   (d) Enterovirus

35. BACTERIAL DISEASES

1. Salmonellosis poultry is characterized by _____ colour of liver.
   (a) Sliver   (b) Gold   (c) Bronze   (d) None
2. Colisepticemia is characterized by _____ in birds.
   (a) Fibrinous pericarditis   (b) Fibrinous hepatitis
   (c) Both   (d) None
3. Hjarre's disease is caused by _____.
   (a) *E.coli*   (b) *Salmonella* sp.
   (c) *Mycobacterium* sp.   (d) None
4. _____ is associated in chronic respiratory disease with mycoplasma.
   (a) *E.coli*   (b) *Salmonella*
   (c) *Pasteurella* sp.   (d) None
5. In omphalitis the yolk becomes _____.
   (a) Thin   (b) Watery
   (c) Coagulated   (d) All of above
6. Infectious coryza is characterized by _____.
   (a) Swollen head   (b) Swollen leg
   (c) Both   (d) None
7. Fowl cholera is caused by _____.
   (a) *Vibrio cholarae*   (b) *Pasteurella* sp.
   (c) *E.coli*   (d) *Salmonella* sp.
8. Necrotic enteritis due to clostridia occurs after _____.
   (a) Colibacillosis   (b) Salmonellosis
   (c) Coccidiosis   (d) None
9. Campylobacter hepatitis is characterized by _____.
   (a) Necrotic hepatitis   (b) Hydropericardium
   (c) Catarrhal enteritis   (d) All of above
10. *Staphylococcus aurues* causes _____ in birds.
    (a) Gangrenous dermatitis   (b) Pustular dermatitis
    (c) Vesicular dermatitis   (d) None

Self Assessment – MCQ

11. Granulomatous nodules are seen in _____ in tuberculous birds.
    (a) Liver (b) Spleen (c) Air sacs (d) All of above
12. Fowl cholera is characterized by _____ colour of comb.
    (a) Red (b) Yellow (c) Blue (d) Pale
13. Pink colony on McConkey agar and white on BGA are seen due to _____ culture.
    (a) *Salmonella* (b) *E.coli* (c) Both (d) None
14. Coligranuloma is characterized by the presence of _____ in intestines.
    (a) Nodules (b) Ulcers (c) Erosions (d) None
15. Salmonellosis is characterized by _____.
    (a) Focal necrosis on liver (b) Marbling in spleen
    (c) Oophoritis (d) All of above

36. CHLAMYDIAL DISEASE

1. Ornithosis is a disease of _____.
   (a) Parrots (b) Pigeons (c) Poultry (d) All of above
2. Chlamydiosis in birds is also known as _____.
   (a) Ornithosis (b) Psittacosis
   (c) Both (d) None
3. Ornithosis is characterized by _____.
   (a) Serofibrinous pericarditis (b) Air sacculitis
   (c) Enteritis (d) All of above
4. In ornithosis, there is _____ colour diarrhoea.
   (a) Brown (b) Red (c) Greenish (d) Black
5. Ornithosis is caused by _____.
   (a) *Chlamydia psittaci* (b) *Chlamydia trachomatis*
   (c) Both (d) None

37. MYCOPLASMAL DISEASES

1. Chronic respiratory disease is caused by _____.
   (a) *Mycoplasma gallisepticum* (b) *E.coli*

(c) Both (d) None
2. Infectious synovitis in birds is caused by _____.
   (a) E.coli (b) Mycoplasma sinoviae
   (c) Both (d) None
3. Avian infectious synovitis is characterized by _____ in joints.
   (a) Cheesy material (b) Serus exudate
   (c) Suppurative mass (d) All of above
4. Chronic respiratory disease occurs in flocks maintained under _____ managemental practices.
   (a) Poor (b) Good (c) Fair (d) Excellent
5. Infectious synovitis is complicated by _____.
   (a) E.coli (b) Pasteurella gallinarum
   (c) Both (d) None

38. SPIROCHAETAL DISEASES

1. Fowl spirochaetosis is caused by _____.
   (a) Leptospira sp. (b) Spirochaeta sp.
   (c) Borrelia sp. (d) None
2. There was _____ diarrhoea in spirochaetosis in birds.
   (a) Redish (b) Yellowish
   (c) Greenish (d) Blackish
3. The spirochaete of fowl are transmitted through _____.
   (a) Mite (b) Tick (c) Lice (d) Fly
4. Fowl spirochaetosis is also known as _____.
   (a) Tick fever (b) Tick paralysis
   (c) Both (d) None
5. There was _____ haemorrhage in proventriculus due to spirochaetosis in birds.
   (a) Petechial (b) Ecchymotic
   (c) Linear (d) All of above

Self Assessment – MCQ

39. FUNGAL DISEASES

1. Aspergillosis in chicks is caused by _____.
   (a) *Aspergillus fumigatus*   (b) *Aspergillus niger*
   (c) *Aspergillus flavus*   (d) All of above
2. Brooder's pneumonia is also known as _____.
   (a) Aspergillosis   (b) Candidiasis
   (c) Favus   (d) Thrush
3. Favus is caused by _____ in poultry.
   (a) *Trichophyton magnini*   (b) *Trichophyton verucosum*
   (c) Both   (d) None
4. Candidiasis is characterized by _____ in birds.
   (a) Turkish towel like crop
   (b) Turkish towel like oesophagus
   (c) Both
   (d) None
5. Histoplasmosis is caused by _____.
   (a) *Histoplasma capsulatum*   (b) *Histomonas meleagredis*
   (c) Both   (d) None
6. Aflatoxicosis is characterized by _____.
   (a) Hepatitis   (b) Immunosuppression
   (c) Cancer   (d) All of above
7. Ochratoxicosis is characterized by _____.
   (a) Nephrosis   (b) Visceral gout
   (c) Pale bone marrow   (d) All of above
8. Aflatoxin(s) is/ are _____.
   (a) B_1 (b) A_1 (c) D_1 (d) All of above
9. Candidiasis is also known as _____.
   (a) Favus   (b) Thrush
   (c) White comb disease   (d) None
10. Candidiasis is caused by _____.
    (a) *Candida albicans*   (b) *Monilia albicans*
    (c) Both   (d) None

40. PARASITIC DISEASES

1. Common round worm of poultry is _____.
   - (a) *Syngamus trachea*
   - (b) *Ascaridia galli*
   - (c) Both
   - (d) None
2. In poultry, this worm is present under the mucosa of crop and causes emaciation and retardation of growth _____.
   - (a) *Syngamus trachea*
   - (b) *Ascaridia galli*
   - (c) *Gongylonema ingluvicola*
   - (d) None
3. Trematods of poultry are _____.
   - (a) *Prosthogonimus macrorchis*
   - (b) *Echinostoma revolutum*
   - (c) Both
   - (d) None
4. The poultry ticks include _____.
   - (a) *Argas persicus*
   - (b) *Aegytianella pullorum*
   - (c) Both
   - (d) None
5. The poultry red mite is _____.
   - (a) *Cytodites nudus*
   - (b) *Dermanyssus gallinae*
   - (c) Both
   - (d) None
6. Caecal coccidiosis is caused by _____.
   - (a) *Eimeria mivati*
   - (b) *Eimeria necatrix*
   - (c) *Eimeria mitis*
   - (d) *Eimeria tennella*
7. Coccidia causes _____ enteritis in birds.
   - (a) Catarrhal
   - (b) Hemorrhagic
   - (c) Fibrinous
   - (d) None
8. Histomoniasis is also known as _____.
   - (a) Black head
   - (b) Swollen head
   - (c) Cyanotic head
   - (d) None
9. Yellow round nodules in oesophagus and crop of pigeons are seen in _____.
   - (a) Histomoniasis
   - (b) Trichomoniasis
   - (c) Both
   - (d) None

10. *Hexamita meleagridis* is _____ shaped parasite of poultry.
   (a) Almond   (b) Bean   (c) Pear   (d) None

41. VICES AND MISCELLANEOUS DISEASE CONDITIONS

1. Cannibalism is a _____ habit of poultry.
   (a) Bad   (b) Good   (c) Fair   (d) None
2. Cannibalism is aggravated by _____.
   (a) Over crowding   (b) Prolapse of cloaca
   (c) Wounds   (d) All of above
3. Egg eating by birds occurs due to _____ in poultry house.
   (a) Presence of broken eggs   (b) Presence of feed
   (c) Presence of water   (d) None
4. Pica occurs as a result of _____ deficiency.
   (a) Calcium   (b) Phosphorus
   (c) Magnesium   (d) None
5. Heat stroke is characterized by _____.
   (a) Open beak   (b) Paralysis
   (c) Both   (d) None
6. Toxic fat syndrome is also known as _____.
   (a) Chick oedema disease   (b) Water belly
   (c) Both   (d) None
7. Gout may occur due to excess of _____.
   (a) Protein   (b) Fat
   (c) Minerals   (d) Vitamin B_1
8. Blue comb disease is also known as _____.
   (a) Monocytosis   (b) Lymphocytosis
   (c) Both   (d) None
9. Fatty liver and kidney syndrome is characterized by _____.
   (a) Pale liver   (b) Hydropericardium
   (c) Pale kidney   (d) All of above

10. Prolapse of cloaca is seen due to _____.
    (a) Aflatoxicosis   (b) Ochratoxicosis
    (c) Fusariotoxicosis   (d) None

42. PATHOLOGY OF DISEASES OF WILD AND ZOO ANIMALS

1. Theileriosis in wild animals is characterized by _____ coloured faeces.
    (a) Red   (b) Clay   (c) Both   (d) None
2. Babesiosis in leopard is characterized by _____.
    (a) Icterus   (b) Hemoglobinuria
    (c) Pulmonary edema   (d) All of the above
3. Anaplasma marginale causes anaplasmosis in leopard characterized by _____.
    (a) Lymphocytosis   (b) Leucocytosis
    (c) Basophilia   (d) None
4. Common disease of pheasants include _____.
    (a) Colisepticemia   (b) Leucosis
    (c) Marek's disease   (d) None
5. Trypanosomiasis in wild animals is characterized by haemorrhages in _____.
    (a) Liver   (b) Kidneys
    (c) Lungs   (d) All of above

43. PATHOLOGY OF DISEASES OF LABORATORY ANIMALS

1. Non infectious disease conditions of rabbit include _____.
    (a) Wool shedding   (b) Mange
    (c) Coccidiosis   (d) None
2. Tapeworm of rabbit is _____.
    (a) *Taenia pisiformes* (b) *Taenia saginata*
    (c) Both   (d) No~

Self Assessment − MCQ

3. Intestinal coccidiosis is rabbit is caused by _____.
   (a) *Eimeria megna*   (b) *Eimeria media*
   (c) Both   (d) None
4. Tyzzer's disease in mouse is caused by _____.
   (a) *Bacillus piliformis*   (b) *Bacillus subtilis*
   (c) Both   (d) None
5. Diarrhoea in infant mouse is caused by _____.
   (a) Clostridia   (b) Coccidia
   (c) Rotavirus   (d) None
6. Reovirus infection in mice cause _____.
   (a) Jaundice   (b) Pneumonia
   (c) Nephritis   (d) None
7. Wet tail disease of hamster is caused by _____.
   (a) *E.coli*   (b) *Salmonella* sp.
   (c) Rotavirus   (d) None
8. In rats hepatitis is caused by _____.
   (a) *E.coli*   (b) *Salmonella* sp.
   (c) Rotavirus   (d) None
9. In guinea pigs the Pasteurellosis is caused by _____.
   (a) *Pasteurella pneumotropica*   (b) *P. multocida*
   (c) *Mannhemia hemolytica*   (d) All of above
10. Labyrinthitis in rat is caused by _____.
    (a) *Streptobacillus* sp.   (b) Mycoplasma
    (c) Both   (d) None

44. CYTOPATHOLOGY

1. Cytopathology is synonymously used with _____.
   (a) Exploited cytology   (b) Histopathology
   (c) Both   (d) None
2. Exploited cytology can be employed on _____.
   (a) Vaginal smears   (b) Rectal washings
   (c) Bronchial washings   (d) All of above

3. Cytopathological diagnosis rests upon alterations in morphology of _____.
   (a) Single cell   (b) Tissue
   (c) Organ   (d) All of above
4. Interventional cytopathology includes the samples obtained from _____.
   (a) Surgical biopsy   (b) Autopsy
   (c) Exfoliated cells (d) None
5. Biopsy is common in diagnosis of _____ in animals.
   (a) Viral diseases   (b) Bacterial diseases
   (c) Tumours   (d) None

SELF ASSESSMENT – KEY

SECTION A – GENERAL VETERINARY PATHOLOGY

1. Introduction
(1) b (2) a (3) b (4) d (5) b (6) a (7) d (8) d (9) a (10) b

2. Etiology
(1) a (2) b (3) c (4) c (5) d (6) d (7) c (8) c (9) a (10) d (11) d (12) b (13) c (14) d (15) c (16) a (17) b (18) d (19) d (20) b

3. General Disorders, Developmental, Anomalies and Monsters
(1) a (2) b (3) c (4) d (5) c (6) a (7) d (8) c (9) b (10) c (11) c (12) a (13) d (14) c (15) c (16) a (17) d (18) c (19) b (20) a

4. Disturbances in Growth
(1) c (2) c (3) a (4) d (5) a (6) a (7) d (8) c (9) a (10) d

5. Disturbances in circulation
(1) a (2) b (3) d (4) d (5) b (6) d (7) d (8) c (9) d (10) c

6. Disturbances in cell metabolism
(1) a (2) c (3) d (4) b (5) a (6) c (7) b (8) d (9) c (10) a

7. Necrosis, Gangrene and post-mortem changes
(1) d (2) d (3) c (4) b (5) a (6) b (7) a (8) b (9) b (10) c

8. Distrubances in calcification and pgment metabolism
(1) d (2) a (3) c (4) b (5) a (6) c (7) b (8) d (9) a (10) d

9. Inflammation and healing
(1) c (2) c (3) b (4) c (5) c (6) a (7) c (8) a (9) c (10) d (11) a (12) d (13) a (14) a (15) a (16) c (17) c (18) a (19) c (20) c

10. Concretions

(1) a (2) c (3) d (4) b (5) b (6) d (7) a (8) b (9) d (10) a

11. Immunity and Immunopathology

(1) c (2) d (3) b (4) c (5) d (6) a (7) b (8) d (9) b (10) a
(11) a (12) c (13) b (14) c (15) a (16) b (17) d (18) d
(19) a (20) a (21) c (22) a (23) b (24) b (25) d (26) a (27) b (28) c (29) c (30) b

SECTION B – SYSTEMIC PATHOLOGY

12. Pathology of Cutaneous System

(1) b (2) c (3) b (4) d (5) a (6) b (7) a (8) a (9) c (10) b

13. Pathology of Musculoskeletal System

(1) b (2) a (3) d (4) b (5) a (6) b (7) b (8) c (9) b (10) a

14. Pathology of cardiovascular system

(1) d (2) a (3) a (4) d (5) d (6) d (7) a (8) a (9) b (10) b

15. Pathology respiratory system

(1) b (2) d (3) a (4) c (5) b (6) c (7) a (8) c (9) d (10) d

16. Pathology of digestive system

(1) a (2) d (3) c (4) d (5) d (6) c (7) a (8) d (9) c (10) a
(11) c (12) c (13) c (14) b (15) c (16) a (17) d (18) d
(19) b (20) c (21) b (22) c (23) b (24) a (25) a

17. Pathology of hemopoitic and immune system

(1) d (2) b (3) a (4) c (5) d (6) b (7) d (8) a (9) d (10) c

18. Pathology of urinary system

(1) b (2) c (3) b (4) a (5) c (6) c (7) a (8) a (9) a (10) d

19. Pathology of genital system female Genital system

(1) d (2) c (3) d (4) a (5) d (6) d (7) a (8) d (9) b (10) b

Self Assessment - MCQ

20. Pathology of nervous system

(1) c   (2) a   (3) b   (4) c   (5) c   (6) b   (7) c   (8) d   (9) b   (10) b

21. Pathology of endocrine system, eyes and ear

(1) b   (2) c   (3) c   (4) d   (5) d   (6) a   (7) d   (8) b   (9) c   (10) a

Section –C (Special Pathology I, Diseases of Animals)

22. Neoplasms

(1) c   (2) b   (3) c   (4) b   (5) b   (6) d   (7) b   (8) b   (9) a   (10) d
(11) a   (12) b   (13) a   (14) c   (15) c   (16) d   (17) c   (18) b
(19) b   (20) b   (21) a   (22) c   (23) c   (24) b   (25) a   (26) d   (27) d   (28) c   (29) c   (30) b

23. Viral Diseases

(1) c   (2) a   (3) c   (4) b   (5) d   (6) d   (7) a   (8) b   (9) c   (10) c
(11) b   (12) c   (13) b   (14) a   (15) d   (16) a   (17) a   (18) d
(19) b   (20) b   (21) c   (22) a   (23) d   (24) a   (25) d   (26) a   (27) d   (28) a   (29) d   (30) d

24. Bacterial Diseases

(1) c   (2) a   (3) d   (4) d   (5) a   (6) d   (7) b   (8) b   (9) d   (10) b
(11) c   (12) a   (13) d   (14) d   (15) a   (16) b   (17) c   (18) a
(19) b   (20) b   (21) b   (22) d   (23) c   (24) c   (25) b   (26) a   (27) a   (28) d   (29) d   (30) b

25. Chlamydial Diseases

(1) a   (2) d   (3) d   (4) c   (5) d

26. Rickettsial Diseases

(1) c   (2) a   (3) a   (4) b   (5) a

27. Mycoplasmal Diseases

(1) a   (2) b   (3) a   (4) c   (5) a   (6) d   (7) b   (8) a   (9) c   (10) c

28. Spirochaetal Diseases

(1) a   (2) d   (3) c   (4) c   (5) c

29. Prion Diseases

(1) d (2) d (3) c (4) b (5) a

30. Fungal Diseases

(1) b (2) d (3) d (4) b (5) d (6) c (7) c (8) a (9) d (10) d
(11) d (12) d (13) b (14) b (15) d

31. Parasitic Diseases

(1) a (2) b (3) c (4) c (5) d (6) a (7) a (8) c (9) a (10) c
(11) b (12) c (13) d (14) c (15) b (16) b (17) c (18) c
(19) b (20) c (21) a (22) c (23) c (24) c (25) a (26) d
(27) c (28) b (29) a (30) d

Section – D (Special Pathology II, Diseases of poultry, wild, zoo and laboratory animals)

32. Avian inflammation

(1) c (2) d (3) b (4) a (5) d

33. Pathology of Nutritional Disorders

(1) a (2) d (3) c (4) b (5) d (6) d (7) c (8) d (9) d (10) c

34. Viral Diseases

(1) c (2) c (3) a (4) b (5) b (6) b (7) a (8) a (9) c (10) b
(11) d (12) a (13) c (14) d (15) b (16) c (17) d (18) a
(19) b (20) b (21) a (22) d (23) b (24) a (25) a (26) a
(27) c (28) b (29) a (30) a

35. Bacterial Diseases

(1) c (2) c (3) a (4) a (5) d (6) a (7) b (8) c (9) d (10) a
(11) d (12) c (13) b (14) a (15) d

36. Chlamydial Disease

(1) d (2) c (3) d (4) c (5) a

37. Mycoplasmal Disease

(1) c (2) b (3) a (4) a (5) b

Self Assessment - MCQ

38. Spirochaetal Diseases
(1) c   (2) c   (3) b   (4) c   (5) c

39. Fungal Diseases
(1) a   (2) a   (3) a   (4) c   (5) a   (6) d   (7) d   (8) a   (9) b   (10) c

40. Parasitic Diseases
(1) b   (2) c   (3) c   (4) c   (5) b   (6) d   (7) b   (8) a   (9) b   (10) a

41. Vices and Miscellaneous Disease Conditions
(1) a   (2) d   (3) a   (4) b   (5) c   (6) c   (7) a   (8) a   (9) d   (10) c

42. Pathology of Diseases of Wild and Zoo Animals
(1) b   (2) d   (3) b   (4) a   (5) d

43. Pathology of Diseases of Laboratory Animals
(1) a   (2) a   (3) c   (4) a   (5) c   (6) a   (7) a   (8) b   (9) d   (10) c

44. Cytopathology
(1) d   (2) d   (3) a   4) a   (5) c

Index

A

Abnormal teeth	31
Abomasitis	194
Abortion	239
Abrachia	44
Abrasions	15
Acanthosis nigricans	142
Acetoacetate	29
Acidophilic	68
Actinobacillosis	371
Actinomyces bovis	157
Actinomycosis	21, 372
Acute myositis	150
Adactylia	44
Adamantinoma	299
Adenocarcinoma	291
Adenoma	291, 295
Adenomatous goiter	255
Adhesive pleuritis	187
Adjuvants	127
Adult rickets	153
Aflatoxicosis	489
African horse sickness	339
Agenesis	233, 265
Agglutinins	129
Agnathia	44
Agrochemicals	27
Air sacculitis	466
Algor mortis	74
Alkali disease	26
Allergen	132
Alveoli	175
Amprolium	33
Amyloid infiltration	64
Anaplasia	266
Anaplasma marginale	81
Anaplasmosis	383
Anchylostomiasis	416
Androgenic hormones	43
Anemia	210, 285
Anencephalia	44
Aneurysm	168
Ankylosing	157
Anoestrus	38
Anophathalmia	44
Anophthalmos	31
Anorexia	35
Anthrax	368
Antioncogenes	273
Aplasia	265
Arteriolosclerosis	167, 168
Arthus reaction	133
Asbestosis	83
Ascariasis	414
Aspergillosis	396, 485
Aspergillus flavus	25
Aspergillus ochracheous	25
Aspiration pneumonia	179
Atelectasis	174
Atresia ani	189
Atresia coli	189
Atrophy	49, 265
Autoimmune hemolytic anemia	213
Autoimmunity	27, 134
Autolysis	73
Autopsy	2
Avian encephalomyelitis	454
Avian inflammation	433
Avian influenza	441
Avian leucosis	444
Avian pox	456
Avian stunting syndrome	451
Azoturia	149
Azurophilic granules	92

B

B- haemolytic streptococci	81
Babesia bigemina	81
Babesiosis	133, 405
Bacillus anthracis	81
Bacterial diseases	349, 463
Balanoposthitis	246
Basal cell carcinoma	290
Benign neoplasms	269
Beryllium granuloma	185
Bile pigments	79
Biliary calculi	122
Bilirubin	79
Biliverdin	79
Biopsy	5
Black disease	378
Black quarter	72, 355
Blast injury	15
Blastomyces sp	180
Blastomycosis	115, 397
Blue tongue	114, 324
Bone marrow atrophy	17
Bordetella bronchiseptica	171
Borrelia ansarina	21
Bos indicus	125
Bos taurus	126
Botriomycosis	373
Botulism	380
Bovine immunodeficiency	321
Bovine leukemia	322
Bovine viral diarrhoea	313
Bradykinin	104, 105
Braxy	358
Bronchial asthma	132
Bronchoconstriction	97
Bronchoconstrictor	96
Bronchopneumonia	176
Brucellosis	22, 352
Brucellosis	22
Bullet wound	15
Bursitis	219

C

Cachexia	284
Calcitriol	31
Campylobacter hepatitis	471
Campylobacteriosis	23, 369
Campylobactor	21
Candidiasis	394, 487
Canine distemper	344
Canine parvoviral infection	346
Canine pellegra	33
Cannibalism	501
Capillaria aerophila	179
Carcinogenesis	272
Cardiac dialation	33
Cardiac temponade	54
Cardiac thrombus	55
Carmine	66
Caseative necrosis	152
Caspases	70
Cataract	258
Catarrhal enteritis	112, 196
Centromere	39
Cephalothoracopagus	47
Cerebrospinal nematodiasis	428
Cervicitis	238
Cestodes	495
Cestodiasis	419
Chediak higashi syndrome	138, 210
Chemical pathology	2
Chemokines	102
Chemotaxis	97
Chicken anemia	461
Chlamydia	157
Chlamydial disease	381, 477
Chlamydiosis	381
Cholangiocellular carcinoma	293
Cholebilirubin	75
Cholecystitis	123, 206
Cholelith	122
Cholelithiasis	82
Chondroma and chondrosarcoma	302

Index

Chromatolysis	67
Chromosomal defects	277
Chronic cardiac failure	161
Chronic enteritis	197
Chronic respiratory disease	479
Chylothorax	187
Cirrhosis	205
Claviceps purpura	25
Cleft palate	189
Clinical pathology	2
Clostridium chauvoei	150
Clostridium toxins	24
Clostriduum hemolyticum	81
Cloudy swelling	61
Coagulative necrosis	67
Coccidioidomyces immitis	181
Coccidioidomyces sp.	157
Coccidioidomycosis	398
Coccidiosis	409, 496
Coccidiostate	33
Coitus	23
Colibacillosis	363, 464
Coligranuloma	466
Colisepticemia	465
Collagenases	97
Colloid goiter	255
Columnar epithelium	51
Comparative pathology	2
Concretions	121
Congenital albinism	141
Congenital alopecia	141
Congenital cutaneous asthenia	142
Congenital icthyosis	141
Congenital immunodeficiency	136
Connective tissue tumours	299
Contagious bovine pleuropneumonia	385
Contagious caprine pleuropenumonia	386
Contagious ecthyma	325
Coproliths	123
Coronavirus infection	318
Corynebacterium diphtheriae	113
Corynebacterium ovis	170
Corynebacterium pseudotuberculosis	151
Cows and sheep	382
Coxiella burnetti	21
Crepitating sound	72
Crush smear cytology	518
Cryptococcosis	399
Cryptorchidism	242
Cryptosporidiosis	414
Curled toe paralysis	33
Cyanocobalamin	32, 34
Cystic ovaries	234
Cysticercosis	420
Cystitis	231
Cytogenetics	40
Cytopathology	3, 515
Cytotoxic reactions	132
Cytotoxicity	103

D

Danish cattle	137
Decreased spermatogenesis	38
Deficiency anemia	212
Delayed type hypersensitivity	144
Deletion	42
Demodectic sp.	144
Dendritic cells	129
Dermatomycosis	512
Dermoid cyst	46
Developmental anomalies	257
Dextrocardia	45
Diamond skin disease	360
Diapedesis	53, 89
Diarrhoea	286
Dicephalus	46
Dictyocaulus viviparous	184
Digestive system	189
Dinobdella ferox	171
Diprosopus	46

Dirofilaria immitis	56
Dirofilariasis	422
Distomiasis	412
Dracunculosis	423
Dry gangrene	71
Dysplasia	266
Dystrophic calcification	77

E

Ear	259
Ecchymoses	54
Echinococcosis	421
Ectopia cordis	45
Egg drop syndrome	460
Egg eating	501
Emo globinurea	37
Emphysema	174
Encephalitis	248
Encephalomalacia	249
Encephalomalacia	32
Endocrine system	253
Endometritis	237
Enteric calculi	123
Enteritis	1, 87, 511
Enterotoxaemia	165, 357
Entomorphthora coronata	146
Enzootic ataxia	37
Eosinophilic granules	93
Eosinophilic inflammation	116
Eosinophilic meningoencephalitis	35
Eosinophils	91, 116
Ephemeral fever	323
Epidermis	16
Epididymitis	244
Epispadias	243
Epistaxis	171
Epithelial pearls	290
Epithelial tumours	289
Epitheliogenesis imperfecta	141
Epithelioid	94
Epithelioid cells	111
Equine cutaneous granuloma	145
Equine encephalomyelitis	336
Equine goiter	255
Equine infectious anemia	335
Equine influenza	334
Equine rhabdomyolysis	149
Equine strongyloidosis	426
Equine viral abortion	340
Equine viral arteritis	337
Erosions	15
Erysipelas rhusiopathae	157
Erysipelothrix rhusiopathe	164
Erythrocytes	34, 55, 106
Erythrophagocytosis	59
Exotoxins	24
Experimental pathology	1
External hazards	23
Eye	257

F

Familial goiter	255
Fat necrosis	69
Fatty animals	73
Favus	486
Feline leukemia	347
Fever	286
Fibrinogen	55
Fibrinopeptides	106
Fibrinous enteritis	199
Fibrinous pneumonia	178
Fibrous osteodystrophy	152
Fine needle aspiration cytology	517
Fissure	146
Flat worms	495
Flu	22
Fluorine	38
Folliculitis	147
Foot and mouth disease	307
Foreign body giant cells	95
Forensic pathology	3
Fowl cholera	469
Freemartinism	43
Fungal diseases	393, 485
Funiculitis	244

Fusarium equiseti	71
Fusarium sp.	145
Fusarium tricinctum	25

G

Gangrene	71
Gangrenous dermatitis	145
Gastritis	195
General pathology	1
Genital system	233
Genital system	1
Glanders	366
Glaucoma	259
Glomeruli	65
Glossitis	33, 88
Goblet cells	62
Goiter	254
Gout	83, 502
Granuloma	90
Granulomatous	112
Granulomatous enteritis	200
Granulosa cell tumour of ovary	296
Guinea pigs diseases	514

H

Haemophilus suis	186
Haemorrhagic myositis	151
Hagman factor	105
Hair cell carcinoma	290
Hair follicles	16
Hamster diseases	514
Haptens	126
Haversian canals	152
Heat stroke	501
Hemangioma and hemangiosarcoma	304
Hematogenous spread	278
Hemicrania	44
Hemoglobinurea.	36
Hemolysis	82
Hemolytic anemia	211
Hemolytic jaundice	81
Hemoperitonium	54
Hemorrhagic anemia	212
Hemorrhagic enteritis	197
Hemorrhagic inflammation	114
Hemorrhagic septicemia	354
Hemosiderosis	78
Hemothorax	187
Hepadna virus	274
Hepatitis	204
Hepatocellular carcinoma	294
Hereditary anemia	209
Hermaphroditism	233
Herpesvirus	275
Herpex simplex virus	23
Heterozygous	40
Hexamitiasis	499
Histomoniasis	498
Histoplasmosis	400, 488
Hjarre's disease	466
Hog cholera	330
Homeostasis	3
Humoral pathology	2
Hyaline membrane pneumonia	179
Hydrocele	57, 243
Hydropericardium	163
Hydropericardium syndrome	458
Hydroperitonium	57
Hydropic degeneration	61
Hydrothorax	58, 187
Hydroxybutyrate	29
Hyperadrenocorticism	256
Hyperbilirubinemia	79
Hypercalcemia	286
Hyperchromasia	52
Hyperchromatic	63
Hyperirritability	36
Hyperkeratinization	142
Hyperlipimia	29
Hyperparathyroidism	78, 256
Hyperpituitarism	253
Hyperplasia	265
Hyperplastic goiter	254
Hypersensitivity pneumonitis	184

Hyperthermia	16
Hyperthyroidism	254
Hypertrophy	265
Hyphomyces destruens	146
Hypoadrenocorticism	256
Hypochromic	37
Hypogammaglobulinemia	137
Hypoglycemia	285
Hypomagnesaemia	36
Hypoparathyroidism	255
Hypopituitarism	253
Hypoplasia	49, 233, 265
Hypospadias	243
Hypostatic congestion	75
Hypothermia	17
Hypothyroidism	254

I

I degree burns	16
Icterus	81
Icterus	79
Idiosyncrasy	14
Ii degree burns	16
III degree burns	16
Immune system	209
Immunodeficiences	136
Immunoglobulins	92
Immunopathology	3, 131
Immunotoxic effects	140
Implantation	279
Imprint cytology	518
In utero	42
Incised wounds	15
Inclusion body hepatitis	457
Incubation period	4
Infectious bovine rhinotracheitis	315
Infectious bronchitis	447
Infectious bursal disease	446
Infectious canine hepatitis	343, 536
Infectious coryza	468
Infectious laryngotracheitis	449
Infectious synovitis	480
Ingluvitis	192

Interleukin	98, 103, 126
Internal hazards	23
Intersexes	43
Interstitial nephritis	226
Interstitial pneumonia	177
Interventional cytopathology	517
Intrinsic causes	13
Iodine	38
Ischiopagus	46

J

Johne's disease	22, 350

K

Kallikrein	104
Karyolysis	67
Karyorrhexis	67
Kennel cough	173
Keratoconjunctivitis	258
Ketosis	29
Kinin system	104
Klebsiella	21

L

Laceration	15
Langhans giant cells	95
Laryngitis	171
Left sided heart failure	161
Leiomyoma and leiomyosarcoma	303
Leptospira ictehaemmorrhagae	81
Leptospirosis	389
Leucocytosis	216
Leucopenia	216
Leucotriene	97
Libido	38
Lincomycin	26
Lipolysis	29
Lipoma and liposarcoma	301
Lipopolysacharide	93
Liquefactive necrosis	68
Listeriosis	361
Livor mortis	75

Lobular pneumonia	177	Microscopic pathology	2
Local anemia	56	Mild irritants	112
Lymphadenitis	218	Mineral deficiency	437
Lymphangitis	169	Monckeberg medial sclerosis	167
Lymphocytes	17	Monday morning disease	149
Lymphocytic infiltration	134	Monoclonal antibody production	282
Lymphocytic thyroditis	255	Monokines	97
Lymphofollicular reaction	134	Monosomy	41
Lymphokines	97	Morbidity rate	5
Lymphoma and lymphosarcoma	306	Mortality rate	5
Lymphosarcoma	43	Mouse diseases	513
Lysins	129	Mucosal disease	313

M

		Mucous mycosis	401
		Multiple deficiencies	27
M. Bovis	181	Mural thrombus	55
Maedi	327	Mural vegetative endocarditis	164
Malabsorption	28	Muscle wasting	28
Male genital system	242	Mycobacterium tuberculosis	21, 24, 151, 186
Malignant catarrhal fever	312		
Malignant melanoma	297	Mycoplasma mycoides	21, 186
Malignant neoplasms	269	Mycoplasma sinoviae	157
Mammary gland	295	Mycoplasmal abortion	387
Managemental diseases	512	Mycoplasmal diseases	385, 479
Mange	432	Myocardium	16
Marble bone disease	154	Myositis	87
Marek's disease	442	Myxoma	300
Marek's disease	139	Myxosarcoma	63, 300
Mastitis	241		

N

Mastocytoma	305		
Medial sclerosis	166	Natural killer	126
Mega colon	189	Natural killer cell	280
Melanosarcoma	14	Necrobacillosis	374
Melena	54	Necrosis	59
Meningitis	250	Necrotic enteritis	198, 470
Mesothelioma	305	Neomycin	26
Metaplasia	51, 266	Neoplasm	263
Metastasis	288	Neoplasms	283
Metastatic calcification	77	Neoplastic cell genesis	272
Metastrongylus apri	179	Neoplastic cell metabolism	275
Metritis	236	Neoplastic cell structure	276
Microbial toxins	24	Neoplastic cells	282
Micrococci	122	Nephrosclerosis	227
Microphthalmos	31	Nephrotoxic	26

Nervous system	247
Neuritis	87, 250
Newcastle disease	439
Niacin	32
Nicotinic	32
Nocardiosis	375
Nutritional disorders	435
Nutritional imbalance	27
Nutritional pathology	2
Nyctalopia	31

O

Occlusive thrombus	55
Ochratoxicosis	490
Oedematous fluid	143
Oesophagostomiasis	418
Oestrus ovis	171
Omasitis	194
Omphalitis	467
Oncogenic viruses	52
Oncology	3
Oophoritis	234
Ophthalmitis	87
Opsonins	109
Opsonization	138
Orchitis	243
Ornithosis	477
Osteoma and osteosarcoma	302
Osteomalacia	153
Osteopetrosis	154
Osteoporosis	154
Otitis	86
Otitis externa	86, 259
Otitis interna	260
Otitis media	260
Ovine pulmonary carcinoma	326
Oxytetracyline	26

P

Pachymeningitis	86
Pale infarct	57
Pancreas	256
Pancreatic calculi	123
Pancreatitis	207

Papilloma	289, 295
Papova virus	274
Parainfluenza-3 infection	320
Paraphimosis	242
Parasitic diseases	403, 493
Parasitic enteritis	199
Paratuberculosis	350
Pasteurella multocida	139
Pasteurellosis	510
Pasteurlla multocida	113
Pathogenicity	5
Pathology of spleen	217
Pavementation	89
Perianal adenoma of dog	292
Pericarditis	162
Perivascular cuffing	115
Perosis	37
Peste de petits in ruminants	329
Petechiae	54
Phagocyosis	106
Phagocytic vacuole	109
Phagocytosis	138
Phallocampsis	243
Phimosis	242
Phlebitis	169
Phlegmon	114
Physiological pathology	2
Phytobezoars	124, 203
Phytoconcretion	121, 124
Piliconcretion	121
Piliconcretions	124, 203
Pineal gland	257
Placentitis	240
Pleurisy	186
Pneumoconiosis	185
Pneumonia	175
Pneumopericardium	163
Pneumothorax	187
Polioencephalomalcia	33
Polybezoars	203
Polyconcretion	121
Polycythemia	214
Polyotia	45
Polysaccharide	64

Polyuria	28
Post-mortem clot	75
Post-mortem emphysema	75
Post-mortem pathology	2
Pox	511
Pregnancy toxaemia	29
Prekallikrein	104
Primary shock	58
Prion diseases	391
Prognosis	5
Prognosis of neoplasms	287
Prosopothoracopagus	47
Prostacylin	96
Prostatitis	246
Protozoan parasites	496
Pseudomelanosis	74
Pseudomonas aeruginosa	16, 164
Pseudomucin	64
Pseudorabies	333
Pseudotuberculosis	376
Psoroptic sp.	144
Pulmonary adenomatosis	51
Pulmonary edema	175
Pulmonary nematodiasis	424
Pulmonary osteoarthropathy	156
Pustule	62
Putrefaction	74
Pyelonephritis	226
Pyknosis	67
Pyknotic	68
Pyometra	236
Pyopagus	46
Pyothorax	187
Pyrethroids	27
Pyridoxine	33

R

Rabbit diseases	509
Rabbit syphilis	511
Rabies	341
Rachipagus	47
Ranikhet disease	439, 536
Rat diseases	513
Reagin	132

Red infarct	57
Renal tubules	16
Renarcuatus	45
Reovirus infection	450
Retained placenta	240
Reticulitis	193
Reticuloendothelial cells	59
Retinitis	259
Retrovirus	274
Rhabdomyoma and rhabdomysarcoma	303
Rheumatism	36
Rhexis	53, 89
Rhinitis	132
Rhinosporidiosis	395
Rhinosporidium sceberi	171
Riboflavin	32
Rickettsia	21
Rickettsial diseases	383
Right-sided heart failure	162
Rigor mortis	74
Rinderpest	310
Ringworm	393
Rotaviral diarrhoea	455
Rotavirus infection	317
Roundworms	493
Rumenitis	193
Ruminal bacteria	37
Russell body	94

S

Saddle thrombus	55
Salivary calculi	123
Salmonellosis	22, 362, 463
Salpingitis	235
Sarcoptes scabei	144
Sarcosporidia spp	151
Sarcosporidiosis	410
Sauce	109
Schistosoma nasalis	172
Schistosomiasis	411
Sebaceous gland adenoma	291
Secondary shock	58
Selenium	37

Seminal vesiculitis	245	**T**		
Seminoma	296			
Septic thrombus	55	T-cytotoxic cells		91
Septicemia	24	T-helper		91
Serum	2	Tape worms		495
Sialolith	123	Telangiectasis		169
Silicosis	83, 185	Tendinitis		88
Skeletal deformities	153	Testicular hypoplasia		242
Sludged blood	59	Tetanus		359
Smoothly homogenous	65	Tetralogy of fallot		160
Snake venom	24	Theileriosis		404
Spasms	35	Thiaminases		28
Species cleansing effect	41	Thiamine deficiency		27
Specific pathology	1	Thoracopagus		47
Spermatocele	242	Thrombocytopenia		285
Spermatozoa	136	Thrombosis		1, 286
Spirocercosis	427	Thymic hyperplasia		219
Spirochaetal disease	389, 483	Thymic hypoplasia		38, 137
Spirochaete	21	Tick fever		483
Splenitis	217	Tnm system		287
Spondylitis	156	Touton giant cells		95
Spongiform encephalopathy	249, 391	Toxic aplastic anemia		213
		Toxic fat syndrome		502
Squamous cell carcinoma	289	Toxic goiter		255
Squamous epithelium	51	Toxopathology		3
Squamous metaplasia	30	Toxoplasmosis		408
Stab wound	15	Transmissible gastroenteritis		332
Staphylococci	16, 114	Trematodes		495
Staphylococcosis	373, 472	Trichinella spp		151
Stargazing	33	Trichinosis		430
Stephanofilariasis	431	Trichomoniasis		407
Strangles	365	Trichomonosis		498
Stratum spinosum	62	Trichostrongylosis		417
Streptococci	16	Trichuriasis		429
Strongylus vulgaris	168	Trisomy		41
Suboestrus	38	True aneurysm		169
Suffusions	54	Trypanosomiasis		403
Superoxide dismutase	110	Trypanosomiosis		133
Sweat gland adenoma	293	Tuberculosis	115, 349,	474
Swine erysepalas	360	Tuberculous lesions		77
Swine fever	330	Tuberculous pneumonia		181
Systemic pathology	1	Tumour antigens		281
		Tumour immunology		280
		Turpentine		114
		Tympany		192

Typhlitis	204
Typhlitis	86
Tyzzer's disease	510

U

Ulcer	147
Unconsciousness	35
United twins	46
Ureteritis	230, 231
Urethritis	88
Urinary calculi	121
Urolithiasis	31, 121, 229
Urticaria	147
Uterus didelphys	234
Uterus unicornis	233

V

Vaginitis	88, 238
Valvular thrombus	55
Van-den-bergh reaction	83
Varicose veins	169
Vasoactive amines	96
Vasoconstrictor	96
Venereal sarcoma	298
Vesicular dermatitis	143
Vesicular exanthema	309
Vesicular stomatitis	308
Vices	501
Viral diseases	307, 439
Viral nephritis	452
Viral oncogenesis	273
Virulence	6
Viscid	62
Visna	327
Vitamin deficiency	435
Vulvitis	89

W

White heifer disease	233
White muscle disease	32, 150
Wild and zoo animals	505

Y

Yersinia	21
Yersiniosis	377

Z

Zeihl neelson	21
Zoonotic diseases	2